Recent Results in Cancer Research

Volume 210

More information about this series at http://www.springer.com/series/392

Ute Goerling · Anja Mehnert
Editors

Psycho-Oncology

Second Edition

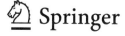 Springer

Editors
Ute Goerling
Charité Comprehensive Cancer Center
Humboldt University of Berlin
Berlin
Germany

Anja Mehnert
Department of Medical Psychology
 and Medical Sociology
University of Leipzig
Leipzig
Germany

ISSN 0080-0015   ISSN 2197-6767   (electronic)
Recent Results in Cancer Research
ISBN 978-3-319-87768-6   ISBN 978-3-319-64310-6   (eBook)
https://doi.org/10.1007/978-3-319-64310-6

Printed on acid-free paper

This Springer imprint is published by Springer Nature
The registered company is Springer International Publishing AG
The registered company address is: Gewerbestrasse 11, 6330 Cham, Switzerland

Contents

About the Editors

Anja Mehnert Ph.D., is chair of the Department of Medical Psychology and Medical Sociology at the University Medical Center Leipzig. She graduated in Psychology from the University of Hamburg. In 2005, she completed her Ph.D. on trauma and stress before being appointed postdoctoral research fellow at the Department of Psychiatry and Behavioral Sciences at Memorial Sloan-Kettering Cancer Center, New York (2007–2008). She completed her Habilitation theses in 2010 on return to work among cancer survivors at the University of Hamburg. Her research topics include cancer survivorship issues, psychological comorbidity and distress screening, as well as psychotherapy and health services research in psycho-oncology. She is coeditor and coauthor of five books and more than 130 academic publications.

Dr. Ute Goerling is currently working as head of the Department of Psycho-oncology at the Charité Comprehensive Cancer Center in Berlin. She has many years of experience in psycho-oncological interventions and research. As a practitioner she is particularly interested in activating resources and promoting adaptive coping with the illness in her clients. She did her Ph.D. at the Humboldt University in Berlin and investigated the efficacy of short-term psycho-oncological interventions for cancer patients. Further special areas of interest in research are the evaluation of need for supportive psychosocial care and specific aspects of quality of life of cancer patients after surgery.

She was the editor of the first edition of the book '*Psycho-oncology*' which was published in '*Recent Results in Cancer Research*'.

Psychosocial Impact of Cancer

Susanne Singer

Abstract

Diagnosis and treatment of malignant diseases affect in many ways the lives of patients, relatives and friends. Common reactions immediately after the diagnosis are shock and denial, frequently followed by depression, anxiety and/or anger. About a third of all cancer patients suffer from a co-morbid mental health condition, requiring professional support by the entire medical team, including psycho-oncologists. Often overlooked issues are financial and social problems due to inability to work or due to out-of-pocket costs for the medical treatment.

Keywords

Distress · Co-morbidity · Burden · Psychosocial aspects · Coping · Financial problems · Return to work

1 Psychological Impact

1.1 Psychological Reaction to the Cancer Diagnosis

After a person hears he or she is diagnosed with cancer, the first reaction frequently is a sort of shock: "It can not be me; they must have mixed up the test results with another person". For many patients, receiving such a diagnosis is associated with

S. Singer (✉)
Division of Epidemiology and Health Services Research, Institute of Medical Biostatistics, Epidemiology and Informatics, University Medical Centre Mainz, Obere Zahlbacher Straße 69, 55131 Mainz, Germany
e-mail: singers@uni-mainz.de

the fear of intense pain, loss of control, stigmatisation and death (Holland and Rowland 1989). Getting such a diagnosis therefore feels like a nightmare. Complex processes of denial and subsequent realisation of the truth, often followed by denial again, are seen in those patients.

After a while, depending on the psychosocial resources a patient has, the truth can be faced more fully by the patient. In this phase of coping with disease, people often start fighting and arguing—with their doctors, their relatives, their fate. It is as if they try to overcome the disease by fighting. When they realise this is not possible, it often results in intense feelings of hope- and helplessness which can turn into depression. Not everybody is able to finally accept the malignant disease as part of his or her life.

These phases of coping described above were conceptualised by Elisabeth Kübler-Ross after she had interviewed numerous dying patients (Kübler-Ross 2008). Her concept has been adapted by many authors, and at the same time criticised for not being empirically valid. Indeed, these "phases" can be seen in many patients (and their relatives). There is, however, no certain order of the "phases" which is why we prefer to call them emotional reactions which can occur consecutively or simultaneously.

1.2 Denial

Denial allows the patient to keep reality away from the consciousness until he or she is able to deal with it. Clinicians should be aware of the fact that this is a natural process of the psyche to keep ones psychological structure alive. At least in the beginning of the cancer trajectory, patients and relatives should get enough time from the medical team until they can refrain from denial. It is not advisable to push them into the truth too fast.

However, continuing denial can be a challenge in oncology, as patients often need to be treated within a short period of time. One should avoid "breaking the denial" by aggressive instructions about the disease and its treatment. This will only result in aggression and anger, be it openly expressed or more silent. Patients may also be in danger of mental decompensation.

Example:

A 58 year old man suffered from a brief reactive psychosis while he was at the intensive care unit. He had a vision of being at a space ship. He was the captain and responsible for the ship, but the cockpit was not functioning, he could neither steer it nor slow it down, it was a nightmare. It turned out that he had been informed about his diagnosis of pancreas carcinoma quite forcefully, and his coping abilities were obviously not strong enough to deal with it at this moment.

A better way of supporting the patient in getting over his denial is to (a) strengthen his psychosocial resources and (b) avoid denial in ones own perspective. Healthcare providers should try to be neutral and not joining the patient in his or her denial. It is often challenging to not do this because it is seductive, especially when treating young patients, to just avoid the idea of pain and potential death. However, if the patient feels that his carers deny his situation he will be even more convinced that his fate is horrible and that he cannot deal with it (if not even the "professionals" can deal with it!). This can also make the patient feel alone with his fears. So, if the healthcare provider can accept the patient in his denial and at the same time be prepared to also talk about distressing topics such as the danger of functional impairment, losses and death, it will support the patient to overcome his denial.

> Example:
>
> My patient is a 40 year old single mother. She received the diagnosis ovarian cancer 5 years ago and I had been seeing her since then. While she first wanted to see a psychologist to identify psychological causes of her disease with the aim of then changing her life accordingly to be cured from cancer, she was faced with multiple metastases in her entire body. Still, she thought that psychotherapy can cure her and she asked me to help her visualize her blood and cancer cells because that is what she had read in a book.
>
> I saw her emotional suffering and wanted to support her, at the same time I knew that she had a tumour with a poor prognosis, she had multiple metastases, and she was admitted to the palliative medicine ward at our hospital. Her daughter was 15 years old, the patient described her ex-husband as being alcohol dependent, so she did not want her daughter to live with him.
>
> The patient seemed torn between the hope of cure and the realisation of nearby death, but the truth was too hard to bear so she denied it and seemed to force all others to share this denial with her. Her physician told me about her refusal to find a solution for her daughter, which needed to be resolved since she was facing death.
>
> During our next session, the patient told me in tears that her parents said to her: "Girl, make sure you get better soon". When she wanted to talk with them about her fears, they both said: "Don't say this, you will get better!" This obviously did not help her, as she felt utterly alone. In this situation, I decided to openly ask the patient about her feelings regarding death and dying. No one from the team had done this before, because of feeling sorry for the patient and because she seemed to refuse any conversation about it. However, the patient now reacted relieved. We talked about dying, her experiences with death, her ideas about what happens thereafter, and finally about her daughter living without her.
>
> The patient deceased two weeks later.

This example shows that, although patients often deny, they can at the same time talk about distressing topics if they experience a supporting relationship with someone they trust and who is not in denial himself.

1.3 Co-morbid Mental Health Conditions

At times, psychological distress can be severe for cancer patients, resulting in clinically relevant mental health conditions. Numerous studies have investigated the frequency of these conditions in cancer patients over the past years.

Several meta-analyses and large multicentre studies have shown that, during the time of cancer diagnosis, about 30% of the patients suffer from a mental health condition (Singer et al. 2010; Mitchell et al. 2011; Vehling et al. 2012; Mehnert et al. 2014; Kuhnt et al. 2016). Less is known however about the course of those conditions during the cancer trajectory. Available evidence suggests that their frequency does not decrease considerably over time (Bringmann et al. 2008; Singer et al. 2016).

Known risk factors for mental disorders in cancer patients are pain, high symptom burden, fatigue, mental health problems in the past and disability (Akechi et al. 2004; Rooney et al. 2011; Banks et al. 2010; Agarwal et al. 2010). There are no consistent correlates of depression in cancer patients (Mitchell et al. 2011).

In some studies, alcohol dependence was more common in men (Matheson et al. 2012; Dawson 1996; Kessler et al. 1994; Bronisch and Wittchen 1992; Krauß et al. 2007) and in patients with malignancies in the head and neck, oesophagus and liver (Shimazu et al. 2012; Freedman et al. 2007; Hashibe et al. 2007; Kugaya et al. 2000).

Not only does psychiatric co-morbidity represent enhanced distress of the patients calling for specific support from the medical team, it also increases the length of hospital stay (Wancata et al. 2001) and negatively affects survival, if not treated adequately (Kissane 2009; Pinquart and Duberstein 2010). It is, therefore, highly important to identify patients suffering from mental health disorders as soon as possible. Unfortunately, healthcare providers often fail in identifying these patients (Singer et al. 2011a; Absolom et al. 2011; Fallowfield et al. 2001; Söllner et al. 2001), resulting in severe under-treatment (Singer et al. 2005, 2011b; Schwarz et al. 2006; Oliffe and Phillips 2008; Stoppe et al. 1999; Werrbach and Gilbert 1987; Wilhelm 2009).

In a large prospective study with cancer patients, we found that of those with mental health conditions, 9% saw a psychotherapist within three months of the diagnosis, 19% after nine months and 11% after 15 months. Mental health care use was higher in patients with children ≤ 18 years (odds ratio 3.3) and somatic co-morbidity (odds ratio 2.6) (Singer et al. 2013a). Interestingly, in this study, uptake of mental health care was equal between men and women, in contrast to findings from studies in the general population (Oliffe and Phillips 2008; Stoppe et al. 1999; Werrbach and Gilbert 1987; Wilhelm 2009). The admission to mental health care did not differ in patients with different educational attainments.

1.4 Potential Positive Impact

During the last decade, increasing interest has been given to potential benefits of the experience of cancer despite it being challenging and often highly distressing, i.e. whether traumatic experiences can lead to emotional growth in patients and relatives (Hungerbuehler et al. 2011; Kahana et al. 2011; Kim et al. 2011; Love and Sabiston 2011; Demirtepe-Saygili and Bozo 2011; Fromm et al. 1996). Such posttraumatic growth has been defined as positive psychological change experienced as a result of the struggle with highly challenging life circumstances (Calhoun et al. 2000; Calhoun and Tedeschi 2001). It describes the experience of individuals whose development has surpassed what was present before the struggle with the crises occurred, i.e. people feel that they did not simply "go back to life as usual" but that they feel enriched, wiser, grown, etc. after the crisis.

According to Tedeschi and Calhoun (2004), positive changes can be found in five dimensions, representing different types of posttraumatic growth: greater appreciation of life and changed sense of priorities; warmer, more intimate relationships with others; a greater sense of personal strength; recognition of new possibilities of paths for one's life; and spiritual development (Tedeschi and Calhoun 2004).

Individuals' experience of posttraumatic growth depends on several predictors. Many facilitating factors have been reported: younger age, female gender, low consumption of alcohol, low levels of pessimism and depression, high life satisfaction, high levels of extraversion, having an active sexual life and receiving counselling (Cormio et al. 2010; Milam 2004; Mols et al. 2009; Paul et al. 2010; Sheikh 2004; Jansen et al. 2011; Barskova and Oesterreich 2009). Benefit finding, a concept similar to posttraumatic growth, depends on the amount of time that has passed since stressor onset, the instrument used and the racial composition of the sample (Helgeson et al. 2006).

To date, only a few studies have investigated whether or not psychosocial interventions can help to increase posttraumatic growth after traumatic events or serious illness. Especially in cancer patients, evidence is scare. Own research has shown that art therapy once weekly over a period of 22 weeks in the outpatient setting did not increase posttraumatic growth (Singer et al. 2013b). This finding is in accordance with scepticism towards the concept of growth in the context of adversity, including serious illness, and towards positive psychology in general (Coyne and Tennen 2010).

2 Social Impact

Human beings are social beings. We all share our lives with others and are closely related to others, willingly or unwillingly. This implies that a malignant disease not only affects the psychological aspects of ones life but also social relations. Both dimensions are closely intertwined.

Being a part of a society implies a certain status within that society. That status shapes the image one has and increases or decreases the possibilities to exchange goods. In high income countries, social status usually is defined by income, educational attainment and employment, which is why the term preferred by sociologists is "socio-economic position". Each of these three factors defining this position can be changed by a malignant disease.

2.1 Socio-economic Position

Low socio-economic position is known to be associated with poor health on the one hand and with less access to health care on the other (Williams 2012; Garrido-Cumbrera et al. 2010; Korda et al. 2009; Habicht and Kunst 2005; Celik and Hotchkiss 2000; Jenkins et al. 2008; Lorant et al. 2007; Weich et al. 2001; Weich and Lewis 1998; Singer et al. 2012). The socio-economic position may even decrease after a cancer diagnosis, especially in younger patients if they lose their jobs due to cancer-caused disability (Banks et al. 2010). On the other hand, it is also possible that social problems may decrease or even disappear after a cancer diagnosis, for example, if a previously unemployed person receives a pension due to disability.

Vocational rehabilitation of cancer patients differs remarkably between countries. For example, while in Scandinavia about 63% of all patients returned to work after a total laryngectomy (Natvig 1983) and 50% did so in France (Schraub et al. 1995) only 11% could return in Spain (Herranz and Gavilan 1999). Predictors of successful return to work are flexible working arrangements, counselling, training and rehabilitation services, younger age, educational attainment, male gender, less physical symptoms and continuity of care (Mehnert 2011).

Similarly, patients' financial burden depends largely on the country's social system and healthcare insurances. Specific problems are the so called "out-of-pocket-health payments". These are expenses the patient has because of the disease and/or its treatment that are not reimbursed by insurance. In the US, breast cancer patients ($n = 156$) who were insured (either by Medicare, Medicaid, or privately) reported that they spent 597 dollars per month for direct medical costs (e.g. stay at a hospital) without reimbursement, 131 dollars for direct non-medical costs (e.g. transport to the hospital, salary for baby sitters etc.) and 727 dollars for indirect costs (e.g. loss of money to do reduced income) (Arozullah et al. 2004).

Regarding the course of financial problems, findings are mixed. In a group of German cancer patients at the time of cancer diagnosis ($n = 799$), 41% reported having financial difficulties due to the disease while this was increased to 52% half a year after diagnosis (Schwarz and Singer 2008). Similar trends were seen in the US (Arozullah et al. 2004) while others found decreasing (Tsunoda et al. 2007; Arndt et al. 2005) or persisting problems (Sullivan et al. 2007).

Financial difficulties can occur not only in the patients but also in the supporters. There are findings showing that especially male support persons and support persons of survivors in active treatment experience increased expenses (Carey et al. 2012).

2.2 Social Relations

Social relations can be a source of great joy and happiness, but also of heavy conflicts and despair. Most patients experience very good social support, especially at the beginning of the cancer treatment trajectory. Family and friends often spend a lot of time and energy to support the patient. If social support is lacking though, it often leads to increased distress (Mehnert et al. 2010).

At times, social support is experienced negatively, especially if relatives or friends are overprotective implying that the patient is not able to care for himself anymore (Bottomley and Jones 1997). This should be kept in mind in clinical practice. For example, if a breast cancer patient has a husband this does not necessarily mean that she receives more support than a single patient. Clinicians should ask patients how they perceive their support and whether they need help with their social life or not.

Another aspect of social relations should be mentioned here: the desire to have children. In younger patients, family planning can be a challenge, especially in patients receiving chemotherapy or anti-hormonal therapy. Doctors should inform them about future possibilities of getting children and about potential alternatives. If patients cannot have children any more although they wished to, this is often experienced as a great loss and the psychosocial and medical team should treat that accordingly.

In conclusion, the impact of malignant diseases on social and psychological aspects of patients' and relatives' daily living can be tremendous. Healthcare professionals should be equipped with the willingness and competence to address these issues and approach patients actively, offering help and support. If patients do not want that help at a given time, it may be wise to offer it later again. Of course, patients should have the freedom to decline psychosocial support from the professionals, however, it might be that they decline out of denial or because it is the only thing they can decline during the time of their cancer treatment. For these reasons, it is good to offer support more than once during the illness trajectory.

References

Absolom K, Holch P, Pini S, Hill K, Liu A, Sharpe M, Richardson A, Velikova G (2011) The detection and management of emotional distress in cancer patients: the views of health-care professionals. Psycho-Oncology 20:601–608

Agarwal M, Hamilton JB, Moore CE, Crandell JL (2010) Predictors of depression among older African American cancer patients. Cancer Nurs 33:156–163

Akechi T, Okuyama T, Sugawara Y, Nakano T, Shima Y, Uchitomi Y (2004) Major depression, adjustment disorders, and post-traumatic stress disorder in terminally Ill cancer patients: associated and predictive factors. J Clin Oncol 22:1957–1965

Arndt V, Merx H, Stegmaier C, Ziegler H, Brenner H (2005) Persistence of restrictions in quality of life from the first to the third year after diagnosis in women with breast cancer. J Clin Oncol 23:4945–4953

Arozullah AM, Calhoun EA, Wolf M, Finley DK, Fitzner KA, Heckinger EA, Gorby NS, Schumock GT, Bennett CL (2004) The financial burden of cancer: estimates from a study of insured women with breast cancer. J Supportive Oncol 2:271–278

Banks E, Byles JE, Gibson RE, Rodgers B, Latz IK, Robinson IA, Williamson AB, Jorm LR (2010) Is psychological distress in people living with cancer related to the fact of diagnosis, current treatment or level of disability? Findings from a large Australian study. Med J Aust 193:S62–S67

Barskova T, Oesterreich R (2009) Post-traumatic growth in people living with a serious medical condition and its relations to physical and mental health: a systematic review. Disabil Rehabil 31:1709–1733

Bottomley A, Jones L (1997) Social support and the cancer patient–a need for clarity. Eur J Cancer Care (Engl) 6:72–77

Bringmann H, Singer S, Höckel M, Stolzenburg J-U, Krauß O, Schwarz R (2008) Longitudinal analysis of psychiatric morbidity in cancer patients. Onkologie 31:343–344

Bronisch T, Wittchen HU (1992) Lifetime and 6-month prevalence of abuse and dependence of alcohol in the Munich follow-up-study. Eur Arch Psychiatry Clin Neurosci 241:273–282

Calhoun LG, Tedeschi RG (2001) Posttraumatic growth: the positive lessons of loss. In: Neimeyer RA (ed) Meaning reconstruction and the experience of loss. American Psychological Association, Washington

Calhoun LG, Cann A, Tedeschi RG, McMillan J (2000) A correlational test of the relationship between posttraumatic growth, religion, and cognitive processing. J Trauma Stress 13:521–527

Carey M, Paul C, Cameron E, Lynagh M, Hall A, Tzelepis F (2012) Financial and social impact of supporting a haematological cancer survivor. Eur J Cancer Care 21:169–176

Celik Y, Hotchkiss DR (2000) The socio-economic determinants of maternal health care utilization in Turkey. Soc Sci Med 50:1797–1806

Cormio C, Romito F, Montanaro R, Caporusso L, Mazzei A, Misino A, Naglieri E, Mattioli V, Colucci G (2010) Post-traumatic growth in long term cancer survivors. Cancer Treat Rev 36: S112–S112

Coyne JC, Tennen H (2010) Positive psychology in cancer care: bad science, exaggerated claims, and unproven medicine. Ann Behav Med 39:16–26

Dawson D (1996) Gender differences in the risk of alcohol dependence: United States, 1992. Addiction 91:1831–1842

Demirtepe-Saygili D, Bozo O (2011) Perceived social support as a moderator of the relationship between caregiver well-being indicators and psychological symptoms. J Health Psychol 16:1091–1100

Fallowfield L, Ratcliffe D, Jenkins V, Saul J (2001) Psychiatric morbidity and its recognition by doctors in patients with cancer. Br J Cancer 84:1011–1015

Freedman ND, Schatzkin A, Leitzmann MF, Hollenbeck AR, Abnet CC (2007) Alcohol and head and neck cancer risk in a prospective study. Br J Cancer 96:1469–1474

Fromm K, Andrykowski MA, Hunt J (1996) Positive and negative psychosocial sequalae of bone marrow transplantation: implications for quality of life assessment. J Behav Med 19:221–240

Garrido-Cumbrera M, Borrell C, Palencia L, Espelt A, Rodriguez-Sanz M, Pasarin MI, Kunst A (2010) Social class inequalities in the utilization of health care and preventive services in Spain, a country with a national health system. Int J Health Serv 40:525–542

Habicht J, Kunst AE (2005) Social inequalities in health care services utilisation after eight years of health care reforms: a cross-sectional study of Estonia, 1999. Soc Sci Med 60:777–787

Hashibe M, Bofetta P, Janout V, Zaridze D, Shangina O, Mates D, Szeszenia-Dabrowska N, Bencko V, Brennan P (2007) Esophageal cancer in Central and Eastern Europe: tobacco and alcohol. Int J Cancer 120:1518–1522

Helgeson VS, Reynolds KA, Tomich PL (2006) A meta-analytic review of benefit finding and growth. J Consult Clin Psychol 74:797–816

Herranz J, Gavilan J (1999) Psychosocial adjustment after laryngeal cancer surgery. Ann Otol Rhinol Laryngol 108:990–997

Holland J, Rowland J (1989) Handbook of psychooncology. Oxford University Press, New York

Hungerbuehler I, Vollrath ME, Landolt MA (2011) Posttraumatic growth in mothers and fathers of children with severe illnesses. J Health Psychol 16:1259–1267

Jansen L, Hoffmeister M, Chang-Claude J, Brenner H, Arndt V (2011) Benefit finding and posttraumatic growth in long-term colorectal cancer survivors: prevalence, determinants, and associations with quality of life. German medical science. doi:10.3205/11gmds213, URN: urn: nbn:de:0183-11gmds2131

Jenkins R, Bhugra D, Bebbington P, Brugha T, Farrell M, Coid J, Fryers T, Weich S, Singleton N, Meltzer H (2008) Debt, income and mental disorder in the general population. Psychol Med 38:1485–1493

Kahana B, Kahana E, Deimling G, Sterns S, VanGunten M (2011) Determinants of altered life perspectives among older-adult long-term cancer survivors. Cancer Nurs 34:209–218

Kessler RC, Mcgonagle KA, Zhao SY, Nelson CB, Hughes M, Eshleman S, Wittchen HU, Kendler KS (1994) Lifetime and 12-month prevalence of Dsm-Iii-R psychiatric-disorders in the United-States—results from the national-comorbidity-survey. Arch Gen Psychiatry 51:8–19

Kim Y, Carver CS, Spillers RL, Crammer C, Zhou ES (2011) Individual and dyadic relations between spiritual well-being and quality of life among cancer survivors and their spousal caregivers. Psycho-Oncology 20:762–770

Kissane D (2009) Beyond the psychotherapy and survival debate: the challenge of social disparity, depression and treatment adherence in psychosocial cancer care. Psycho-Oncology 18:1–5

Korda RJ, Banks E, Clements MS, Young AF (2009) Is inequity undermining Australia's 'universal' health care system? Socio-economic inequalities in the use of specialist medical and non-medical ambulatory health care. Aust NZ J Public Health 33:458–465

Krauß O, Ernst J, Kuchenbecker D, Hinz A, Schwarz R (2007) Prädiktoren psychischer Störungen bei Tumorpatienten: Empirische Befunde. Psychother Psychosom Med Psychol 57:273–280

Kübler-Ross E (2008) Interviews mit Sterbenden. Kreuz, Stuttgart

Kugaya A, Akechi T, Okuyama T, Nakano T, Mikami I, Okamura H, Uchitomi Y (2000) Prevalence, predictive factors, and screening for psychologic distress in patients with newly diagnosed head and neck cancer. Cancer 88:2817–2823

Kuhnt S, Brähler E, Faller H, Härter M, Keller M, Schulz H, Wegscheider K, Weis J, Boehncke A, Hund B, Reuter K, Richard M, Sehner S, Wittchen H-U, Koch U, Mehnert A (2016) Twelve-month and lifetime prevalence of mental disorders in cancer patients. Psychother Psychosom 85:289–296

Lorant V, Croux C, Weich S, Deliege D, Mackenbach J, Ansseau M (2007) Depression and socio-economic risk factors: 7-year longitudinal population study. Br J Psychiatry 190:293–298

Love C, Sabiston CM (2011) Exploring the links between physical activity and posttraumatic growth in young adult cancer survivors. Psycho-Oncology 20:278–286

Matheson FI, White HL, Moineddin R, Dunn JR, Glazier RH (2012) Drinking in context: the influence of gender and neighbourhood deprivation on alcohol consumption. J Epidemiol Commun Health 66:e4

Mehnert A (2011) Employment and work-related issues in cancer survivors. Crit Rev Oncol Hematol 77:109–130

Mehnert A, Lehmann C, Graefen M, Huland H, Koch U (2010) Depression, anxiety, post-traumatic stress disorder and health-related quality of life and its association with social support in ambulatory prostate cancer patients. Eur J Cancer Care 19:736–745

Mehnert A, Brähler E, Faller H, Härter M, Keller M, Schulz H, Wegscheider K, Weis J, Boehncke A, Hund B, Reuter K, Richard M, Sehner S, Sommerfeldt S, Szalai C, Wittchen HU, Koch U (2014) Four-week prevalence of mental disorders in patients with cancer across major tumor entities. J Clin Oncol 32:3540–3546

Milam JE (2004) Posttraumatic growth among HIV/AIDS patients. J Appl Soc Psychol 34:2353–2376

Mitchell AJ, Chan M, Bhatti H, Halton M, Grassi L, Johansen C, Meader N (2011) Prevalence of depression, anxiety, and adjustment disorder in oncological, haematological, and palliative-care settings: a meta-analysis of 94 interview-based studies. Lancet Oncology 12:160–174

Mols F, Vingerhoets AJJM, Coebergh JWW, van de Poll-Franse L (2009) Well-being, posttraumatic growth and benefit finding in long-term breast cancer survivors. Psychol Health 24:583–595

Natvig K (1983) Laryngectomees in Norway. Study No. 4: social, occupational and personal factors related to vocational rehabilitation. J Otolaryngol 12:370–376

Oliffe JL, Phillips MJ (2008) Men, depression and masculinities: a review and recommendations. J Mens Health 5:194–202

Paul MS, Berger R, Berlow N, Rovner-Ferguson H, Figlerski L, Gardner S, Malave AF (2010) Posttraumatic growth and social support in individuals with infertility. Hum Reprod 25:133–141

Pinquart M, Duberstein PR (2010) Depression and cancer mortality: a meta-analysis. Psychol Med 40:1797–1810

Rooney AG, McNamara S, Mackinnon M, Fraser M, Rampling R, Carson A, Grant R (2011) Frequency, clinical associations, and longitudinal course of major depressive disorder in adults with cerebral glioma. J Clin Oncol 29:4307–4312

Schraub S, Bontemps P, Mercier M, Barthod L, Fournier J (1995) Surveillance et rehabilitation des cancers des voies aero-digestives superieures. [Surveillance and rehabilitation of cancers of upper respiratory and digestive tracts]. Rev Prat 45:861–864

Schwarz R, Singer S (2008) Einführung in die Psychosoziale Onkologie. Ernst Reinhardt Verlag, München

Schwarz R, Rucki N, Singer S (2006) Onkologisch Kranke als Patienten der psychotherapeutischen Praxis: Beitrag zur Qualitätserkundung und psychosozialen Versorgungslage. Psychotherapeut 51:369–375

Sheikh AI (2004) Posttraumatic growth in the context of heart disease. J Clin Psychol Med Settings 11:265–273

Shimazu T, Sasazuki S, Wakai K, Tamakoshi A, Tsuji I, Sugawara Y, Matsuo K, Nagata C, Mizoue T, Tanaka K, Inoue M, Tsugane S (2012) Alcohol drinking and primary liver cancer: A pooled analysis of four Japanese cohort studies. Int J Cancer 130:2645–2653

Singer S, Schwentner L, van Ewijk R, Blettner M, Wöckel A, Kühn T, Felberbaum R, Flock F, Janni W; BRENDA Study Group (2016) The course of psychiatric co-morbidity in patients with breast cancer–results from the prospective multi-centre BRENDA II study. Psychooncology 25:590-596

Singer S, Herrmann E, Welzel C, Klemm E, Heim M, Schwarz R (2005) Comorbid mental disorders in Laryngectomees. Onkologie 28:631–636

Singer S, Das-Munshi J, Brähler E (2010) Prevalence of mental health conditions in cancer patients in acute care—a meta-analysis. Ann Oncol 21:925–930

Singer S, Brown A, Einenkel J, Hauss J, Hinz A, Klein A, Papsdorf K, Stolzenburg J-U, Brähler E (2011a) Identifying tumor patients' depression. Support Care Cancer 19:1697–1703

Singer S, Hohlfeld S, Müller-Briel D, Dietz A, Brähler E, Schröter K, Lehmann-Laue A (2011b) Psychosoziale Versorgung von Krebspatienten - Versorgungsdichte und -bedarf. Psychotherapeut 56:386–393

Singer S, Lincke Th, Gamper E, Schreiber S, Hinz A, Bhaskaran K, Schulte Th (2012) Quality of life in patients with thyroid cancer compared with the general population. Thyroid 22:117–124

Singer S, Ehrensperger C, Briest S, Brown A, Dietz A, Einenkel J, Jonas S, Konnopka A, Papsdorf K, Langanke D, Löbner M, Schiefke F, Stolzenburg J-U, Weimann A, Wirtz H, König HH, Riedel-Heller SG (2013a) Comorbid mental health conditions in cancer patients at working age—prevalence, risk profiles, and care uptake. Psychooncology 22:2291–2297

Singer S, Götze H, Buttstädt M, Ziegler C, Richter R, Brown A, Niederwieser D, Dorst J, Jäkel N, Geue K (2013b) A non-randomized trial of an art therapy intervention for patients with haematological malignancies to support post-traumatic growth. J Health Psychol 18:939–949

Söllner W, DeVries A, Steixner E, Lukas P, Sprinzl G, Rumpold G, Maislinger S (2001) How successful are oncologists in identifying patient distress, perceived social support, and need for psychosocial counselling? Br J Cancer 84:179–185

Stoppe G, Sandholzer H, Huppertz C, Duwe H, Staedt J (1999) Gender differences in the recognition of depression in old age. Maturitas 32:205–212

Sullivan PW, Mulani PM, Fishman M, Sleep D (2007) Quality of life findings from a multicenter, multinational, observational study of patients with metastatic hormone-refractory prostate cancer. Qual Life Res 16:571–575

Tedeschi RG, Calhoun LG (2004) Posttraumatic growth: conceptual foundations and empirical evidence. Psychol Inq 15:1–18

Tsunoda A, Nakao K, Hiratsuka K, Tsunoda Y, Kusano M (2007) Prospective analysis of quality of life in the first year after colorectal cancer surgery. Acta Oncol 46:77–82

Vehling S, Koch U, Ladehoff N, Schön G, Wegscheider K, Heckl U, Weis J, Mehnert A (2012) Prävalenz affektiver und Angststörungen bei Krebs: Systematischer Literaturreview und Metaanalyse. Psychother Psychosom Med Psychol 62:249–258

Wancata J, Benda N, Windhaber J, Nowotny M (2001) Does psychiatric comorbidity increase the length of stay in general hospitals? Gen Hosp Psychiatry 23:8–14

Weich S, Lewis G (1998) Poverty, unemployment, and common mental disorders: population based cohort study. BMJ 317:115–119

Weich S, Lewis G, Jenkins SP (2001) Income inequality and the prevalence of common mental disorders in Britain. Br J Psychiatry 178:222–227

Werrbach J, Gilbert LA (1987) Men, gender stereotyping, and psychotherapy—therapists perceptions of male clients. Prof Psychol Res Prac 18:562–566

Wilhelm KA (2009) Men and depression. Aust Fam Physician 38:102–105

Williams J (2012) Geographic variations in health care utilization: effects of social capital and self-interest, and implications for US Medicare policy. Socio-Econ Rev 10:317–342

Fear of Progression in Cancer Patients and Survivors

Andreas Dinkel and Peter Herschbach

Abstract

Fear of progression (or fear of recurrence) is an appropriate, adequate response to the real threat of cancer. However, elevated levels of fear of progression can become dysfunctional, affecting well-being, quality of life, and social functioning. Research has shown that fear of progression is one of the most frequent distress symptoms of patients with cancer. As a clear consensus concerning clinically relevant states of fear of progression is still lacking, it is difficult to provide a valid estimate of the rate of cancer patients who clearly suffer from fear of progression. Current evidence suggests that probably 50% of cancer survivors experience moderate to severe fear of progression. Furthermore, many patients express unmet needs in dealing with the fear of cancer spreading. These results underscore the need to provide effective psychological treatments for clinical states of fear of progression. Some psychosocial interventions for treating fear of progression have been developed. Our own, targeted intervention study showed that clinical fear of progression can be effectively treated with brief group therapy.

This is an updated version of the chapter: Herschbach P, Dinkel A (2014) Fear of progression. In: Goerling U (Ed). Psycho-Oncology (Recent Results in Cancer Research 197). Berlin: Springer; p. 11-29.

A. Dinkel (✉)
Department of Psychosomatic Medicine and Psychotherapy, Klinikum rechts der Isar, Technical University of Munich, Langerstraße 3, Munich 81675, Germany
e-mail: a.dinkel@tum.de

P. Herschbach
Roman-Herzog-Cancer Center (RHCCC), Klinikum rechts der Isar, Technical University of Munich, Trogerstraße 26, Munich 81675, Germany
e-mail: p.herschbach@tum.de

13

Keywords
Fear of progression · Fear of recurrence · Cancer worry · Distress

1 Introduction

There is sound evidence today that about 30% of all cancer patients suffer from some form of mental disease (Mehnert et al. 2014; Mitchell et al. 2011; Singer et al. 2010; Vehling et al. 2012). The most prevalent diagnoses are depression, anxiety, and adjustment disorders.

These diagnoses are based on a thorough assessment of cancer patients, using some kind of structured clinical interview for diagnosing mental disorders. These measures relate to the current psychiatric classification systems, i.e., DSM or ICD, which were primarily developed for the assessment of (more or less) physically healthy patients with psychological problems. However, there are some limitations of the psychiatric model in medical illness, and the criteria of mental disorders might not generally apply to cancer patients. The psychological symptoms of cancer patients, and other medical patients, sometimes do not fit the usual descriptions and the criteria of common mental disorders. As Gurevich et al. (2002, p. 259) noticed, "the personal tragedy of serious medical illness is not necessarily captured within the bounds of psychiatric illness".

In the field of psycho-oncology, one way to resolve this dilemma was to introduce the concept of distress. This is a broadly defined umbrella term that encompasses a wide range of psychological problems, ranging from severe psychopathological symptoms to mild forms of irritation. According to the US-American National Comprehensive Cancer Network Clinical Practice Guideline, distress is "a multifactorial unpleasant emotional experience of a psychological (cognitive, behavioral, emotional), social, and/or spiritual nature that may interfere with the ability to cope effectively with cancer, its physical symptoms and its treatment. Distress extends along a continuum, ranging from common normal feelings of vulnerability, sadness, and fears to problems that can become disabling, such as depression, anxiety, panic, social isolation, and existential and spiritual crisis" (see NCCN Guideline Distress Management 2013). Distress can be measured by self-report, which is one methodological advantage compared to the interviewer-based assessment of mental disorders.

There are plenty of studies that demonstrate the relevance and frequency of various distress symptoms. In our own work we found that the fear of the cancer spreading was one of the most frequent and important problems of patients. In a sample of 1721 patients with different cancer diagnoses, about one-third of the patients acknowledged that being afraid of disease progression was a serious or very serious problem to them. Indeed, this problem received the highest severity rating (Herschbach et al. 2004).

In the following, we will provide a description and definition of fear of disease progression; report on its prevalence, course and correlates; and refer to the psychological treatment of clinical levels of fear or progression.

2   Fear of Disease Progression

It is not unusual for physically ill patients to suffer from fears that are related to various aspects of the illness itself. We referred to these kinds of illness-related fears as *fear of progression* (FoP; Dankert et al. 2003).

FoP should be differentiated from the psychiatric concept of anxiety disorders. A central and common characteristic of neurotic anxiety disorders (such as generalized anxiety disorder, panic disorder, and agoraphobia) is that these problems are unreal or irrational. In the context of cancer, however, patients are confronted with real threats; their reactions are neither irrational nor inappropriate. Yet, patients can experience long-lasting and exaggerated realistic fears that affect their well-being and quality of life.

Thus, we define FoP as patients' fear that the illness will progress with all its biopsychosocial consequences, or that it will recur. Patients are fully aware of this reactive, non-neurotic fear response. The fear is based on the personal experience of a life-threatening or incapacitating illness. Like other anxieties, FoP is experienced in emotional, cognitive, behavioral, and physiological qualities. Basically, FoP is an adequate response to the real threats that are associated with diagnosis, treatment, and course of illness. In our view, the level of FoP can range between functional and dysfunctional ends. Elevated levels of FoP that become dysfunctional, i.e., affecting coping, treatment adherence, quality of life or social functioning, are in need for treatment.

2.1   Excursion: Fear of Progression Versus Fear of Recurrence

The fear of chronically or severely ill patients about the illness getting worse is not a new phenomenon. It seems plausible that this kind of fear is inextricably linked with the experience of severe physical illness.

Northouse (1981) provided one of the earliest empirical accounts of cancer patients' fear that the illness might recur. More than a decade later, Lee-Jones et al. (1997) summarized the available, still sparse literature on that topic, and developed a cognitive-behavioral model to explain the exacerbation and maintenance of recurrence fears in cancer patients.

These authors, as well as others, coined the term *fear of recurrence* when speaking of realistic, illness-related fears of cancer patients and survivors. So, is there any difference between the two concepts, *fear of progression* and *fear of recurrence*?—Basically, the two concepts are nearly identical.

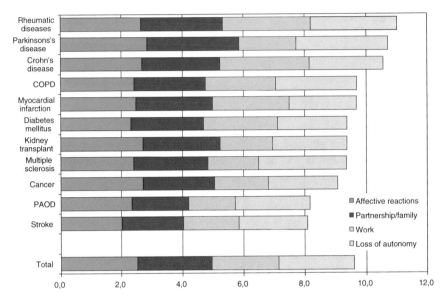

Fig. 1 Fear of progression in different diseases according to subscales and total score of the Fear of Progression Questionnaire (FoP-Q), adapted from Berg et al. (2011). Abbreviations: *COPD* chronic obstructive pulmonary disease; *PAOD* peripheral artery occlusive disease

Our own research on illness-related fears has not been restricted to cancer patients. As our early work revealed, FoP was evident in patients with cancer, rheumatoid arthritis, and diabetes mellitus (Dankert et al. 2003). Furthermore, we discovered that the content of patients' illness-related fears was quite comparable across the studied diseases, with slight nuances concerning predominant fears within each disease group (Dankert et al. 2003). Thus, we conceptualized FoP as a generic concept. To be applicable across a wide range of chronic diseases, we used the term *fear of progression*. This label allows adequately including various diseases with a different disease course, e.g., constantly progressing or remitting-recurring. A further study with more than 800 patients who belonged to 11 disease groups confirmed that FoP is widespread across different diseases (see Fig. 1). Although the disease groups were not fully comparable with regard to sociodemographic and clinical character-istics, the results suggested that FoP is a serious concern in rheumatic diseases and some neurologic diseases, too (Berg et al. 2011).

The concept of *fear of recurrence* was mainly developed in the field of psycho-oncology. From early days on, it was mainly used to refer to cancer patients in remission, or disease-free cancer survivors, who worried about the cancer coming back (e.g. Northouse 1981). Today, fear of recurrence is defined as "the fear or worry that cancer will return, progress or metastasise" (Crist and Grunveld 2013, p. 978). Another frequently cited definition is usually traced back to the work of Vickberg (2003), although she did not provide this definition verbatim in her paper. It states that fear of recurrence is "the fear that cancer could return or progress in the same place or in another part of the body" (see Koch et al. 2013; Thewes et al. 2012a). It is obvious that despite the different labeling, the two constructs *fear of progression* and *fear of recurrence* share relevant defining features and are, basically, comparable. This is reflected in the definition recently proposed by an expert panel: "Fear, worry, or concern about cancer returning or progressing" (Lebel et al. 2016). Therefore, we included studies using either one of these two concepts in the writing of this chapter.

2.2 Theoretical Models

As early as 1997, Lee-Jones and colleagues proposed a theoretical model incorporating the empirical evidence that was available at that time. Since then, most of the research on fear of recurrence in cancer was atheoretical. A systematic review by Fardell et al. (2016) identified only 16 papers that explicitly referred to a theoretical approach. The one that was mentioned most often was the Common Sense Model, which already had been used and adapted by Lee-Jones et al. (1997). Apart from that, several other models have been applied, like Protection Motivation Theory, the Extended Parallel Process Model or the Uncertainty in Illness Theory (see Fardell et al. 2016; Simonelli et al. 2016). Based on their review, Fardell et al. (2016) proposed a synthesis of theories. In their model, they focus on the role of cognitive processing and propose that unhelpful beliefs about the importance, impact, and control of worry, i.e., metacognitive beliefs, play a central role in the transformation of adequate emotional, cognitive, and behavioral responses to real threats to a dysfunctional state of heightened fear of cancer recurrence.

3 Assessment of Fear of Progression

As fear of progression is conceptually different from anxiety disorders and general anxiety, traditional anxiety measures, such as the State-Trait Anxiety Inventory (STAI; Spielberger et al. 1983) or the Beck Anxiety Inventory (Beck and Steer 1993), cannot adequately measure FoP. During the past years, several self-report measures have been developed that focus specifically on FoP. Thewes et al. (2012b) provided a systematic review on current multi-item self-report questionnaires and subscales that assess FoP in cancer patients. They identified 20 multi-item assessment tools, six of which being subscales of more comprehensive instruments. Ten measures were classified into the group of brief instruments with 2–10 items. Most of these measures had only limited reliability and validity data available. The remaining four measures fell into the group of longer tools with more than 10 items. These latter measures were judged as reliable and valid. One of these longer self-report measures that had proved reliable and valid is the Fear of Progression Questionnaire (FoP-Q). Actually, the FoP-Q received the highest total quality rating of all instruments, together with the Concerns about Recurrence Scale by Vickberg (see Thewes et al. 2012b).

The FoP-Q is a multi-dimensional self-reporting questionnaire that was developed in our research group, using samples of patients who were suffering from cancer, rheumatic diseases, and diabetes mellitus (Herschbach et al. 2005). The questionnaire contains 43 items that are rated on a five-point scale, ranging from *never* to *very often*. The items relate to the five dimensions *affective reactions*, *partnership/family issues*, *occupation*, *loss of autonomy*, and *coping with anxiety*. The total score is calculated as the sum of the subscales' mean scores, *excluding* the coping subscale. The questionnaire has high internal consistency (Cronbach's $\alpha = 0.95$), as well as high test-retest reliability over one week ($r_{tt} = 0.94$) (Herschbach et al. 2005).

Apart from this full version, Mehnert et al. (2006) developed a unidimensional short form, using a sample of breast cancer patients. This abbreviated version, FoP-Q-SF, comprises 12 items pertaining to four of the five subscales (excluding coping). The short form showed adequate reliability ($\alpha = 0.87$); correlational analyses with other psychosocial measures suggested validity. A recent psychometric study with a large sample of cancer patients with different diagnoses supported reliability and validity of the short form (Hinz et al. 2015).

Furthermore, the questionnaire was adapted for use with parents of chronically ill children (Fidika et al. 2015; Schepper et al. 2015) and partners of chronically ill patients (Zimmermann et al. 2011).

Moreover, the Fear of Progression Questionnaire was translated into two further languages. Shim et al. (2010) provided a Korean version of the full FoP-Q, based on research with a heterogeneous cancer sample. Kwakkenbos et al. (2012) adapted the short form and developed a Dutch version of the FoP-Q-SF, using a sample of patients with systemic sclerosis. Thus, the FoP-Q and the FoP-Q-SF proved to be applicable and useful measures of fear of progression, or fear of cancer recurrence.

Most researchers acknowledge that FoP is an adequate response to the suffering from cancer that, nonetheless, might become dysfunctional. Therefore, it would be highly desirable to identify patients who experience heightened, clinically relevant levels of FoP. However, to date none of the available self-report measures, including FoP-Q and FoP-Q-SF, provides a validated cut-off for the classification of dysfunctional FoP. One reason for this unsatisfying condition is the lack of established external criteria. To date, we do not have a well-established definition of a clinical state of dysfunctional FoP, analogous to the definition of common mental disorders. Furthermore, it does not seem appropriate to use one of the common anxiety measures as a gold standard, and to conduct sensitivity and specificity analyses of FoP measures in order to establish a clinical cut-off score. Therefore, most researchers who need to define clinical FoP use cut-off scores that are based on statistical considerations, taking into account the distributional characteristics of the measure. Alternatively, cut-off scores are defined based on theoretical considerations.

This shortcoming of the current state of research on FoP has far reaching consequences. As Thewes et al. (2012b) and Lebel et al. (2017) point out, the lack of diagnostic criteria limits comparison between studies, the development of specific interventions, the evaluation of the criterion validity of measures, as well as the development of screening tools indicative of clinical states of FoP.

4 Frequency and Correlates of Fear of Progression

Research on FoP in cancer patients has grown rapidly during the recent years, and the research literature has accumulated. In fact, there are already several systematic reviews on different aspects of FoP in cancer (Crist and Grunveld 2013; Fardell et al. 2016; Koch et al. 2013; Simard et al. 2013). Most of this research was conducted with breast cancer patients. For instance, only 2 of the 17 articles in the systematic review by Koch et al. (2013) included patients who were not diagnosed with breast cancer. In the most comprehensive systematic review, so far, Simard et al. (2013) included 130 papers. The majority of these studies focused on a specific cancer site, primarily breast cancer (42 studies). However, studies also looked at patients with prostate, ovarian, hematological, or colorectal cancer, among others. Most of the research on FoP was conducted in the United States, but there are also several studies from the UK, Canada, or Germany (see Simard et al. 2013).

In the following, we will briefly refer to the main empirical results on prevalence and correlates of FoP.

4.1 Prevalence and Course

FoP is an appropriate, adequate response to the diagnosis of cancer and its treatment. Accordingly, nearly all patients acknowledge feelings of FoP, ranging from very mild upset to severe worries. In Table 1, we present the responses of cancer patients to the items of the Fear of Progression Questionnaire-Short Form (FoP-Q-SF) in women with breast cancer and in a sample with mixed cancer diagnoses. The results show that the vast majority experiences fears and worries. Breast cancer patients, as well as patients with other diagnoses, stated that they are mainly bothered by thoughts about the cancer spreading, worries about severe medical treatments, worries about the next physical examination, and fear of pain.

As there is no clear consensus on clinically elevated FoP, different definitions were applied. This limits the comparability of the available data concerning the prevalence of clinical levels of FoP. Prevalence was reported to amount to 47% in women newly diagnosed with gynecological cancers (Myers et al. 2013), or 56% in a sample of patients with first-ever cancer diagnosis (Savard and Ivers 2013). Dysfunctional FoP is also high in cancer survivors: 24% (Mehnert et al. 2009) to 70% (Thewes et al. 2012a) in breast cancer survivors, 35% in head and neck cancer survivors (Ghazali et al. 2013), 31% in testicular cancer survivors (Skaali et al. 2009), and 50% in colorectal cancer survivors (Fisher et al. 2016). In contrast,

Table 1 Reponses to the items of the Fear of Progression Questionnaire-Short Form (FoP-Q-SF) in two different samples; mean (M), standard deviation (SD), and percent of patients (% positive) experiencing the item at least seldom (scoring at least 2 in the FoP-Q-SF item)

	Breast cancer patients; cancer registry $(N = 1.083)^a$			Mixed diagnoses; inpatient rehabilitation $(N = 482)^b$		
	M	SD	% positive	M	SD	% positive
I become anxious if I think my disease may progress	2.71	1.12	85.0	3.02	1.06	92.6
I am nervous prior to doctors' appointments or periodic examinations	3.28	1.34	86.9	3.22	1.06	91.1
I am afraid of pain	2.93	1.25	85.0	2.95	1.07	92.1
The thought that I might become less productive at my job disturbs me	2.14	1.39	49.1	2.10	1.31	51.2
When I am anxious, I have physical symptoms, e.g. rapid heartbeat, stomach ache	2.91	1.30	81.4	2.88	1.20	85.9
The possibility of my children contracting my disease disturbs me	2.81	1.54	67.0	2.86	1.42	85.2
It disturbs me that I may have to rely on strangers for activities of daily living	3.08	1.34	84.0	2.88	1.25	85.2
I am worried that at some point in time, because of my illness I will no longer be able to pursue my hobbies	2.38	1.22	69.0	2.46	1.18	75.4
I am afraid of severe medical treatments in the course of my illness	2.80	1.26	82.2	3.08	1.10	91.4
I worry that my medications could damage my body	2.83	1.31	79.7	2.86	1.19	85.0
I worry about what will become of my family if something should happen to me	2.88	1.31	81.0	3.01	1.33	82.0
The thought that I might not be able to work due to my illness disturbs me	2.09	1.32	50.4	2.20	1.24	59.0

Note Item wording of the FoP-Q-SF is taken from Herschbach et al. (2005)
[a]Mehnert et al. (2006)
[b]Herschbach (unpublished data)

Koch-Gallenkamp et al. (2016) found that only 13% of the survivors in a mixed sample of breast, prostate, and colorectal cancer survivors suffered from moderate to high fear of recurrence.

In their review, Simard et al. (2013) found that, across different cancer sites and assessment strategies, on average 49% of cancer survivors reported moderate to high degree of FoP, and on average 7% reported high degree.

Several researchers found that FoP is quite stable over time, with slight decreases in the first months after diagnosis (Savard and Ivers 2013) or during rehabilitation (Mehnert et al. 2013). Simard et al. (2013) report that of 22 longitudinal studies on the course of FoP, eight studies showed that FoP decreased after diagnosis or cancer treatment and then remained stable. The other studies reported no change, or even increase over time. Thus, these results clearly underscore that FoP is a constant companion of cancer patients.

4.2   Correlates and Consequences

Research has looked at many potential variables that might correlate and predict FoP. Among potential demographic characteristics, the strongest evidence is for younger age to predict FoP (Crist and Grunveld 2013; Koch et al. 2013; Simard et al. 2013). In contrast to many research results from the field of psychiatry that typically report an association between gender and distress, there is no clear evidence that women experience higher FoP. Similarly, the evidence concerning marital status and FoP is mixed (Crist and Grunveld 2013; Koch et al. 2013; Simard et al. 2013). Some studies suggest that having children is associated with higher FoP (Mehnert et al. 2009, 2013), but there is also contrasting evidence (Thewes et al. 2012a).

Although some studies reported significant associations among cancer type, disease stage and treatment-related factors, especially chemotherapy, and FoP, these variables typically did not predict FoP in multivariate analyses (Koch-Gallenkamp et al. 2016; Simard et al. 2013; van de Wal et al. 2016). With regard to physical symptoms, there is strong evidence that more frequent or higher number of somatic symptoms are related to higher FoP (Koch et al. 2013; Simard et al. 2013). Thus, the evidence to date suggests that medical and treatment-related factors are of only minor relevance for patients' FoP, except for the presence of somatic complaints.

Overall, mixed evidence exists for the influence of psychological factors (Koch et al. 2013; Simard et al. 2013). Some results suggest that FoP is higher among cancer patients with high neuroticism, low optimism, low social support (see Simard et al. 2013) or low health literacy (Halbach et al. 2016), but these results need further replication as they were investigated in only a few studies, so far.

FoP is significantly correlated with distress, depression, anxiety, and traumatic stress symptoms (Simard et al. 2013). These associations are moderately high, showing that FoP is distinct from more general distress or common psychopathological conceptions of emotional disorder.

With regard to the consequences of FoP, there is strong evidence that FoP is related to reduced quality of life and social functioning (Simard et al. 2013). Furthermore, there is some evidence that FoP relates to healthcare use and health behaviors after cancer diagnosis. Higher FoP predicted more unscheduled visits to the general practitioner (Thewes et al. 2012a) and visits to the emergency department (Lebel et al. 2013). Colorectal cancer survivors with high fear of recurrence showed poorer health behaviors, i.e., higher rates of smoking and lower physical activity levels (Fisher et al. 2016). Among breast cancer patients, higher FoP was associated with higher frequency of breast self-examination but, interestingly, a lower participation rate in formal medical surveillance, e.g., mammograms or ultrasound. The authors of this study suggest that this behavior pattern is consistent with a cognitive-behavioral model of general health anxiety which postulates that high anxiety is associated with both excessive threat monitoring and avoidance behaviors (Thewes et al. 2012a).

Taken together, despite many research efforts, our knowledge concerning the most potent and relevant predictors of FoP is still limited. The results show that FoP is common and long lasting, and that it has a negative impact on patients' lives. However, apart from two or three variables for which there is a quite consistent results pattern, there is mainly mixed evidence regarding the predictive relevance of demographic, illness/treatment-related, and psychological factors.

4.3 Couple and Family Perspective

Some investigations on FoP also looked at partners and family caregivers. One study with relatives of cancer, rheumatoid arthritis, and migraine patients showed that 49% of the relatives suffered from clinical levels of FoP (Zimmermann et al. 2012). Studies that included cancer patients as well as their caregivers revealed that FoP was even higher among the family caregivers than in the patient group (Hodges and Humphris 2009; Mellon et al. 2007).

Furthermore, as might be expected, FoP is not only influenced by individual factors, but also by partner effects. One study showed that caregivers' FoP is higher if the patient is in poorer physical health (Kim et al. 2012). Another investigation revealed an effect for age; survivors with younger caregivers, as well as caregivers with younger survivors experienced higher levels of FoP (Mellon et al. 2007). Furthermore, one longitudinal study showed that patients' FoP 3 months after diagnosis of head/neck cancer predicted caregivers' FoP at 6 months after diagnosis. No effects of family caregivers' FoP on patients' level emerged (Hodges and Humphris 2009).

Thus, these results remind us that cancer is a family affair, and that it is fruitful to adopt a family perspective on FoP. Notably, the fact that caregivers express levels of FoP higher than patients should motivate researchers to develop treatment approaches that also include or are specifically targeted at family caregivers.

5 Psychological Treatment Approaches

5.1 Clinical Relevance of Dysfunctional Fear of Progression

Like other researchers, we conceptualize FoP as an adaptive response that can become dysfunctional. As already shown, the prevalence of FoP is rather high among newly diagnosed cancer patients and among cancer survivors. However, are there any empirical hints that justify the assumption that these are clinically relevant states?

In our view, there is convincing evidence that FoP in cancer patients can reach levels that are in need of treatment. First, as stated above, FoP is often experienced as the most severe distress symptom (Herschbach et al. 2004). Second, FoP is among the most important concerns cancer patients would like to discuss during their consultation with their oncologist. Research with head and neck cancer patients showed that about 40% of the patients indicated FoP as their main concern (Kanatas et al. 2013; Rogers et al. 2009). Third, FoP is a main reason for the uptake of psychological treatment. As Salander (2010) reports, anxiety and worries caused by the disease represented the leading cause for consulting a psychologist. Finally, research has shown that FoP is the most commonly identified unmet psychosocial need of cancer patients, during treatment as well as in the posttreatment phase (Armes et al. 2009; Harrison et al. 2009).

Only very few studies investigated whether high levels of fear of recurrence are associated with the diagnosis of a mental disorder. Simard and Savard (2015) as well as Dinkel et al. (2014) found that some patients with elevated fear of recurrence also suffered from a mental disorder. However, there also seem to be patients with isolated clinical fear of progression who do not suffer from a comorbid anxiety disorder but who experience symptom burden similar to patients with an anxiety disorder. These results suggest that clinical fear of progression appears to be a distinct phenomenon (Dinkel et al. 2014).

These results underscore the need to identify patients who suffer from dysfunctional FoP and to develop and provide appropriate treatments. In the following, we will present, in some detail, a group-based treatment approach that was developed in our research group.

5.2 The Munich Approach

The psychotherapeutic treatment of realistic problems—such as FoP—does not have many predecessors in the professional literature (see Moorey 1996, for an exception). Usually, psychotherapeutic interventions are theoretically related to and developed for psychosomatic or mental disorders. Thus, it seemed inevitable to develop a special psychotherapeutic intervention for dysfunctional FoP in physically ill patients.

This new intervention was developed with the guideline that the intervention would be applicable in an inpatient rehabilitation setting. Therefore, it seemed most appropriate to design a brief group-based intervention. The group-based intervention is based on the principles of cognitive-behavioral psychotherapy (CBT). It is prescriptive and specific, which are the main general features. The aim is to confront the patients with their recurrence fears and supporting patients learning to cope with them. One further treatment goal was to strengthen patients' self-awareness regarding the elicitation and experience of fear. The treatment followed the well-established concepts of cognitive restructuring and worry exposure. Educational elements and homework assignments were also included.

Eventually, this approach comprised four sessions of group psychotherapy. It is a manualized intervention (Waadt et al. 2011). Each of the sessions lasted 90 min. The session topics are self-awareness and self-assessment, fear exposure, and behavior change and problem solving. Homework assignments, diary keeping, and relaxation exercises were used as accompanying interventions.

In the beginning, patients identify key personal triggers of FoP. In addition, they report on their subjective experience of FoP. Patients are instructed to differentiate cognitive, behavioral, emotional, and physiological characteristics of their fear response. They are educated that experiencing FoP is an adequate response to the real threat of being ill, and that it is necessary to differentiate between functional aspects of FoP and dysfunctional fear levels. The actual cognitive exposure intervention is called "To-Think-the-Fear-to-an-End" (*Zu-Ende-Denken* in German). This intervention resembles the worry exposure, which is used in the treatment of generalized anxiety disorder (Hoyer et al. 2009). Patients are to choose a personally relevant situation that elicits high levels of FoP. In the next step, patients are asked to imagine this situation and to elaborate on all aspects and possible consequences —a task that was usually avoided in daily life. One such scenario might be losing one's hair during chemotherapy. An example of a therapeutic dialogue with a female patient suffering from the fear of losing her hair is presented in Box 1.

Box 1: Example of cognitive exposure of FoP

Therapist: How will you notice that you start losing your hair?

Patient: I will find hair on my pillow… and in the basin, after hair combing.

Therapist: What will happen in the worst case, what do you think?

Patient: I will also lose my eyebrows.

Therapist: What will be the consequences in your every day life?

Patient: I will feel unfeminine. I will stay at home. I won't go out because people will see that I am a cancer patient. It will be embarrassing for my child, in school when others ask her about her mom.

Therapist: How would you like to react? What do you think would be a competent response, a response you feel well with?

Patient: I'd like to face my cancer, feeling confident, not to hide at home.

Therapist: How could you prepare for this situation?

Patient: I will cut my hair gradually beforehand…I will try wigs and head-scarves… I will show myself only to good friends first.

It is assumed that confronting the patient with the possible consequences leads to an increase in perceived control and a reappraisal of the feared consequences. The consequences might get clearer, and the patient might develop helpful ways to deal with the feared consequences.

At the end, patients are asked to think about personal changes in coping with FoP as well as changes they would like to implement in their daily lives. Patients are encouraged to choose specific goals that they would like to reach in the next 4 weeks after the end of the group intervention.

As mentioned initially, this group-based intervention was developed for use in inpatient rehabilitation (Waadt et al. 2011). This is a time-limited setting where patients receive multidisciplinary, multimodal therapeutic treatment. It seems reasonable to make necessary adaptations to the treatment protocol, depending on the specific circumstances. For instance, we developed a slightly modified protocol for use with cancer patients who are treated in our outpatient department. Here, we provide a six-session group therapy (Rudolph et al. 2017).

In routine clinical practice, it is essential to inform patients beforehand about the treatment rationale, as this kind of therapy is not suited for all cancer patients. There are patients who feel heavily burdened by clinically elevated FoP but who refrain to join this CBT-based group treatment. Typically, these patients cannot believe that they might tolerate the confrontation with their recurrence fears. These patients will very likely drop out of the therapy if they are not adequately informed about the exposure-based treatment. Obviously, alternative treatments should be offered in this case.

5.2.1 Evaluation

This brief group-based psychotherapeutic treatment was evaluated in a (partially-) randomized controlled trial. As this treatment approach was conceptualized as a generic intervention, applicable to diverse populations, the trial included patients with cancer and patients with rheumatoid arthritis. In the following, we will briefly summarize the trial and the main results, with a special focus on the cancer patients (see Herschbach et al. 2010a, b).

Study Design and Procedure

This was a multi-center, longitudinal (partially-)randomized controlled study. Patients were sampled consecutively during the study, which was conducted in three rehabilitation clinics. Cancer patients were approached in two clinics, arthritis patients came from one clinic. In Germany, admission to inpatient rehabilitation is not necessarily a sign of exacerbation or dramatic worsening of symptoms. Many patients with acute or chronic illness get inpatient rehabilitation treatment in order to reestablish vocational capability, to prevent work disability or to increase vocational and community participation.

To be eligible for the study, patients had to be at least 18 years old and had to suffer from dysfunctional FoP, i.e., they had to score above a predefined cut-off. The cut-off score for dysfunctional FoP was derived in a separate investigation, conducted before this intervention study, with $N = 130$ arthritis and $N = 150$ cancer inpatients. These patients filled in the short form FoP-Q-SF. In addition, they indicated whether they felt in need of treatment for FoP and would participate in a psychotherapeutic intervention ("yes"/"no"). As there were no external criteria to validate the cut-off score, we followed the conventional strategy of using the median score in a first step. Next, we stratified the sample according to their self-reported treatment need. 38% of the arthritis patients and 36% of the cancer patients scored above the median and felt in need of treatment. About 10% in both groups scored above the median and did not express a need for treatment, and about 30% scored below the median but said they were in need of treatment. These results qualified the median score as a pragmatic cut-off for dysfunctional FoP. The consequence of this approach, which leads to a corresponding rate of treatment need in the two diagnostic groups, was the use of two different cut-off scores. Thus, the predefined FoP-Q-SF cut-off scores (summary score) for this intervention study were 38 for the arthritis patients and 34 for the cancer patients.

Patients were randomized into two interventions. Patients in both intervention groups received four sessions of group psychotherapy, each lasting 90 min. The intervention groups were specific to each diagnosis. Groups were designed for a maximum of 10 participants. Both group interventions were conducted as a manualized treatment. The CBT intervention was highly manualized with regard to structure and content. The second intervention was a supportive-experiential group intervention (SET). It was manualized with regard to structure, but less prescriptive regarding content. It was based on a client-centered concept and was characterized by nondirectiveness. This intervention aimed at facilitating the expression of personal experiences and emotions, it did not specifically focus on the management of FoP. In each session, the patients decided which topic they would like to discuss. They were supported in reflecting the issues they had selected with regard to FoP. Patients from both intervention groups received two booster phone calls 6 and 9 months after discharge from the clinic. The groups were led by psychotherapists who had at least 3 years of clinical experience and/or who had accomplished or were in the final phase of their therapeutic training.

Originally, the SET intervention was conceptualized as the control condition. However, to exclude that improvement in outcomes was related to overall improvement through the rehabilitation program, a treatment-as-usual control group was sampled after the completion of the intervention phase. These patients did not receive either of the two interventions for reducing FoP. The control group was sampled one year after the intervention phase in the same clinics; the same research staff conducted the recruitment using the same eligibility criteria.

Of 457 cancer patients screened, 210 patients were eligible. Of those, 174 (82.8%) agreed to participate and were assigned to one of the two interventions. In addition, 91 patients were recruited for the control group, resulting in a total sample of $N = 265$ patients. Although patients were not randomly assigned to the control group, our procedure resulted in no relevant systematic differences between the intervention groups and the control group in the measured variables.

FoP was the primary outcome of the study and was assessed using the FoP-Q (full version). Secondary outcomes were anxiety, depression, health-related quality of life, and life satisfaction. Patients from the intervention groups provided data on all outcome measures prior to the initial group therapy session (T1), shortly before discharge from the clinic (T2), 3 months (T3), and 12 months (T4) after discharge. Patients from the control condition only reported on T1, T2, and T4, and they only provided data on the primary outcome FoP.

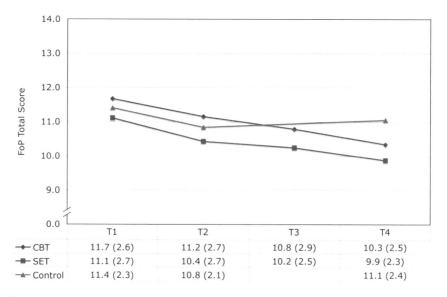

Fig. 2 Course of fear of progression in different intervention groups during 12 months; total score of the Fear of Progression Questionnaire (FoP-Q) (see Herschbach et al. 2010a). Abbreviations: *CBT* cognitive-behavioral group therapy; *SET* supportive-experiential group therapy

Results

The mean age of the cancer patients was 53.7 years (SD = 10.2), 83% were women. Not surprisingly, breast cancer was the most frequent diagnosis (58.9%). 13.1% of the patients had metastases. The mean illness duration was 19.2 months (SD = 30.6).

The results revealed that, compared with treatment-as-usual (TAU), both group therapies were effective in reducing dysfunctional FoP, but only among cancer patients. The effect sizes were 0.54 for the CBT intervention, 0.50 for the SET intervention, and 0.14 for the TAU group (Herschbach et al. 2010a). As is shown in Fig. 2, the FoP total score significantly declined from pre to post intervention, and continued to decline until 12 months after discharge. In contrast, FoP declined in the TAU group during inpatient stay, but reached the initial level after 12 months. The interventions (CBT, SET) also were not differentially effective in reducing the secondary outcomes.

In a secondary analysis, we aimed to uncover treatment effects beyond the mere reduction of FoP at the group level and, thus, investigated the long-term response to group therapy using the Reliable Change Index (RCI) as response criterion. The results showed that 39.5% of the cancer patients experienced reliable (though not necessarily clinically significant) improvement 12 months after the intervention. The rate of reliable improvement did not differ according to intervention type. Higher educational level emerged as a significant predictor of reliable change after 12 months (OR 2.53, 95% CI 1.33-4.81; $p = 0.005$) (Dinkel et al. 2012).

Furthermore, an economic cost-effectiveness evaluation with about 60 patients from the CBT and the SET group, respectively, revealed that group CBT, compared with group SET, is cost-effective without the need for additional costs to payers (Sabariego et al. 2011).

In light of our very brief four-session treatment, the effect sizes as well as the proportion of over one-third of patients who showed a reliable improvement 12 months after the group interventions can be regarded as very promising.

One of the patients who had participated in the CBT intervention provided a vivid account of the helpful experience of this intervention: "*Through 'Thinking-the-Fear-to-an-End' I am not so fearful anymore, I became calmer…The exercise was a 'transformation'. The greatest fear was that I would have to go to a nursing home if the cancer recurs. This is quite unlikely now… However, in case it recurs - I have registered at a nursing home… I do not like to go there but it is an option*".

However, there was no difference in the effectiveness between our newly developed, highly structured CBT intervention and the less prescriptive SET intervention (except for the economic cost-effectiveness analysis). The reasons are unclear. Yet, there seems to be more than just one single way to reduce dysfunctional FoP in cancer patients.

5.3 Further Treatments

In the recent years, some conceptual publications and trial descriptions on specific interventions for elevated FoP were published. These protocols describe interventions that are primarily based upon a CBT framework (Butow et al. 2013; Humphris and Ozakinci 2008; Maheu et al. 2016; van de Wal et al. 2015; van Helmondt et al. 2016). Recent feasibility studies showed promising results and suggest that these interventions might be effective (Lebel et al. 2014; Smith et al. 2015). Furthermore, the RCT by Dieng et al. (2016) showed that psychoeducation significantly reduced fear of recurrence in melanoma survivors. In addition, some interventions did not specifically focus on elevated FoP but included it as a secondary outcome. For instance, Lengacher et al. (2009, 2016) investigated the effects of mindfulness-based stress reduction (MBSR) for breast cancer survivors. They found that a 6-week MBSR program, compared to standard care, significantly reduced FoP.

Finally, one intervention study focused on couples. This study investigated the effects of a couple-based skills program for women recently diagnosed with breast or gynecological cancer and their partners on FoP and other individual and dyadic outcomes. The effects of the couple-skills intervention were compared to couple cancer education. The results showed that the skills intervention was superior compared to the education intervention in reducing FoP, but only in the short-term. The effect was not maintained over the follow-up period of 16 months (Heinrichs et al. 2012). Thus, this research provides initial evidence for short-term effectiveness of a couple-based intervention in reducing FoP levels in women with cancer.

Undoubtedly, as cancer and FoP are also a family affair, more research on the development and evaluation of dyadic and family interventions seems necessary.

6 Conclusion

Many researchers and clinicians have realized that it is necessary and promising to pay special attention to cancer patients' fear of progression. The recent years witnessed a marked increase in research on fear of progression. Several assessment tools were developed, with some instruments reaching high-quality ratings. Research revealed some relevant predictors, correlates, and consequences of fear of progression. A few psychosocial interventions for treating fear of progression were developed. Results on the efficacy of such interventions are sparse; some trials are under way, some research showed that dysfunctional fear of progression could be effectively treated.

So what are the main future tasks in research on fear of progression in cancer patients? In our view, the priorities are first, to reach consensus on the definition and measurement of clinical levels of fear of progression; second, to better understand the relevance of illness-related and personal/social factors for dysfunctional fear of progression; and third, to develop, further elaborate and evaluate individual and family-oriented psychological treatments for clinical fear of progression (see also Lebel et al. 2017). Accumulating knowledge on these topics should help to provide even better psychosocial care to our patients.

References

Armes J, Crowe M, Colbourne L et al (2009) Patients' supportive care needs beyond the end of cancer treatment: a prospective, longitudinal study. J Clin Oncol 27:6172–6179

Beck AT, Steer RA (1993) Beck anxiety inventory. Manual. Psychological Corporation, San Antonio

Berg P, Book K, Dinkel A et al (2011) Progredienzangst bei chronischen Erkrankungen [Fear of progression in chronic diseases]. Psychother Psychosom Med Psychol 61:32–37

Butow PN, Bell ML, Smith AB et al (2013) Conquer fear: protocol of a randomised controlled trial of a psychological intervention to reduce fear of cancer recurrence. BMC Cancer 13:201

Crist JV, Grunfeld EA (2013) Factors reported to influence fear of recurrence in cancer patients: a systematic review. Psychooncology 22:978–986

Dankert A, Duran G, Engst-Hastreiter U et al (2003) Progredienzangst bei Patienten mit Tumorerkrankungen, Diabetes mellitus und entzündlich-rheumatischen Erkrankungen [Fear of progression in patients with cancer, diabetes mellitus and chronic arthritis]. Rehabilitation 42:155–163

Dieng M, Butow PN, Costa DS et al (2016) Psychoeducational intervention to reduce fear of cancer recurrence in people at high risk of developing another primary melanoma: results of a randomized controlled trial. J Clin Oncol 34:4405–4414

Dinkel A, Herschbach P, Berg P et al (2012) Determinants of long-term response to group therapy for dysfunctional fear of progression in chronic diseases. Behav Med 38:1–5

Dinkel A, Kremsreiter K, Marten-Mittag B et al (2014) Comorbidity of fear of progression and anxiety disorders in cancer patients. Gen Hosp Psychiatry 36:613–619

Fardell JE, Thewes B, Turner J et al (2016) Fear of cancer recurrence: a theoretical review and novel cognitive processing formulation. J Cancer Surviv 10:663–673

Fidika A, Herle M, Herschbach P et al (2015) Fear of disease progression questionnaire for parents: psychometric properties based on a sample of caregivers of children and adolescents with cystic fibrosis. J Psychosom Res 79:49–54

Fisher A, Beeken RJ, Heinrich M et al (2016) Health behaviours and fear of cancer recurrence in 10 969 colorectal cancer (CRC) patients. Psycho-Oncology 25:1434–1440

Ghazali N, Cadwallader E, Lowe D et al (2013) Fear of recurrence among head and neck cancer survivors: longitudinal trends. Psycho-Oncology 22:807–813

Gurevich M, Devins GM, Rodin GM (2002) Stress response syndromes and cancer: conceptual and assessment issues. Psychosomatics 43:259–281

Halbach SM, Enders A, Kowalski C et al (2016) Health literacy and fear of cancer progression in elderly women newly diagnosed with breast cancer—a longitudinal analysis. Patient Educ Couns 99:855–862

Harrison JD, Young JM, Price MA et al (2009) What are the unmet supportive care needs of people with cancer? A systematic review. Support Care Cancer 17:1117–1128

Heinrichs N, Zimmermann T, Huber B et al (2012) Cancer distress reduction with a couple-based skills training: a randomized controlled trial. Ann Behav Med 43:239–252

Herschbach P, Berg P, Dankert A et al (2005) Fear of progression in chronic diseases. Psychometric properties of the fear of progression questionnaire (FoP-Q). J Psychosom Res 58:505–511

Herschbach P, Berg P, Waadt S et al (2010a) Group psychotherapy of dysfunctional fear of progression in patients with chronic arthritis or cancer. Psychother Psychosom 79:31–38

Herschbach P, Book K, Dinkel A et al (2010b) Evaluation of two group therapies to reduce fear of progression in cancer patients. Support Care Cancer 18:471–479

Herschbach P, Keller M, Knight L et al (2004) Psychological problems of cancer patients: a cancer distress screening with a cancer-specific questionnaire. Br J Cancer 91:504–511

Hinz A, Mehnert A, Ernst J et al (2015) Fear of progression in patients 6 months after cancer rehabilitation—a validation study of the fear of progression questionnaire FoP-Q-12. Support Care Cancer 23:1579–1587

Hodges LJ, Humphris GM (2009) Fear of recurrence and psychological distress in head and neck cancer patients and their carers. Psychooncology 18:841–848

Hoyer J, Beesdo K, Gloster AT et al (2009) Worry exposure versus applied relaxation in the treatment of generalized anxiety disorder. Psychother Psychosom 78:106–115

Humphris G, Ozakinci G (2008) The AFTER intervention: a structured psychological approach to reduce fear of recurrence in patients with head and neck cancer. Br J Health Psychol 13:223–230

Kanatas A, Ghazali N, Lowe D et al (2013) Issues patients would like to discuss at their review consultation: variation by early and late stage oral, oropharyngeal and laryngeal subsites. Eur Arch Otorhinolaryngol 270:1067–1074

Kim Y, Carver CS, Spillers RL et al (2012) Dyadic effects of fear of recurrence on the quality of life of cancer survivors and their caregivers. Qual Life Res 21:517–525

Koch L, Jansen L, Brenner H et al (2013) Fear of recurrence and disease progression in long-term (≥ 5 years) cancer survivors—a systematic review of quantitative studies. Psycho-Oncology 22:1–11

Koch-Gallenkamp L, Bertram H, Eberle A et al (2016) Fear of recurrence in long-term cancer survivors—do cancer type, sex, time since diagnosis, and social support matter? Health Psychol 35:1329–1333

Kwakkenbos L, van den Hoogen FHJ, Custers J et al (2012) Validity of the fear of progression questionnaire-short form in patients with systemic sclerosis. Arthritis Care Res 64:930–934

Lebel S, Maheu C, Lefebvre M et al (2014) Addressing fear of cancer recurrence among women with cancer: a feasibility and preliminary outcome study. J Cancer Surviv 8:485–496

Lebel S, Ozakinci G, Humphris G et al (2016) From normal response to clinical problem: definition and clinical features of fear of cancer recurrence. Support Care Cancer 24:3265–3268

Lebel S, Ozakinci G, Humphris G et al (2017) Current state and future prospects of research on fear of cancer recurrence. Psycho-Oncology 26:424–427

Lebel S, Tomei C, Feldstain A et al (2013) Does fear of recurrence predict cancer survivors health care use? Support Care Cancer 21:901–906

Lee-Jones C, Humphris G, Dixon R et al (1997) Fear of cancer recurrence—a literature review and proposed cognitive formulation to explain exacerbation of recurrence fears. Psycho-Oncology 6:95–105

Lengacher CA, Johnson-Mallard V, Post-White J et al (2009) Randomized controlled trial of mindfulness-based stress reduction (MBSR) for survivors of breast cancer. Psycho-Oncology 18:1261–1272

Lengacher CA, Reich RR, Paterson CL et al (2016) Examination of broad symptom improvement resulting from mindfulness-based stress reduction in breast cancer survivors: a randomized controlled trial. J Clin Oncol 34:2827–2834

Maheu C, Lebel S, Courbasson C et al (2016) Protocol of a randomized controlled trial of the fear of recurrence therapy (FORT) intervention for women with breast or gynecological cancer. BMC Cancer 16:291

Mehnert A, Berg P, Henrich G et al (2009) Fear of cancer progression and cancer-related intrusive cognitions in breast cancer survivors. Psycho-Oncology 18:1273–1280

Mehnert A, Brähler E, Faller H et al (2014) Four-week prevalence of mental disorders in patients with cancer across major tumor entities. J Clin Oncol 32:3540–3546

Mehnert A, Herschbach P, Berg P et al (2006) Progredienzangst bei Brustkrebspatientinnen— Validierung der Kurzform des Progredienzangst-fragebogens PA-F-KF [Fear of progression in breast cancer patients—validation of the short form of the Fear of Progression Questionnaire (FoP-Q-SF)]. Z Psychosom Med Psychother 52:274–288

Mehnert A, Koch U, Sundermann C et al (2013) Predictors of fear of recurrence in patients one year after cancer rehabilitation: a prospective study. Acta Oncol. doi:10.3109/0284186X.2013.765063

Mellon S, Kershaw TS, Northouse LL et al (2007) A family-based model to predict fear of recurrence for cancer survivors and their caregivers. Psycho-Oncology 16:214–223

Mitchell AJ, Chan M, Bhatti H et al (2011) Prevalence of depression, anxiety, and adjustment disorder in oncological, haematological, and palliative-care settings: a meta-analysis of 94 interview-based studies. Lancet Oncol 12:160–174

Moorey S (1996) When bad things happen to rational people: cognitive therapy in adverse life circumstances. In: Salkovskis PM (ed) Frontiers of cognitive therapy. Guilford, New York, pp 450–469

Myers SB, Manne SL, Kissane DW et al (2013) Social-cognitive processes associated with fear of recurrence among women newly diagnosed with gynecological cancers. Gynecol Oncol 128:120–127

NCCN Guideline Distress Management, Version 2.2103. http://www.nccn.org/professionals/physician_gls/pdf/distress.pdf. Accessed 01 June 2013

Northouse LL (1981) Mastectomy patients and the fear of cancer recurrence. Cancer Nurs 4:213–220

Rogers SN, El-Sheikha J, Lowe D (2009) The development of a Patients Concerns Inventory (PCI) to help reveal patients concerns in the head and neck clinic. Oral Oncol 45:555–561

Rudolph B, Wünsch A, Herschbach P et al (2017) Ambulante verhaltenstherapeutische Gruppentherapie zur Behandlung von Progredienzangst bei Krebspatienten [Cognitive-behavioral group therapy addressing fear of progression in cancer outpatients]. Psychother Psychosom Med Psychol. doi:10.1055/s-0043-107774

Sabariego C, Brach M, Herschbach P et al (2011) Cost-effectiveness of cognitive-behavioral group therapy of dysfunctional fear of progression in cancer patients. Eur J Health Econ 12:489–497

Salander P (2010) Motives that cancer patients in oncological care have for consulting a psychologist—an empirical study. Psycho-Oncology 19:248–254

Savard J, Ivers H (2013) The evolution of fear of cancer recurrence during the cancer care trajectory and its relationship with cancer characteristics. J Psychosom Res 74:354–360

Schepper F, Abel K, Herschbach P et al (2015) Progredienzangst bei Eltern krebskranker Kinder: Adaptation eines Fragebogens und Korrelate [Fear of progression in parents of children with cancer: adaptation of the Fear of Progression Questionnaire and correlates]. Klin Pädiatr 227:151–156

Shim EJ, Shin YW, Oh DY et al (2010) Increased fear of progression in cancer patients with recurrence. Gen Hosp Psychiatry 32:169–175

Simard S, Savard J (2009) Fear of Recurrence Inventory: development and initial validation of a multidimensional measure of fear of cancer recurrence. Support Care Cancer 17:241–251

Simard S, Savard J (2015) Screening and comorbidity of clinical levels of fear of cancer recurrence. J Cancer Surviv 9:481–491

Simard S, Thewes B, Humphris G et al (2013) Fear of cancer recurrence in adult cancer survivors: a systematic review of quantitative studies. J Cancer Surviv 7:300–322

Simonelli LE, Siegel SC, Duffy NM (2016) Fear of cancer recurrence: a theoretical review and its relevance for clinical presentation and management. Psycho-Oncology. doi:10.1002/pon.4168

Singer S, Das-Munshi J, Brähler E (2010) Prevalence of mental health conditions in cancer patients in acute care—a meta-analysis. Ann Oncol 21:925–930

Skaali T, Fosså SD, Bremnes R et al (2009) Fear of recurrence in long-term testicular cancer survivors. Psychooncology 18:580–588

Smith AB, Thewes B, Turner J et al (2015) Pilot of a theoretically grounded psychologist-delivered intervention for fear of cancer recurrence (Conquer Fear). Psycho-Oncology 24:967–970

Spielberger CD, Gorsuch RL, Lushene R et al (1983) Manual for the state-trait anxiety inventory. Consulting Psychologists Press, Palo Alto

Thewes B, Butow P, Bell ML et al (2012a) Fear of cancer recurrence in young women with a history of early-stage breast cancer: a cross-sectional study of prevalence and association with health behaviors. Support Care Cancer 20:2651–2659

Thewes B, Butow P, Zachariae R et al (2012b) Fear of cancer recurrence: a systematic literature review of self-report measures. Psycho-Oncology 21:571–587

van de Wal M, Gielissen MFM, Servaes P et al (2015) Study protocol of the SWORD-study: a randomised controlled trial comparing combined online and face-to-face cognitive behaviour therapy versus treatment as usual in managing fear of cancer recurrence. BMC Psychology 3:12

van de Wal M, van de Poll-Franse L, Prins J et al (2016) Does fear of cancer recurrence differ between cancer types? A study from the population-based PROFILES registry. Psycho-Oncology 25:772–778

van Helmondt SJ, van der Lee ML, de Vries J (2016) Study protocol of the CAREST-trial: a randomised controlled trial on the (cost-) effectiveness of a CBT-based online self-help training for fear of cancer recurrence in women with curatively treated breast cancer. BMC Cancer 16:527

Vehling S, Koch U, Ladehoff N et al (2012) Prävalenz affektiver und Angststörungen bei Krebs: Systematischer Literaturreview und Metaanalyse [Prevalence of affective and anxiety disorders in cancer: systematic literature review and meta-analysis]. Psychother Psychosom Med Psychol 62:249–258

Vickberg SMJ (2003) The concerns about recurrence scale (CARS): a systematic measure of women's fears about the possibility of breast cance recurrence. Ann Behav Med 25:16–24

Waadt S, Duran G, Berg P et al (2011) Progredienzangst. Manual zur Behandlung von Zukunftsängsten bei chronisch Kranken [Fear of Progression. Treatment manual]. Schattauer, Stuttgart

Zimmermann T, Alsleben M, Heinrichs N (2012) Progredienzangst gesunder Lebenspartner von chronisch erkrankten Patienten [Fear of progression in partners of chronically ill patients]. Psychother Psychosom Med Psychol 62:344–351

Zimmermann T, Herschbach P, Wessarges M et al (2011) Fear of progression in partners of chronically ill patients. Behav Med 37:95–104

Gender Opportunities in Psychosocial Oncology

Matthew Loscalzo and Karen Clark

Abstract

So much has happened since the original publication of this chapter. In some ways, the progress made in appreciating the full spectrum of sexual and gender expression has been uneven and in some nations, there has been serious regression and resulting repression. But overall, especially in the industrialized countries, there is much greater awareness of sex and gender and its importance in health and well being. In this updated chapter, we put sex and gender into a historical context that is relevant to psycho-oncology and that openly accepts that society overall, is highly conflicted when it comes to how women and men get the best out of each other, never mind how to best integrate lesbian, gay, bisexual, and transgender (LGBT) communities. With the advent of more tailored treatments and strategic medicine, sex becomes much more important as a variable and this has led to greater scientific requirements to create protocols that integrate sex into all aspects of health from prevention, diagnosis, treatment, survivorship, and death. But we still have a very far way to go. There is a serious dearth of data on sex and gender in science overall and in cancer medicine specifically. Avoidance of discussions of sex and gender in medicine reflects the larger lingering societal discomfort with any discussion that links potential sex and gender differences with superiority. The data shows that there is more

---

"Sex does matter. It matters in ways that we did not expect. Undoubtedly, it also matters in ways that we have not begun to imagine." Mary-Lou Pardue, p. X. IOM 2001.

M. Loscalzo (✉)
City of Hope, 1500 East Duarte Road, Main Medical Bldg Suite Y-1,
Duarte, CA 91010-3000, USA
e-mail: Mloscalzo@COH.org

K. Clark
City of Hope, 1500 East Duarte Road, Main Medical Bldg Suite Y-8,
Duarte, CA 91010-3000, USA
e-mail: kclark@coh.org

© Springer International Publishing AG 2018
U. Goerling and A. Mehnert (eds.), *Psycho-Oncology*, Recent Results
in Cancer Research 210, https://doi.org/10.1007/978-3-319-64310-6_3

intrasexual than intersexual variation in men and women. When speaking about sex and gender the literature reflects that, on average, there are many differences, and although they are small, that when taken together, the impact may be quite robust. Sex and gender differences are relevant to how individuals, couples, and families experience and cope with serious illness; however these important and obvious variables are seldom taken into account when counseling seriously ill patients and their families. Cancer is a complex disease that brings into sharp relief the potential alignments and misalignments in the sexes. In this chapter we have attempted to communicate the imperative for and importance of understanding people under stress within the context of sex and gender. Gender-specific medicine is a very young movement for scientific study but one that has great potential to maximize adaptation and mutual respect at a time when men and women are redefining themselves and adapting to new social realities and challenges.

Keywords
Gender · Sex · Coping with cancer

1   Sex, Gender Health, and Illness in Context

At the very essence of our being, sex is important because every cell has a sex which means that every bodily organ does as well (de Vries and Forger 2015). Sex matters, a lot. Biology is bathed in sex but societies, from the very beginning of written history, have imbued sex with multiple complex rational and supernatural meanings. Avoidance of discussions of sex and gender in medicine reflects the larger lingering societal discomfort with any discourse that links potential sex and gender differences with superiority. At the same time, there are few topics that are of more interest to people (scientists, clinicians, educators, and the public) then how sex and gender influence our daily lives. It has been shown and is now widely accepted that women and men are equally intelligent (Halpern 2000) though the underlying neural mechanisms are clearly different and may in fact be added support for the co-evolution of the sexes (Haier et al. 2005). Recognizing the unique adaptations and resulting strengths and contributions of women and men have a particular significance for coping with illness, for the patient and the caregiver (Loscalzo et al. 2010). The data shows that there is more intrasexual than intersexual variation in men and women (IOM 2001). When speaking about sex and gender the literature reflects that, on average, there are many differences, and although they are small, that when taken together, the impact may be quite robust. Ironically, the general public, and this is most clearly seen in movies, novels, websites, etc., have always assumed that women and men are different. Paradoxically, it has been in universities, where open and provocative discussions are expected (and need to) take place, that have been the most restrictive as it relates to the implications of sex and gender (McCallister 2017). In some ways, the sexual revolution of the 1960s and 1970s resulted in much needed demands (and real progress) for gender equality that somehow resulted in an intolerance to even discuss the realities and implications of what makes women and men different. Fortunately, science is all about reality: asking difficult, unsettling, complex, and provocative questions.

The evolving field of gender-specific medicine in cancer care has been growing rapidly and is gaining additional momentum from the larger interest in and ability to personalize medical care. (for example see, Kim and Loscalzo 2018, in press). But first, it will be helpful to understand the recent genesis of gender-specific medicine as this history reveals why some of the barriers persist and how this rich, yet ambiguous, past can infuse the future with excitement and passion for this topic.

2 Psychiatry and Psychology Meets Sex and Gender

Even as scientific explanations gained acceptance over supernatural and religious ones, it was inevitable that deep-seated societal values would influence how sex and gender would be understood and explored. For example, in the DSM 1 published in 1952, there were no actual findings related to sex ratios, updated in 1962, DSM II mentioned sex ratios one time (in the pediatric section) (Narrow 2007). DSM III released in 1980 and the subsequent revision in 1987 would, for the first time, offer different criteria for women and men with an increasing emphasis on sex and gender, but this was clearly important progress (DSM-III 1980 and DSM-III-R 1987). In the DSM V released in 2013, there are multiple references to and comprehensive descriptions of sex, gender, and related information. Clearly, sex and gender is coming into its own in the psychiatric literature and has begun to reveal its influence in mental illness, adaptation to life's stressors, and wellness. Interestingly, the DSM V uses the terms gender differences as a general term given the complexity of the topic: "The term 'gender *differences*' is used...because...the differences between men and women are the result of both biological sex and individual self-representation. However, some of the differences are based on only biological sex."

The politically tumultuous 1970s saw growing unrest with traditional values and systems. Sex and gender were major issues for women now demanding the equal rights which they had been for too long denied. Women's rights and civil rights became synonymous and each empowered the other. Science and funding are always influenced by the community zeitgeist. Within the context of exuberant challenging of the system, the lack of, and in many cases, an absence of medical research that included women in both clinical and laboratory research became obvious and in some cases shocking. Rationalizations for the omission of women in clinical trials was multi-determined and complex. The scientifically naïve (and convenient) attitude that women and men were so similar that simply studying men would benefit both sexes obviated the need to deal with the "complexity" that women presented to clinical trials. Paradoxically, women were simultaneously seen as both simple (same as men) and too complex (pregnancy, monthly, and long-term hormonal changes, etc.), to enroll in carefully controlled expensive studies that often spanned numbers of years. In essence, women were messy. The 1980s saw that the major changes experienced in many industrialized societies begin to influence health care initially and then finally research. Increasing patient consumerism, the AIDS epidemic, the women's movement, breast cancer advocates taking lessons from the successful gay men's advocacy groups like Act Up, community-based hospice and palliative care movements, demands for pain management and increasing numbers of women in health and science, all began to coalesce into greater awareness and ultimately fertile firmament for change. In health care, initial advances, as it relates to sex and gender did (and still), has not emanated from cancer care or research.

Mariane J. Legato, MD published the first of a number of highly popular books for the lay public, *The Female Heart: The Truth About Women and Coronary Artery Disease* (Legato and Colman 1992). Dr. Legato was a true pioneer in the scholarly creation of the field of gender-based medicine (Legato and Bilezikian 2004). The importance of evidence-based information was a watershed moment at the time and had serious political and scientific implications, as it does now, for the awareness and need for precision medicine. But still little has changed in terms of new funding or programs. It is only now that the reality for clinical care or research an essential and first question to be asked almost always must be must be: Is it XX, XY, or other. Needless to say, this more realistic, comprehensive, accurate, and ethical perspective had and has important implications for the biobehavioral and supportive care needs of patients, families, and communities. Legato's pioneering textbook (Legato and Bilezikian 2004) was a catalyst for the rapidly evolving scientific field of gender medicine that is only now being appreciated for its importance for the health benefits of women, men, and society (Foundation for Gender-Specific Medicine, https://gendermed.org).

In 1998, the IOM report on gender susceptibility to environmental exposures emphasized that responses to chemicals and stress are related to sex. But it would be in 2001 that the influential IOM Consensus Report: *Exploring the biological contributions to human health: Does sex matter?* that the scientific community was confronted, not only with the challenges of sex- and gender-based gaps but with unique opportunities for research. It is difficult to overestimate the ongoing impact of this IOM report. The Chair and Committee Members were scientists of high international regard for large bodies of high-quality research. The IOM report cogently presented a level of specificity of the data, persuasiveness of the importance of sex differences, and recommendations for future research that was credible and overwhelming. The Chair, Mary-Lou Pardue, Ph.D. summed up the main and compelling quoted call to action of the Committee: "*Sex does matter. It matters in ways that we did not expect. Undoubtedly, it also matters in ways that we have not begun to imagine…. Until the question of sex is routinely asked and the results—*

positive or negative—are routinely reported, many opportunities to obtain a better understanding of the pathogenesis of disease and to advance human health will surely be missed."

The *womb-to-tomb* call for biobehavioral research of sex and gender differences by the IOM 2001 made the study of sex and gender a legitimate area for systematic exploration and discovery. Organizations such as Society for Women's Health Research (http://swhr.org/), the FDA Office of Women's Health (especially see CME course https://sexandgendercourse.od.nih.gov/), American Association of Sexuality Educators, Counselors and Therapists (AASECT) (www.aasect.org), and journals, Journal of Sex Specific Medicine, Journal of Men's Health and Gender and books.

An additional benefit of the IOM report was that the authors made the objective discussion of sex differences (and by extension gender characteristics) an acceptable topic for scientific and social examination at a time when "political correctness" reflexively misinterpreted any discussion of sex differences as sexist, derogatory, and potentially oppressive. Unfortunately, this was and is in many cases still prevalent in health care and especially university settings. Although sexism against women is still an undeniable reality in the world today and is wrong, the women and men who resist the knowledge of the unique contributions of the sexes also lose the opportunity to benefit from the knowledge and wisdom that has been essential to the amazing evolutionary successes of the human race. It is also important to manage the resistance to identifying, understanding, and acknowledging the realities of sexual differences, inclinations, and unique contributions of the sexes because within the emotionally charged and stressful clinical context, sex and gender-based characteristics are more likely to be exaggerated, behaviorally manifested, and most obvious. Here lies the opportunity for the skilled clinician to use what comes most naturally to patients, families, and colleagues therapeutically at a time when they may be most open to influence.

But to be clear, sex and gender inequalities have real-life implications as there is high-quality cancer research that continues to document disparities that negatively affect women in particular (Amri et al. 2014). Genomics, age, sex, gender, personality, behavior, education, and environmental factors all relate to health and illness. There are very few things that can be reliably said about men and women without multiple qualifiers. However, men and women are different and these differences go beyond hormones and genetics. There is still the misperception that sex is primarily or solely related to reproductive functions. As referred above, the highly influential and provocative 2001 IOM Report: "Exploring the Biological Contributions to Human Health: Does Sex Matter?" documented important sex differences that demonstrate the complexity of sex differences that go far beyond the reproductive system alone. These include sex chromosomes, immune function, symptom manifestation to same diseases, responses to toxins, brain organization, pain prevalence, and response to medications (IOM 2001). Within this reality, sex and gender differences have significant implications for high-risk populations, screening, assessments, diagnosis, therapy, response, and survival.

Given that men and women are by far much more similar than they are different, questions about why there are sex differences at all are as intriguing as they are provocative and are beyond the focus of this chapter (Buss 2011). In some ways, the influences of sex and gender may be so rapid, multisensory, subtle, and reflexive that the experience feels as natural and essential as inhaling the invisible air we breathe to keep us alive. The prevailing view proposed by Buss and others is from evolutionary psychology and postulates that women and men have had to adapt to different problems (relating to food, habitat, defense, mate selection, social structures, etc.) (Buss 1995). Over many thousands of years, the survival advantages resulting from the successful adaptations sculpted the biology and behavior of the most successful humans—our common progenitors. But as with many other human potentials, the behaviors resulting from these adaptations, and associated with one sex more than the other, are highly flexible, with none, other than reproductive functions, being limited solely to either sex. Evolutionary psychology therefore accurately predicts, across many cultures, that the gatherer (more closely associated with women) would have superior spatial location memory and that the hunter (more closely associated with men) would have a keener sense of spatial rotation (Silverman and Peters 2007). That the potential for women and men solving ongoing problems together, but at times in different ways, is as evident as it is exciting from a strengths-based perspective. The diversity of perceptions, behaviors, and solutions is evident once there is a willingness to perceive access, activate, and build on these innate human potentials. Needless to say, there are other explanations relating to sex differences but none have the empirical support of evolutionary psychology (Buss and Schmitt 2011). In fact, Vandermassen in her book, *Who is Afraid of Charles Darwin? Debating Feminism and Evolutionary Theory* attempts to bridge the empirical chasm between feminist sex role perspectives and that of evolutionary psychology and makes a significant contribution to this complex and evolving field (Vandermassen 2005). Regardless of theoretical perspectives, it would be hard to find any reasonable clinician or scientist who would argue that sex and gender are not relevant to the full biopsychosocial experience. For within this context lie many fruitful areas for much needed research on sex and gender as primary outcomes.

3 Sex and Gender Matters

From the moment of conception there is a defined sex. But sex is anything but simple. Exceptions to clearly defined sex status as female or male are more common than most people realize. For example, the prevalence of disorders of sex development (DSD) (also known as intersex, atypical sex, pseudohermaphroditism) is 1 in 4000 live births and has gained increasing clinical and public attention (Calleja-Agius et al. 2012). Readers with an interest in this area are referred to the Consensus Statement on Management of Intersex Disorders as this topic is beyond the focus of this chapter (Lee et al. 2006). What is important about DSD is that it demonstrates that both sex and gender are complex and multi-determined and must be seen on a continuum that transcends clearly defined boundaries. But for the vast majority of newborns male or female sex is defined by their genetics. Unfortunately, even in some scientific and medical literature the terms sex and gender continue to be used interchangeably. This has lead to confusion. It is generally agreed that the boundaries between sex and gender are unclear but there are standard definitions that take the overlap into consideration and that lead to greater clarity and credible empirical investigation. In essence, *sex* is seen as biologically determined at birth, one time, by XY chromosomes in males and XX chromosomes in women, while *gender* is a social construct that may change over time. The World Health Organization's definitions of sex and gender are relevant to this discussion and provide insight into the territory, a sense of the complexities involved and a practical common language to understand and address the topic. Sex is defined as "…genetic/physiological or biological characteristics of a person which indicates whether one is female or male…" While gender relates to "women's and men's roles and responsibilities that are socially determined." (page 10) (World Health Organization 1998). This description of sex and gender naturally leads to the necessity of understanding "…sex and gender as a single system in which social elements act with biological elements to produce the body has important consequences for medical treatment…genes, physiology, and the physical and social environments operate in concert to produce a phenotype" (P.19) (IOM 2001). This context is the foundation for all that follows in this chapter.

4 Sexual Dimorphisms Is Only Part of the Story but an Important Part

Sex and gender implications for health are most clearly seen at the beginning and end of life. Women outsurvive men at birth and also live longer by about 6 years. In the United Sates, this finding has been upheld across all of the 12 ethnic groups measured (National Center for Health Statistics 2012). There is now a very large international literature demonstrating the reality, implications, and importance of sexual dimorphisms and gender differences (Buss et al. 2011). For example, even from the time of birth, although more males are born, 120 males die in the first year for every 100 females. In fact, in the perinatal period males suffer higher rates of morbidity than females in: stillbirths, premature birth, congenital malformations, pulmonary hemorrhage, intracranial hemorrhage, respiratory distress, perinatal asphyxia, perinatal infection, cerebral palsy, developmental delay, Sudden Infant Death Syndrome, Attention Deficit Hyperactivity Disorder, and neurobehavioral difficulties (Rosen and Bateman 2004). There can be no question that these early serious challenges have the potential to negatively impact physical, cognitive, and social development. But sex differences are not limited to early life. Later in life there are also significant sex differences in morbidity and mortality. For example, women are more likely than men to suffer from the following serious illnesses:

cardiovascular disease, autoimmune disorders, obesity/diabetes, Post Traumatic Stress Disorder, depression, and anorexia nervosa (Becker et al. 2008). While men are more likely to be diagnosed with cancer, dementias, Parkinson's, mental retardation, autism spectrum disorders (including schizophrenia) substance abuse, and addiction.

It is essential to note that that "sex differences exist at the population level, and as such they should not be used for making inferences about a single individual" and that "...sex differences in the brain and behavior refer to average differences between men and women and that differences between individuals within each sex are much greater than the average differences between sexes" (Resnick and Driscoll 2008). Although in some areas the intersex differences may be small taken together they are very important as it relates to clinical care. In the clinical setting, the manifestations of sex and gender are always influenced to varying degrees and at different times by biology, anthropology, psychology, and societal supports and constraints.

Almost all people see themselves as either men or women regardless of sexual preference. That sex and gender differences are relevant to how individuals, couples, and families experience and cope with serious illness would seem to be apparent, these important and obvious variables are seldom taken into account when counseling seriously ill patients and their families. The very complexity of sex and gender and how it plays out in society, and is reflected in the clinical setting may be a deterrent as an open topic for discussion. This is unfortunate and may be a lost opportunity for meaningful communication and joint problem-solving that is at the heart of patient- and family-centered care. Fortunately, there is an increasing openness in science, medicine, and psychology to empirically understand the complexities of sex and gender. There is also an interest in the general public about how men and women have coevolved and want to better understand each other. In fact, in many ways, the general public has been more open to the reality of sex and gender differences than having some in the academic community.

5 Getting the Sexes Straight

It may seem paradoxical to say that the differences in the sexes are small but still very important in part because these variations change over time and may be most pronounced during extreme situations. But because these differences may be most obvious under stressful conditions, within a gender-sensitive therapeutic context, these variations are most easy to see and to reframe as immediate opportunities for enhanced mutual understanding, personal growth, and decreased interpersonal conflict. It is also essential to note that although across large populations, average sex differences may be small, individual differences in couples, families, or culturally defined groups may be quite robust with high levels of time-sensitive malleability. The cancer experience always involves a larger biopsychosocial context than merely the person diagnosed with cancer and this more realistic perspective, when therapeutically managed, is a unique opportunity to build on internal and external resources that may not have been identified, acknowledged, understood, or utilized.

It is hard to talk about sex or gender differences in the abstract and across large groups, but in the clinical setting it is much more obvious and easier to identify and to give voice to the perceptual, attitudinal, and behavioral elements that influence how people struggle to emotionally connect with each other at a core atavistic level. In our Couples Coping with Cancer Programs Together, we now have years of experience in screening couples and applying this knowledge to help newly diagnosed and advanced cancer patients and their partners work together as a team. This gender-strengths-based approach maintains a strictly *here-and-now* perspective to focus on strengths in actively working with the couples in a number of modalities (Loscalzo et al. In press, Spring 2018; Bitz et al. 2014).

For those men and women who are largely in sync in the manner in which they regulate emotions, respond to threat, and adapt to a rapidly changing environments, the relationship will be comforting but may be overly restricted in the diversity of their coping repertoire. Their motivation for exploration and change may also be decreased. A tailored program of psychoeducation may be best suited for this group. In the context of a man and woman who manifest different responses and adaptations to challenges that are different but compatible, there is the greatest opportunity for a wide range of coping responses and just enough stress to promote openness to growth. A general program of psychoeducation may be best suited for this group. In the extreme group where the woman and man have gender inclinations that have become a foundation for their life-story, their relationships and a rigid character structure, distress may be high while motivation will be low and psychotherapy will be the intervention of choice. Ultimately, it is the ability of two or more people to emotionally connect that will influence the level of distress experienced but it is not, with the level of data now available, possible to confidently state the quality of healthy adaptation to the cancer experience overall. This is an area of research that needs to be addressed.

Men and women are too complex to compartmentalize. But it would be disingenuous to ignore compelling paradigms that have empirical support and their relevancy to this discussion—how to help women and men to best support each other during a cancer crisis and beyond. The sexes need to be seen on a continuum. The intra- and intersexual differences must always be assessed but when helping individuals it is always a one–to-one interaction. Many women (as compared to men) may naturally manifest inclinations (e.g., circling the wagons, verbally sharing vulnerabilities and emotional concerns) that can be clearly identified personally, socially, and culturally as feminine. However, there are many women who do not fit this generalization and who will manifest characteristics that have been traditionally thought of as masculine. While many men (as compared to women) may naturally manifest inclinations (e.g., turning inward, ruminating about fixing the problem, and minimizing the danger through humor) that are associated, identified personally, socially and culturally with masculinities, this is not necessarily an accurate reflection of the male reality. As with women, there are many men who do not match with what historically has been considered to be the masculine expectation, never mind, the societal ideal. Women, who manifest, what has been traditionally masculine traits, are women, and men who manifest what has historically been seen as feminine traits are men. The diversity and overlap of human adaptations, by sex specifically, to millennia of dangers and opportunities, is an inherent strength that is far greater than either sex in isolation. This is no less true when men and women confront life-threatening disease together. We will now share some key information about sex and gender and how it affects patients and couples within the setting of coping with cancer and quality of life.

6 Clinical Challenges and Opportunities Within the Context of Cancer

Although the data reviewing sex and or gender as a primary variable in cancer is quite limited, there is a body of literature that is highly informative and is worth a brief review. For example, in a series of important studies, Hagedoorn and colleagues have been extremely productive in elucidating some of the more nuanced aspects of sex and gender within the complex context of cancer (Hagedoorn 2008; Revenson et al. 2016).

As it relates to psychological distress, the majority of studies suggest that women overall report more psychological distress than men. This information has been confirmed by many international studies using a wide variety of screening instruments and in diverse cancer populations (Loscalzo et al. In press, Spring 2018; Loscalzo and Clark 2014; Hagedoorn et al. 2008; Zabora et al. 2001). There is no convincing data that can answer the question if women simply feel emotions more intensely, or, if overall, men simply experience emotions less intensely than do women. In our clinical experience, however, the strong impression is that both may be true. In terms of willingness to report vulnerabilities based on gender, women do report more requests for help (Merckaert et al. 2010) and accept more help (Curry et al. 2002). Women tend to report more distress and unmet needs as it relates to emotional concerns while men tend to focus on more physical problems. However when gender is looked at by age groups, new trends have emerged in the data. In a recent study of three age groups of cancer patients, including Adolescent and Young Adults (AYAs) (18–39 years), middle-aged patients (40–64 years), and older patients (65 + years), it indicated that AYA males expressed more distress than AYA females. Further, both AYAs and middle-aged male patients requested to talk to a member of the medical team for support more frequently than female patients in same age groups. Written information was more often requested by AYA patients, while older patients more likely requested to talk to a member of the medical team for support (Clark et al. 2016). It should be noted however, regardless of the sex of the patient and the country studied, caregivers report higher distress than do cancer patients (Matthews 2003; Kim et al. 2007). Also within the groups of caregivers, women report more emotional distress than do men (Curry et al.

2002). The essential clinical caveat here is that there is great variation and that every individual needs to be assessed carefully. In the clinical setting, sex and gender are seen as potential *inclinations* that open deeper and more meaningful understandings, but not *determinations* that reinforce stereotypes and restricts personal options. But ultimately, the evidence is unequivocal that supportive interpersonal relationships matter, both emotionally and physiologically, and for most people, at least some of these key relationships will be with the opposite sex (Zaider and Kissane 2010). Sex and gender matter because both are very powerful influences (seen and unseen) on the quality of interpersonal relationships and social support. Men and women who have been diagnosed with cancer report that their partners play a key role in their ability to cope and to manage the challenges of the cancer experience. It is a given that spouses or partners are a major support to people diagnosed with cancer. In an important study investigating the partner relationship in response to breast cancer, Pistrang and Barker found that male partner support (high empathy and low withdrawal) plays a pivotal role in the woman's adaptation and psychological well-being (Pistrang and Barker 1995). While Fergus and Gray (2009) reported that even when women had other strong social supports in place, this did not compensate for an unsupportive male partner. Significantly, in a large study of caregivers, Kim et al. (2006) reported that female cancer patients felt that their male partners were very supportive when it came to practical tasks, but that they did not provide the emotional support that was so important to them. In essence, men were much more comfortable with demanding and ongoing practical and physical tasks than with the emotional components of the experience. This misalignment has significant implications not only for couples but whenever men and women try to support and connect with each other during times of stress or crisis. The interdependence of spouses and partners highlights the struggles of men and women to identify and to meet each other's expectations, and the value that they place on the supportive efforts they manifest. In fact, the authors suggest that the focus on deficit psychology and prevalence of distress overall (as a natural and seductive extension of the medical model) has hindered a more com-plete picture of people affected by serious illness and their capacities to cope and evolve as individuals and as social systems.

In studies of resiliency, emotional growth and finding benefit in the cancer experience, relationships have been shown to be particularly crucial. For example, Stanton has summarized a number of studies focusing on what led to benefit-finding or emotional growth in cancer patients. The interpersonal realm, specifically enhanced personal relationships and intimacy (social support) were consistently the most endorsed variables across a number of studies (Stanton 2010). Benefit-finding and resiliency research is important to psychosocial oncology because it represents a strengths-based approach that can be used to tease out the essential elements of best coping practices. It can be argued that the coevolution of women and men represents a strength-based process in which the two sexes (including the benefits of heterosexual and same sex orientation) have adapted to each other's needs to insure the short-term and long-term survival of the species. However, the skills that were once essential for the physical survival of the human species have dramatically (and quite suddenly in evolutionary time frames) changed from responding to dangers, challenges, and opportunities in the immediate environment (fast limbic reactions) to highly complex social interactions (slower but more complex pre-frontal cortical processes) aimed at emotional regulation, accurate interpretation of social cues, socially acceptable and effective social interactions, and problem-solving (Kahneman 2011). In the stressful clinical setting, it is helpful to the counselor and therapeutic for the patient and their family caregivers to be able to understand and to reflect these multilevel innate resources in the clinical work.

We will now focus on some gender-specific approaches to helping patients and their caregivers to benefit from understanding the importance of focusing on *motivation over behavior interpretation* and *leveraging natural inclinations.*

7 Getting Women and Men to Understand Each Other at Their Core: Accessing Motivations and Leveraging Natural Inclinations

Approximately 65% of women (ages 25–64) now work outside the home (Bureau of Labor Statistics 2011). Within the context of the demanding workplace, these are primarily competitive rather than the collaborative relationships that have comprised women's relationships for many millennia. This has been a double stressor for women as they no longer can depend on the support and feedback from other women on a consistent basis to manage their stress. This may leave women feeling emotionally unfulfilled, isolated, diluted, and frustrated. Within the context of cancer, women may turn to men to provide the kind of support which they have historically received from their sisters, mothers, grandmothers, aunts, and female friends. Men are seldom equipped to intuitively respond in a helpful way or to comprehend what women need from them. One of the well-documented gender differences found in the literature is the stress response. When under stress, women have been shown to reach out to others and to "tend and befriend," (Taylor et al. 2000) as an initial response to control their sense of danger and fear. Women feel secure in reaching out to others when trying to manage the stress associated with their vulnerability and do not experience any diminution of self-esteem by asking for help. For women, their level of self-efficacy (i.e., confidence that she can be a good caregiver) has been shown to be an indicator of how they manage stress related to chronic illness (Hagedoorn et al. 2002).

For men, who have traditionally gained their sense of purpose and direction in a highly competitive action oriented environments, such as work, recent social demands focusing on high levels of verbal communication, collaborative team work, and sensitivity to their emotional impact on others has created stress and confusion. Within the context of cancer, both as care recipients and caregivers, many men are confronted with demands from their loved ones that do not come naturally to them and lead to a sense of shame and guilt that encourages their natural inclination to withdraw. When men experience stress, there is an innate tendency to react with the fight-or-flight response. When confronted with stressors that are not manageable by immediate action, there is a strong inclination to turn inward to access internal resources and for reflection related to problem-solving. Unlike women, men may experience a sense of diminished self-esteem by sharing their vulnerabilities with others. Although women are adept at prospectively sharing their emotional concerns to reduce their immediate sense of threat, it is only in retrospect that men are generally comfortable sharing their fears and concerns with others, once the sense of threat is reduced to manageable levels. The ways in which many women and men manage their vulnerabilities (women seeking emotional connection and men seeking space and time to think) have significant implications within the context of caregiving. Although female caregivers report higher levels of emotional distress, (Hagedoorn et al. 2008), male caregivers may express their distress by becoming rebellious or aggressive, or by smoking and drinking more (Hagedoorn et al. 2002). At first impression, it would appear that the mismatches of women and men in regulating stress are misaligned and maladaptive. For women, reaching out to a variety of others, verbally processing, sharing detailed internal vulnerabilities, and not expecting resolutions or fixes are natural inclinations for managing stress. For men, turning inward, self-reliance, taking action, outcome orientation, and problem resolution are natural inclinations for managing stress. The changing social demands on women and men when confronted with serious life-threatening illness are different than the more predatory obvious and external dangers for which men and women have had to adapt together throughout history. Cancer is a complex disease that brings into sharp relief the potential alignments and misalignments in the sexes.

What is now expected from women and men in the face of serious threat, such as a cancer diagnosis, may be new to both. In essence, the focus of gender-based interventions is the premise that men and women have the capacity to effectively support each other but that these propensities have not been activated at such an advanced social and psychological level until very recently in evolutionary time. A part of the clinical work is to teach women and men to be open to understanding the evolution of men and women successfully working together over many thousands of years, and then for them to learn how to be open to broadened perceptions and to activate other innate behaviors that may be less familiar. Sex and gender go well beyond committed sexual partners and often includes parents, siblings, friends, bosses, and co-workers. Being able to understand potential gender-based responses, and to reframe them to therapeutic benefit, has the potential to reduce confusion, frustration, and isolation while simultaneously creating an environment of mutual understanding, respect and active problem-solving, ultimately coping. It is a given that when people are under stress, they are more likely to revert to their habitual behavioral patterns. In essence, they become more like caricatures of themselves. There are some common behaviors that men and women produce in different frequencies that are generalizations (to be at least considered but never assumed) in the clinical setting. Teaching men and women to get beyond the subjective interpretation of behaviors and to reach for and understand the underlying motivations of their partner can be a potent therapeutic exercise in itself.

7.1 Understanding and Accessing Motivations

The truism that *actions speak louder than words* is only helpful if the actions are interpreted accurately and ultimately leads to a deeper understanding of the behaviors of the actor. For example, in general, humor may be used to deflect the emotional intensity of the situation or to minimize the seriousness of the situation. But a partner may easily see the behavior as disrespectful and emotionally distancing. Making assurances that may not be realistic can also result in a serious misalignment or incongruence (lack of understanding of the other's perspective resulting in increased conflict) (Lewis et al. 2006; Ezer et al. 2011). Our experience has shown us that these are tactics more often used by men. In this situation, the woman may feel that the man is not strong enough and may not be able to be counted on to be there for her when she really needs him. Likewise, when a woman feels confident that she "knows" (because she intuitively feels it so intensely) what her partner is experiencing ("I know that you are angry at me.") and shares her perceptions with her already stressed partner, this may be easily experienced by him as a boundary violation (as well as being incorrect). In this situation, again, everyone loses. The man, feeling powerless and frustrated, may retreat further into the very isolation that the woman was trying to avoid in the first place, which results in her feeling even more alone. These are two very common scenarios that occur within the context of coping with cancer because there is an overreliance on subjective interpretations that is endemic to the mental modeling that all people do in their everyday lives to deal with the multitude of repetitive situations that have to be efficiently managed. But being diagnosed with cancer is not a repetitive experience which most people can delegate to a lower level of reflection. The stress of illness and the potential crisis of cancer require a very large investment of higher cortical functions to emotionally regulate, solve complex problems, make meaning of the situation within a life being lived, and to maintain deep committed emotional connections with others.

Understanding the motivations (what the individual was trying to *achieve* in that specific situation) is a skill that women and men can be taught. Rather than interpreting (making educated/intuitive guesses based on other experiences), teaching women and men how to reach for (and listen with an open mind and an open heart), to the stated motivations of the other person can lead to a positive realignment of the relationship and in the individuals. By putting complex emotions, expectations (rational/irrational), and concerns into language that both people can understand leads to deeper and more authentic communication and emotional connections, even if they disagree. The strengths-based assumption here is that when a behavior is being repeated, it is serving some purpose (even if only for the primitive release of physical tension). It is the core purpose (the motivation) that is most important. In most cases the behavior is a signpost but not the destination. Here are some examples of actual scripts that men and women have used in our gender counseling sessions, support and problem-solving groups, and psycho-educational workshops to give voice to their partner's motivations:

- When you spend hours on the Internet or watching television, I get confused. Can you please teach me how this helps you to cope with this situation? I want to understand; so I do not read into things that will make me feel worse. I need your help to understand.
- When you talk about your cancer in detail to people we hardly know it confuses me and makes me uncomfortable. Can you please teach me how this helps you to talk with strangers about our private matters? I want to be supportive. I really need your help to understand what benefits you get out of this. How does this help you?
- When you make jokes about your cancer and dying, it makes it hard for me to understand what you are going through. It also makes the children and me feel more distant from you. Can you please teach me how humor helps you? I really want to understand. How does this help you?
- I am confused and I need your help please. You tell me not to come with you to your doctor appointments. But then when I do not go with you, as you ask, you get enraged at me. What are you trying to achieve by giving me these no-win messages. Please teach me what this is like for you? I care about you and I want to know what you are trying to achieve with these different messages.

Given the emotional intensity and complexity of the life-space in which patients and their caregivers find themselves, and the psychological, physical, and spiritual investments to be made over extended periods of time, building on existing behaviors and the natural inclinations of the individual has potential for more positive outcomes. We will now discuss how teaching women and men, how to leverage their natural inclinations builds on their existing innate strengths and resources.

7.2 Natural Inclinations

In the classic song Professor Higgins sings, "Why Can't a Woman be More Like a Man?" (My Fair Lady, 1964 song by Frederick Loewe &y Alan Jay Lerner), the stage (a theme repeated too many times in multiple media) is set and so is the trap. By the end of the movie, it is the "Professor" who is educated not only about women but also what it means to be a complete man—the emotional and the intellectual are appreciated. Women and men seldom fit into neat categories—they are both intellectual and have rich emotional lives. In fact, in many parts of the western world, women are now going to colleges and are getting advanced degrees in larger numbers than are men (Aliprantis et al. 2011). The impact of these imminent changes is beyond the scope of this discussion but the need to understand the evolving expectations of the genders is not. In most societies around the world dramatic changes are occurring in the roles, opportunities, and expectations for women and men. For example, although women are still the primary caregivers for seriously ill family members, men are increasingly taking on the role as primary caregiving role from 25% in 1987 to 39% in 2004, (Kim et al. 2006, 2007). Given the larger numbers of women attaining college and advanced degrees and the decrease in men pursuing higher education in job markets requiring highly skilled labor, dramatic role shifts are expected to accelerate. Within the context of these rapid social changes, men and women will have to be highly adaptable in redefining the roles they value and are prepared to assume in this changing environment. Within the context of cancer, we have seen how in the face of serious life-threatening illness men and women can make major changes in their lives, at times, literally overnight.

The perceptions, attitudes, and behaviors to which people naturally gravitate (the default) when sensing danger can be used as a catalyst for expanding the repertoire of adaptive responses. It is helpful to label these behaviors as "natural inclinations" (Legato 2008) which, as a term, may be less judgmental and stigmatizing and can provide a sense of emotional distance and safety that is essential for the therapeutic context. There is also a connection to a much larger group of known and unknown individuals (in this case women and men), who may share traits and behaviors in common. The added benefit of teaching patients and their caregivers about gender-based natural inclinations is that they can quickly and easily see this process in their own lives and this may lead to a greater openness to learn about and accept the perceptions and responses of others. When people do not perceive the fit into gender-based generalizations, this can be reframed into the unique adaptability and flexibility of people to manage the many challenges individuals are forced to manage in their lives as an evolved blend across the sexes; that men or women fit into the generalizations is not important. What is important is that they see their lives as connected to the many courageous and adaptable generations who have come before them and that they have the benefit of building on this legacy, to help them today.

8   Sex and Gender in the Real World

In our work, we have focused on teaching men and women to go beyond their subjective interpretations of the behaviors of their loved ones and to try to learn about the subjective *intentions* or *motivations* of the other person. Statements that create an open and honest discussion of the behaviors being manifested are reframed as conversation openers. For example, men and women are taught to ask about behaviors and to not assume or interpret without giving the other person the benefit of the doubt. For instance, we teach men and women to ask specific questions such as; what are you trying to achieve by doing what you are doing? Such as, telling me not to worry, minimizing my concerns, drinking alcohol, bringing up past hurts, making jokes, withdrawing from me physically and emotionally. The men and women are then encouraged to practice this process in the actual session to insure the fidelity of the process and to be sure that they are actually getting to the intention or motivation of the behavior. It will probably not come as surprise to the reader that learning the intention or motivation of the specific behavior reflexively manifested by the man and woman may seem like novel information to them and can enhance motivation to continue the process independent of their work with the clinician. Table 1 lists examples of direct quotes from participants of our gender-specific programs. While Table 2 lists some examples of the guidelines for the men and women who participate in the gender-specific programs and Table 3 lists clinical implications of gender-specific interventions.

Table 1 Examples of quotes from the gender-specific programs	"…oh, is that why he does that, I never would have guessed…"
	"…how can she not know that I love her, I am here…"
	"…we have been married for 50 years and we never had a conversation like this…"
	"…if I would have known how to talk like this I might still be married…"
	"…enough of him sharing his feelings, I want my man back…I have feelings too"

Table 2 Women and men solving problem together

What you can do as a Partner that is Helpful for the Woman in your life:
Reflect before reacting to your partner
Communicate with each other in a way that you will be proud of in the future
Actively encourage the sharing of emotional concerns and fears
Be open to help the woman with her physical post surgery care
Listen to concerns without trying to "fix" or minimize them
Be a good listener by listening twice as much as you speak
Only give reassurances that are firmly based in reality (for e.g. "You can count on me")
Be physically present at all medical appointments even when not asked
Learn about the illness and treatments
Help the woman get through the information she needs to read
Take notes and ask questions at medical appointments
Help the woman get things done when the woman can not
Respect and support the woman's right to make her own decisions
Remember that the woman is still a capable individual
Help the woman share information to others she wants to keep informed
Advocate for the woman if needed (whether with health care providers or other family members)
Offer advice only when specifically requested
Be open to listening to the woman expressing her concerns as long as she needs to
What you can do as a Woman to get the best out of your partner or family member:
Reflect before reacting to your partner
Be honest and direct about how you feel, especially about your fears
Avoid testing-be specific about what you want from others

(continued)

Table 2 (continued)

Stay in the present-no past hurts or conflicts
No mind-reading-if confused about the behavior of your partner, ask about their motivation
Avoid proving points-focusing on who is right means that you both lose
Tell your partner when you need for them to just listen or when you are seeking advice
Respect that you and your partner might cope with things differently
Access support from peers and/or professionals when needed
Accept help

Table 3 Clinical implications of gender-specific interventions	Creating therapeutic environments where women and men can more fully appreciate the others individual natural inclinations while celebrating their unique contributions unrestrained by sex or gender
	Transcending gender roles can have multiple benefits
	Some sex differences become manifest in extreme circumstances only or at certain time (s) only
	Identifying, supporting and building on the foundation of natural inclinations of both sexes
	Expanding men's skill repertoire to include those used by women
	Expanding women's skill repertoire to include those used by men
	Benefitting from the inherent synergies of men and women working together

9　Summary and Future Directions

In this updated chapter, we have attempted to communicate the imperative for and importance of understanding people under stress within the context of sex and gender. Gender-specific medicine is a very young movement for scientific study but one that has great potential to maximize adaptation and mutual respect at a time when men and women are redefining themselves and adapting to new social realities and challenges. In fact, since the original publication of this chapter, much has changed as tailored or strategic cancer treatments increasingly must take sex into account as every cell has a sex. In addition, the National Institutes of Health/National Cancer Institute in the United States and other funding organizations now have as a standard that women and men be part of relevant trials (https://grants.nih.gov/grants/guide/notice-files/NOT-OD-15-102.html). This is a very big advance in the struggle for fairness and quality science with direct implications for improved cancer care.

Fortunately, women and men have been adapting to serious challenges since the beginning of time-together. Most significantly, men and women have insured to survival of the species by coevolving. For the first time, women and men can be aware of what was a set of complex unconscious processes to one that is now conscious and intentional and this can lead to an acceleration of creative adaptations and emotional growth.

With this appreciation of gender differences in coping and the reciprocal strengths each gender can provide, future research should focus on interventional studies that focus on getting the best out of each gender. These studies are now absent but we are getting closer. Such data is important because of the implications for public health, especially mental health, as the world becomes much more complex, automated, and less personally interactive. There is also a need to gain a better understanding of how sex differences lead to vulnerabilities for some and growth for others. The great biopsychosocial complexity of studying sex and gender (and political sensitivities) that have frustrated scientific exploration now creates many exciting opportunities. Ultimately, sex and gender, if for no other reason is worthy of scientific study, because it is the most fascinating of stories and it is a story that is still being written, by people like you.

References

Aliprantis D, Dunne T, Fee K (2011) The growing difference in college attainment between women and men. Federal Reserve Bank of Cleveland. http://www.clevelandfed.org/research/commentary/2011/2011-21.cfm. Accessed 28 Sept 2012

American Psychiatric Association (1980) Diagnostic and statistical manual of mental disorders, 3rd edn. American Psychiatric Association, Washington, DC

American Psychiatric Association (1987) Diagnostic and statistical manual of mental disorders, 3rd edn revised. American Psychiatric Association, Washington, DC

Amri R, Stronks K, Bordeianou L et al (2014) Gender and ethnic disparities in colon cancer presentation and outcomes in a US universal health care setting. J Surg Oncol 109:645–651

Becker JB, Berkley KJ, Geary N et al (2008) Sex differences in the brain: from genes to behavior. Oxford University Press, New York

Bitz C, Clark K, Vito C et al (2014) Partners' clinic: an innovative gender strengths-based intervention for breast cancer patients and their partners immediately prior to initiating care with their treating physician. Psycho-Oncol 24:355–358

Bureau of Labor Statistics (2011) Women in the labor force. Available at http://www.bls.gov/cps/wlf-table1-2011.pdf. Accessed 1 Oct 2004

Buss DM (1995) Psychological sex differences: origins through sexual selection. Am Psychol 50:164–168

Buss DM (2011) Evolutionary psychology: the new science of the mind, 4th edn. Allyn & Bacon, Needham Heights

Buss DM, Schmitt DP (2011) Evolutionary psychology and feminism. Sex Roles 64:768–787

Calleja-Agius J, Mallia P, Sapiano K et al (2012) A review of the management of intersex. Neonatal Netw 31:97–103

Clark K, Bergerot CD, Philip EJ et al (2016) Biopsychosocial problem-related distress in cancer: examining the role of sex and age. Psycho-Oncol. doi: 10.1002/pon.4172

Curry C, Cossich T, Matthews JP et al (2002) Uptake of psychosocial referrals in an outpatient cancer setting: improving service accessibility via the referral process. Support Care Cancer 10:549–555

de Vries G, Forger N (2015) Sex differences in the brain: a whole body perspective. Biol Sex Diff 6:15–16

Ezer H, Rigol Chachamovich JL, Chachamovich E (2011) Do men and their wives see it the same way? Congruence within couples during the first year of prostate cancer. Psycho-Oncol 20:155–164

Fergus KD, Gray RE (2009) Relationship vulnerabilities during breast cancer: patient and partner perspectives. Psycho-Oncol 18:1311–1322

Hagedoorn M, Sanderman R, Buunk BP et al (2002) Failing in spousal caregiving: the 'identity-relevant stress' hypothesis to explain sex differences in caregiver distress. Br J Health Psychol 7:481–494

Hagedoorn M, Sanderman R, Bolks HN et al (2008) Distress in couples coping with cancer: a meta-analysis and critical review of role and gender effects. Psychol Bull 134:1–30

Haier JR, Jung RE, Yeo RA et al (2005) The neuroanatomy of general intelligence: sex matters. NeuroImage 25:320–327

Halpern DF (2000) Sex differences in cognitive abilities, 3rd edn. Erlbaum, New Jersey

Institute of Medicine (2001) Exploring the biological contributions of human health: does sex matter?. National Academy Press, Washington, DC

Kahneman D (2011) Thinking fast and slow. Farrar, Straus and Giroux, New York

Kim Y, Loscalzo M, Wellisch D et al (2006) Gender differences in caregiving stress among caregivers of cancer survivors. Psycho-Oncol 15:1086–1092

Kim Y, Baker F, Spillers RL (2007) Cancer caregivers' quality of life: effects of gender, relationship, and appraisal. J Pain Symp Manage 34:294–304

Kim Y, Loscalzo M (eds) (In press, Spring 2018) Gender-oriented psycho-oncology research and practice. Oxford University Press, Oxford

Lee PA, Houk CP, Ahmed FS et al (2006) Consensus statement on management of intersex disorders. Pediatrics 118:488–500

Legato MJ, Colman C (1992) The female heart: the truth about women and coronary artery disease. Simon and Schuster, New York

Legato MJ, Bilezikian JP (2004) Principles of gender-specific medicine (vol 2). Gulf Professional Publishing, Houston

Legato MJ (2008) Why men die first. Palgrave MacMillan, New York

Lewis MA, McBride CM, Pollak KI et al (2006) Understanding health behavior change amnion couples: an interdependence and communal coping approach. Soc Sci Med 62:1369–1380

Loscalzo MJ, Kim Y, Clark K (2010) Gender and Caregiving. In: Holland J (ed) Psycho-oncology, 2nd edn. Oxford

Loscalzo M, Clark K (2014) Gender opportunities in psychosocial oncology. In: Goerling (ed) Psycho-oncology (Recent results in cancer research). Springer, Berlin, 197, pp 31–48

Loscalzo M, Clark K, Bitz C, Rosenstein D, Yopp J (In press, Spring 2018). When the invisible screen becomes visible: sex and gender matters in biopsychosocial interventions and programs. In: Kim Y, Loscalzo M (eds) Gender-oriented psycho-oncology research and practice. Oxford University Press, Oxford

Matthews BA (2003) Role and gender differences in cancer-related distress: a comparison of survivor and caregiver self-reports. Oncol Nurs Forum 30:493–499

McCallister K (2017) Unwanted advances: sexual paranoia comes to campus. 95–95

Merckaert I, Libert Y, Messin S et al (2010) Cancer patients' desire for psychological support: prevalence and implications for screening patients' psychological needs. Psychooncology 19:141–149

Narrow WE (ed) (2007) Age and gender considerations in psychiatric diagnosis: a research agenda for DSM-V. American Psychiatric Pub Incorporated

National Center for Health Statistics. Health, United States (2012) With Special Feature on Socioeconomic Status and Health. Hyattsville, Maryland

Pistrang N, Barker C (1995) The partner relationship in psychological response to breast cancer. Soc Sci Med 40:789–797

Resnick S, Driscoll I (2008) Sex differences in brain aging and alzheimer's disorders. In: Becker JB et al (eds) Sex differences in the brain: from genes to behavior. Oxford University Press, New York

Revenson TA, Griva K, Luszczynska A, Morrison, V et al (2016) Gender and caregiving: the costs of caregiving for women. In Caregiving in the illness context (pp 48–63). Palgrave Macmillan, UK

Rosen TS, Bateman D (2004) The role of gender in neonatology. In: Legato M (ed) Gender-specific medicine. Elsevier Academic Press, London

Silverman I, Choi J, Peters M (2007) The hunter-gatherer theory of sex differences in spatial abilities: data from 40 countries. Arch Sex Behav 36:261–268

Stanton AL (2010) Positive consequences of the experience of cancer: perceptions of growth and meaning. In: Holland J (ed) Psycho-oncology, 2nd edn. Oxford University Press, New York

Taylor SE, Klein LC, Lewis BP et al (2000) Biobehavioral responses in stress in females: tend and-befriend, not fight-or-flight. Psychol Rev 107:411–429

Vandermassen G (2005) Whos afraid of charles darwin? Debating feminism and evolutionary theory. Rowman & Littlefield, Maryland

World Health Organization (1998) Gender and health. Technical Paper, Geneva

Zabora J, Brintzenhofeszoc K, Curbow B et al (2001) The prevalence of psychological distress by cancer site. Psychooncology 10:19–28

Zaider TI, Kissane DW (2010) Psychosocial interventions for couples and families coping with cancer. In: Holland J (ed) Psycho-oncology, 2nd edn. Oxford University Press, New York

Psycho-Oncology: A Patient's View

Patricia Garcia-Prieto

Abstract

Culturally the most important, valued, and less stigmatized part of cancer care is the medical part: The surgeon cutting the tumors out and the oncologist leading the strategic decision-making of the medical treatments available. The least valued and stigmatized part of cancer remains the psychosocial care. This chapter describes—through the eyes of an academic, psychologist, stage IV melanoma patient, and patient advocate—how one patient navigated changing psycho-oncological needs from early stage-to-stage IV through a whole range of psychological interventions available. Her voice joins that of all cancer patients around the world whom are urgently calling for psycho-oncological care to be fully recognized as a central part of cancer treatment.

Keywords

Melanoma · Psycho-oncology · Patient · Mindfullness

P. Garcia-Prieto (✉)
Centre Emile Berhneim, Solvay Brussels School of Economics and Management, Université Libre de Bruxelles, Brussels, Belgium
e-mail: alexandre@chevalier-garciaprieto.org

P. Garcia-Prieto
Melanoma Independent Community Advisory Board, European Cancer Patient Coalition, Brussels, Belgium

© Springer International Publishing AG 2018
U. Goerling and A. Mehnert (eds.), *Psycho-Oncology*, Recent Results in Cancer Research 210, https://doi.org/10.1007/978-3-319-64310-6_4

1 A Disclaimer

I need to start with a disclaimer. This chapter represents one patient's view on psycho-oncology. I am a stage IV metastatic melanoma patient, president and founder of the Melanoma Independent Community Advisory Board,[1] a pilot project of the European Cancer Patient Coalition (ECPC, Brussels). I am also a psychologist and an academic living in Brussels. I started writing this chapter one week after my latest PET-CT scan showed again continued progressive disease. My objective here is to illustrate how my psycho-oncological needs have greatly varied throughout the different stages—Ib to IVc—and describe how I responded to those needs as a function of the psychosocial care that was available to me in my path.

2 Psycho-Oncology?

Psycho-oncology was suggested to me when the first tears welled up during one of my early diagnosis consults in 2008. After an early stage Ib "caught in time" melanoma I had progressed to a stage IIIc by March 2009. I sat in that small stuffy room while my husband told me *it* would be fine, and the dermatologists and an intern were telling me they would help me take care of *it*, while the nurse was changing the dressing on *it*. Like in a bad B movie time stood still and we all did our best to play according to very scripted roles. The hope we all had was that a psycho-oncologist referral would take care of the emotional distress part, which clearly seemed a separate section of cancer care. It was also the one part of my care that we were all the most uncomfortable with. In retrospect, psycho-oncology was presented as a different chapter—if not a different volume—of my cancer story. I did not know at the time that psycho-oncology was in fact a subspecialty of oncology with its own body of knowledge contributing to cancer care. I now know research in this area addresses both (a) patients' psychological reactions to cancer and (b) the psychosocial and behavioral factors that may lead to cancer (Holland 2001). As a patient I have high expectations about (a); and as a researcher I remain skeptical but curious about (b)...

3 Cancer as My New Psychology Lab

I was trained as an experimental social psychologist at the University of Queensland in Australia, and I did a Ph.D. in the area of cognitive appraisal theories of emotion at the University of Geneva in Switzerland. When I became "the patient experiencing emotional distress" because of cancer I must confess I initially amused myself by applying well-known stress theories to myself (especially the model of

---

[1]M-ICAB activities are now currently carried on by the melanoma patient.

Lazarus and Folkman 1984). I noted the different appraisals that would drive my new cancer emotional landscape including emotions such as numbing fear, anxiety, sadness and despair and anger and hostility. In fact my Ph.D. thesis was about how our social identities (group memberships) can affect our appraisals and emotions (Garcia-Prieto 2004). I have often used social identity theory strategies (Tajfel and Turner 1986) to counter social identity threats. For example, by creatively redefining my cancer social identity in counter stereotypical ways, or by bringing attention to my professor dimension and away from the patient dimension during an interaction with a doctor, or by engaging in cancer patient advocacy and activism, just to see what would change in me and others. I just have fun with this. After all, even today the cancer social identity remains highly stigmatized by our society and the discrimination one may experience because of the cancer membership can actually lead to increased levels of stress and damage health even more. In a way, with cancer, it feels like you have to pay your bill twice as you have to deal with the cancer and you have to deal with the stigma of cancer! So many of my multiple group identities (being an academic, a psychology professor, trained as an experimentalist, working in an economics and business school, co-director of a research center, etc.) represent a great psychosocial resource on which I draw when I am confronted with any hint of discriminatory behavior due to cancer. Of course, the stereotyping of cancer patients is not just done by others (she is a young mother fighting cancer for her children, she is a terminal patient, she is a difficult patient) but also by ourselves (I am an activist battling tooth and nail to join a trial, or I am a resilient cancer patient, I am cancer patient who believes in euthanasia, etc.). There is enough research on how social identities and all the stereotyping and intergroup-related processes can positively and negatively affect health (Hardwood and Sparks 2003). For me, it has become an art form to strategically negotiate my way through the many available cancer social identities.

In response to stressful cancer-related situations I have used both problem-focused coping (navigated my care across the best specialties in 5 hospitals, researching the potential clinical trials I could access before going for my appointments, enquiring about my health rights as a EU citizen, etc.) and emotion-focused coping (binging on dark Belgian chocolate when I would have thoughts of recurrence, purchasing a very expensive leather jacket right after a "bad" PET-CT scan). Truth be told, in that first year after the diagnosis I naïvely thought I knew enough about the psychological aspects of distress to go at it alone. Until the day came that I physically collapsed on the floor in front of my two young kids, exhausted from the interferon injections and trying to keep up being an academic, mother, wife and "know it all of the psychology of cancer" patient, I accepted that I was strong enough to search for my first psycho-oncological consultation.

4 Psycho-Oncology as a Side Dish

Luzia Travado [current treasurer[2] of International Psycho-Oncology Society (IPOS)] has reported that there is a great variation in access to psychological services in oncological centers in Europe: if you look at national cancer plans only 19 countries have psycho-oncological services (Beishom 2011). I live in Brussels and thanks to the work of Prof. Darius Razavi, the "tracks" of psycho-oncology in Belgium are well defined. I found a great psycho-oncologist and felt comforted by familiar methodologies set clinical goals and experienced results quickly. I wanted a cognitive-behavioral perspective. I did not want a group therapy. I did not want a psychiatrist. I wanted to feel in control, to know the independent variables, mediators, and dependent variables of "my experiment of one". Part of me believed that the psycho-oncological intervention in combination with a good anticancer diet and attitude (Servan-Schreiber 2007) could actually reduce my chances of relapse. At the very least I hoped it would prevent some sort of posttraumatic stress or depression. I did well for a beginner I guess. I knew the cognitive-behavioral approach was sound and evidence based, proven to be just as good as antidepressants and I felt it worked…at least for a while. I then started finding the relief of "relapse-anxiety" would only last the time between consults, and I did not like the feeling of being dependent on the psychologist and on the occasional low-dose Xanax my oncologist could prescribe. Interestingly, like the rest of my medical team (surgeon, dermatologist, oncologist and nurses) I too perceived my psychological needs as a separate issue, the side dish or dessert, but clearly not as the sauce of the main course! Now I can look back and say without a doubt: psychosocial issues in cancer are grossly underestimated.

I have never heard of the "distress thermometer" or sixth vital sign around me, and I suspect given the amount of distress I have seen in hospital staff; it is clearly not yet measured among oncologists and nurses, surgeons, etc. It has taken me a long time to integrate that the psycho-oncological needs are not "a separate" part; it was the same "me" that was living with the cancer and responding with distress. How could part of me have surgery, radiotherapy, and injections of low-dose interferon and another part of me sit down and cry in the shower hiding from my kids? But that is exactly how we all proceed with psychosocial needs on an implicit and sometimes explicit level. Culturally the most important and valued and less stigmatized part of cancer care is the medical part: The surgeon cutting the tumors out, the dermatologist doing skin follow-up, and the oncologist leading the strategic decision-making of medical treatments. The least valued and stigmatized part of cancer remains the psychosocial care, an option only to be activated "if need be", maybe even for those who are not strong enough. Though it seems that in the US the science of psychosocial care in oncology and of caring for the whole patient is evolving (Jacobsen et al. 2012), I have not experienced this myself.

---

[2]As of 2013. She is currently president of IPOS, 2014–2017.

5 Embodying Cancer: Mindfulness-Based Stress Reduction (MBSR)

As per text book, I have gone through denial, despair and anger, graduated to bargaining, and depression and have experienced many different levels of acceptance (Kübler-Ross and Kessler 2005). And though I know the theory, nothing prepared me for what the phases of grief would "feel" like in the body. And that was the turning point for me. I was initially caught up in "thinking" about the thoughts and feelings about living with cancer, and despite autohypnosis and relaxation body techniques, I was clearly not embodying my cancer experience. This felt like a bit of a paradox: in the case of metastatic melanoma your body gets "intervened" with a lot through surgery. Being an academic did not help. I thought of that well-known movie "Wit" where Emma Thompson plays a professor with stage IV ovarian cancer and how she succeeds in doing a full dose of an innovative chemotherapy cocktail in a trial. She masters that like any other academic project and gains the admiration of her doctors, and then she dies after a trial *well done*. I have approached cancer and the thoughts and experiences of the life of a patient with advanced melanoma much like I would have approached an experiment too. But in those early years I was not paying attention to the subject's body.

My first attempts to understand the psychological aspects of embodying the cancer experience lead me again to theories and research I knew. Toward the end of my Ph.D. I had seen research on long-term meditators coming out of the prestigious lab of Richard Davidson at the University of Wisconsin-Madison. Two of my best friends had in fact moved from Geneva to Davidson's lab and were there when the study took place and we had talked about it at the time, so I read anything I could find on mindfulness-based stress reduction (MBSR; Kabat-Zinn 1993) and especially as it related to cancer (Kabat-Zinn et al. 1998; for a good summary see Carlson and Speca 2010 or Shennan et al. 2010) and the immune system more specifically (Davidson et al. 2003; Carlson et al. 2007). I was impressed.

In September 2009 I was still struggling with being an over-anxious IIIc melanoma patient in fear of relapse. I signed up for an 8-week MBSR course at my local hospital. I practiced and asked no questions. I started to become aware of how I felt in my body while I was doing the cancer follow-up routines (medical visits, blood test, follow-up scans, adjuvant treatment, etc.). I noticed the breathing changes, the tensions, the thoughts that would come and go, and the emotions that would visit me quite often. MBSR gave me a new perspective that allowed me to distinguish the thoughts about the cancer situation from the actual experience in the body of those situations. I was able to see that my awareness of my distress was not distressed, which my awareness about fear was not afraid. Work, family life, my couple, and medical experiences all became a perfect lab to test the utility of this new approach. I amazed others and myself at how good I could be at surfing the waves of cancer and at managing to go deep down when the waves became too rough. But had I yet embodied my experience of cancer? Not really.

While I was out surfing a follow-up scan I experienced my own Hokusai great wave. On December 18, 2009, a few days before I drove down to Switzerland with my little family for Christmas, I found out I was stage IV and progressing fast. No treatment existed for stage IV melanoma in Belgium. Subcutaneous tumors were popping up like popcorn over the next weeks while my family was worried about the foie gras and the champagne. For the first time I started looking myself for a clinical trial and when I found out that there was one across the border from Brussels (in Paris) but that my health insurance was denying me the right of cross-border health agreements I experienced the most incredible rage I have ever felt in my life. The appraisals of injustice and of high control driving my rage were the fuel of my first steps in patient advocacy mobilizing local media, lawyers, and EU politicians. I won that battle with the support of ECPC and others but the trial I fought for could not include me because my tumor burden was too low. I came back to Brussels with a new sense of despair. All throughout this ordeal I held on to MBSR.

The MBSR methodology was easy to follow and I did not need to adhere to any belief system. It was simple and I embraced the new feeling of autonomy and mastery that MBSR practice gave me compared to classic psycho-oncological sessions where I was much more passive and in demand of guidance. With MBSR the guidance was there "online" as things developed, all that I did was show up for what was already there and through each moment of attention given to breath, bodily sensation, thought or emotion I experienced a strong sense of mastery. Paradoxically, the more I surrendered to what was already happening (tumors coming out, surgery, change of treatment, side effects), the more I felt this sense of mastery. Saki Santorelli describes this beautifully:

> Inwardly speaking, via meditation practice, mastery is cultivated through attending to thoughts, emotions and physical sensations and events in the field of awareness—by allowing these events to arise, be seen, honoured the way they are, and eventually dissipate or dissolve rather than dominate the mind (Santorelli 2011, p. 209).

I did not necessarily like what I experienced and felt, as I was terrified and angry and anxious, or in pain from the surgeries, but the difference was that this time I turned toward those experiences, which were already there anyways, and did not try to change them. Practicing presence or simply "showing up" for whatever the day threw at me radically changed my quality of life, not just life with cancer, but all of my life. I changed my attitude as a teacher, for better or for worse I changed as a wife, mother, daughter, and colleague. But during this period I recognize now that there was also a lot of bargaining with the cancer. I gave myself authority to engage in large projects and accepted increasing responsibility and accepted academic leadership challenges I would have never taken. I know now that it was a way for me to set future goals that I still needed to achieve before I was "done". And as if by magic, things got done, and I am still setting future goals. My relationship with psycho-oncology changed. I was still heavily relying on help from a psychiatrist for my couple, which was suffering, and sometimes more than my body, but I relied less and less on psycho-oncological consults.

It was also in early 2010 that I started working with a group of like-minded people in Brussels that includes cancer patients like myself, Reliable Cancer Therapies,[3] Association pour le Development du Mindfulness (ADM); The Université Libre de Bruxelles; Institut Jules Bordet; UZ Brussels; UZ Gent; Institute for Attention and Mindfulness, Sint Elisabeth Ziekenhuis (ZNA), and The Chirec Cancer Institute and a few private sponsors on a long-term project that aims at better integrating mindfulness into oncology centers in Belgium. This work is ongoing and holds great promise on seeing one-day mindfulness-based interventions become standard part of care in oncology centers, and we hope this also becomes reality for the medical/nursing staff.

6 Meaning and Posttraumatic Growth

As the illness has progressed into a stage IV *life-limiting illness*, and I continue to navigate through clinical trials to extend survival I must confess classic problem- and emotion-focused coping are not enough. MBSR practice without any meaning or spiritual context is also not enough. I am not religious, nor have I been one to search for the "meaning" of life. Thus as I reach the end I feel I am starting my spiritual awakening from scratch.

I have started more and more to experience what Susan Folkman (1997) has described as meaning-based coping. She has suggested that positive emotions play an important function in stress, and are related to coping mechanisms that are different from those that regulate distress (Folkman 2008). What is interesting in this perspective is that it seems that the coping mechanisms that decrease the negative emotions might be different than those that increase the positive emotions. She talks about the importance of creating the situations that allow for positive emotion. Indeed I am happier now than I have ever been before, and what is interesting is that I feel a quality and intensity of positive emotions that is totally different from pre-cancer positive emotions. I have indeed experienced that it is possible to experience stress from the stage IV situation, yet feel both positive and negative emotions during the stress.

Another concept that describes well what I am experiencing now is posttraumatic growth or PTG (Tedeschi and Calhoun 1995). The main idea is that the experience of a highly stressful or traumatic event such as stage IV diagnosis violates one's basic beliefs about the self and the world and that some type of meaning-making or cognitive processing is activated to rebuild these beliefs and goals, resulting in perceptions that one has grown through the process (Tedeschi and Calhoun 2004). A recent meta-analysis of PTG following cancer or HIV/AIDS patients has shown that PTG is related to better positive mental health and self-reported physical health, and less negative mental health (Sawyer et al. 2010).

---

[3] Anticancer Fund since 2014.

I have also recently engaged in a process of rediscovering my whole mind–body–spirit dimension. I can imagine this is not the sort of approach that may be readily available in most oncology centers. Yet for me, living with advanced disease, it is the most groundbreaking. I confess that I do not have all the psychological concepts to describe it in much detail here. But the process involves interacting with a therapist that enables me to embody thoughts and emotions, and to perceive what I will call—for lack of a better term—"my sensitive body". I suspect many people discover this dimension and their sensitive body through yoga, reiki, qi gong, tai chi, music or art therapy or faith. For me this exploration started with meeting and experiencing a session with Jean Paul Resseguier, a French kinésitherapist who developed this method almost 30 years ago. He was influenced by the phenomenology movement (through authors like Edmund Husserl, Maurice Merleau-Ponty and more recently Francisco Varela) and its understanding of the body not as a machine but as a dynamic "living" body that is constantly in a state of "creative" homeostasis interacting within and outside of the body. The Resseguier method has been applied to many medical conditions in Europe and Brasil—including cancer—and patients systematically report better quality of life and enhanced pain management and reduction of side effects during treatment. Unfortunately, there is no published research for cancer patients. The major feature of this method is the creation of an empathic relationship ("nouage empathique" in French) between the therapist and the patient through hand touch in the moment to moment. Basically, you both "show" up for what is there as it unfolds. Concretely for me as an advanced cancer patient it enables me to silently witness the dynamic and sensitive nature of mind–body–spirit. During a session I may experience online physical readjustments that seems to me to occur outside of my conscious "cognitive pilot". These readjustments may be not only physically felt and observed to the naked eye, but also confirmed via medical imagery (in my case the physical readjustments have been recorded via ultrasound and in one case via PET/CT scans). This work, which I continue with a person trained by him Brigitte Maskens in Brussels, has brought me clearly out of my academic comfort zone and for now I am just purely enjoying the ride…

Personally, I must conclude that the awareness of my own death as inevitable leads me to see the absence of all lived possibilities and to hold on to the present as the only place to be. In the words of Merleau-Ponty "…present without a future, or an eternal present, is precisely the definition of death" (1945 p. 388).

7 Conclusion

For us, the patients, psycho-oncology should not be presented as a side dish or separate chapter of cancer treatment to be activated only "if need be". Psycho-oncology is a cancer treatment. If empirical evidence of the impact of psychological intervention on overall survival is hard to demonstrate but it is there (see Andersen et al. 2008), there is ample evidence of its positive effect on quality of life, pain reduction, and cancer treatment side-effect management. For patients it is clearly not about just extending overall survival, but about living well the time that we live with cancer. Psycho-oncology holds a central place in each step of the path from diagnosis to recovery, and for those who like me live with advanced disease, all the way to the terminal phases of cancer. This central place needs to be recognized and integrated into existing cancer centers, hospitals, and national health systems and cancer plans. Recent reviews leave us with hope that access to psycho-oncological care being facilitated not only in the US but also around the world, and in great part this is due to better-organized patient advocacy and greater inclusion of the patient view in decision-making and debates (Beishom 2011). This chapter is a clear testimony to this.

8 Post-Scriptum (2016)

Patricia Garcia-Prieto Chevalier passed away on July 2, 2013. After more than 5 years fights against melanoma, and about 4 years as a stage IV patient, she leapt over to the other side. We updated some of the information (in footnote) but this is a testimony and state of thought and research as of 2013.

References

Andersen BL, Hae-Chung Yang WBF, Golden-Kreutz D, Emery C, Thorton LM, Young DC, Carson WE III (2008) Psychologic intervention improves survival for breast cancer patients a randomized clinical trial. Cancer 113(12):3450–3458

Beishom M (2011) Luzia Travado: improving outcomes for patients by attending their distress. Cancer World

Carlson LE, Speca M (2010) Mindfulness-based cancer recovery: a step-by-step MBSR approach to help you cope with treatment and reclaim your life. New Harbinger, Oakland, CA

Carlson LE, Speca M, Patel K, Faris P (2007) One year follow-up of psychological, endocrine, immune, and blood pressure outcomes of mindfulness-based stress reduction (MBSR) in breast and prostate cancer outpatients. Brain Behav Immun 21(8):1038–1049

Davidson R, Kabat-Zinn J, Schumacher J, Rosenkrantz M, Muller D, Santorelli S, Urbanowski F et al (2003) Alterations in brain and immune function produced by mindfulness meditation. Psychosom Med 65:564–570

Folkman S (1997) Positive psychological states and coping with severe stress. Soc Sci Med 45:1207–1221

Folkman S (2008) The case for positive emotions in the stress process. Anxiety Stress Copin 21 (1):3–14

Garcia-Prieto P (2004) The influence of social identity on appraisal and emotion. Doctoral dissertation. University of Geneva, Faculty of Psychology and Education Sciences, Switzerland. http://www.unige.ch/cyberdocuments/theses2004/Garcia-PrietoP/meta.html

Hardwook J, Sparks L (2003) Social identity and health: an intergroup communication approach to cancer. Health Comm 15(2):145–159

Holland JC (2001) Improving the human side of cancer care: psycho-oncology's contribution. Cancer J 7(6):458–471

Jacobsen PB, Holland JC, Steensma DP (2012) Caring for the whole patient: the science of psychosocial care. J Clin Oncol 30(11):1151–1153

Kabat-Zinn J (1993) Mindfulness meditation: health benefits of an ancient buddhist practice. In: Goleman D, Gurin J (eds) Mind/body medicine, consumer reports books. Yonkers, NY

Kabat-Zinn J, Massion AO, Hebert JR, Rosenbaum E (1998) Meditation. In: Holland JC (ed) Textbook of psycho-oncology. Oxford University Press, Oxford, pp 767–779

Kübler-Ross E, Kessler D (2005) On grief and grieving: finding the meaning of grief through the five stages of loss. Scribner, New York

Lazarus RS, Folkman S (1984) Stress, appraisal and coping. Springer, New York

Merleau-Ponty M (1945) Phénoménologie de la perception. Gallimard, Paris

Shennan C, Payne S, Fenlon D (2010) What is the evidence for the use of mindfulness-based interventions in cancer care? A review. Psycho-Oncol 20(7):681–697

Santorelli S (2011) Enjoy your death: leadership lessons forged in the crucible of organizational death and rebirth infused with mindfulness and mastery. Contemporary Budism 12:199–217

Sawyers A, Ayers S, Field AP (2010) Posttraumatic growth and adjustment among individuals with cancer or HIV/AIDS: a meta-analysis. Clin Psychol Rev 30(4):436–447

Servan-Schreiber D (2007) Anticancer - Prévenir et lutter grâce à nos défenses naturelles. Éditions Robert Laffont, S.A

Tajfel H, Turner JC (1986) The social identity theory of intergroup behaviour. In: Worschel S, Austin WG (eds) Psychology of intergroup relations. Nelson Hall, Chicago, pp 7–24

Tedeschi R, Calhoun L (1995) Trauma and transformation: growing in the aftermath of suffering. Sage Publications, Thousand Oaks

Tedeschi R, Calhoun L (2004) Posttraumatic growth: conceptual foundations and empirical evidence. Psychol Inq 15:1–18

The Oncological Patient in the Palliative Situation

Steffen Eychmueller, Diana Zwahlen and Monica Fliedner

Abstract

Palliative care approaches patients and their suffering with a bio-psycho-social-spiritual model. Thus, it is the strength of palliative care to complement the diagnosis driven approach of medical cancer care by a problem and resources-based assessment, participatory care plan and person-directed interventions. Interventions need to reflect timely prognosis, target population (the patient, the family carer, the professional) and level of trust and remaining energy. In palliative care the relevance of psycho-oncological aspects in the care of the terminally ill is considerable in the understanding of the overall suffering of patients approaching death and their loved ones and in their care and support. There is little evidence to date in terms of clinical benefit of specific psycho-oncological interventions in the last months or weeks of life, but there is evidence on effects of stress reduction and reduced anxiety if locus of control can stay within the patient as long as possible. One major challenge in psychosocial and palliative care research, however, is defining patient relevant outcomes.

Keywords

Palliative care · Person-centered assessment in oncology · Multi-professional team

S. Eychmueller (✉) · M. Fliedner
University Center for Palliative Care, Inselspital Bern, Bern, Switzerland
e-mail: steffen.eychmueller@insel.ch

D. Zwahlen
Department of Oncology, University Hospital Basel, Bern, Switzerland

© Springer International Publishing AG 2018
U. Goerling and A. Mehnert (eds.), *Psycho-Oncology*, Recent Results
in Cancer Research 210, https://doi.org/10.1007/978-3-319-64310-6_5

67

A Patient's Journey: Mrs. B

Mrs. B. is a 58 years formerly very active and athletic woman whose husband died some years ago from cardiac arrest. We, the palliative care inpatient interprofessional consultancy service team and the patient, met for the first time on a surgical ward where she was hospitalized for abdominal pain and vomiting both due to progressive cholangiocarcinoma. Unintended she broke out into tears when telling about the recent months: after primary surgery she underwent chemotherapy. Despite experiencing severe fatigue she felt pretty well, continued to play tennis and met with friends and family regularly. She did not at all expect her cancer to grow during this phase of treatment, and now she feels dramatically disappointed: not only that her cancer was growing again, but also that she misjudged her body's condition. The sudden change in body condition and the new perspective of life-limited disease lead to an overall weakness and break down. Being a former nurse she saw herself for the first time in the new role of a patient, more and more depending on the help of others and most of all as being a burden for her daughter.

We discussed her preferences ("going home, no additional chemotherapy"), her worries ("becoming a burden for her daughter and the whole issues of dying"), her network at home ("nice home, living on my own, daughter with small children living closed by, son abroad for work"), and potential support needs for the future ("most important, providing psychological support for my daughter"). It was proposed to discuss the issues such as role changes in the family and the fear of being a burden and not being able to support others anymore, respectively, together with the psycho-oncologist.

After referral to the palliative care ward we organized a family conference using "skype-link™" to her son who was at that time working abroad. It was the patient herself who finally lead the family conference based on a structured problem-based prompt sheet ("SENS"-structure, i.e. discussion regarding Symptom management, End of life decisions based on individual preferences, Network-organization issues for the future care at home and Support needs of family carers). Abdominal pain and vomiting improved through medication, complementary therapy and nutritional counselling.

Mrs. B. returned home, stayed there for several weeks managing symptoms on her own, with little support by her general practitioner, managing her household with external support twice a week and—most important—meeting regularly with her daughter and grandchildren. Several sessions with the psycho-oncologist lead to open and honest discussions between mother and daughter about family roles, needs, fears and finally to a better acceptance of role changes and support. The daughter herself wished further psychotherapeutic support and was referred to a psychotherapist in private practice.

Three days before she died, Mrs. B. returned to our palliative care ward accompanied by her entire family, requesting for professional help for these last days of life, recognizing that no energy was left to survive any longer. She was greatly satisfied to have the opportunity to spend valuable time together with her family, experiencing security through the "net" around her and the opportunity of "the final growth, the completion of her life's symphony" even if the end was far too early.

1 Background and Definitions

"Palliative care" or the "palliative situation" is still poorly defined and the concept remains vague. Ellen Fox wrote in 1997 a remarkable editorial in the JAMA highlighting the "predominance of the curative model of medical care", as a "residual problem" (Fox 1997; Holland et al. 2007). Mrs. B.'s last weeks could have been easily filled with several medical interventions, which would have resulted in spending most of her remaining lifetime in the hospital. She was in a "palliative situation" and chose the model of care provided by palliative care. Fox continued: "…on a basic level, the curative model conflicts with the notion of a good death". There is a certain danger to omit individual values and goals and the "tendency to perceive patients in terms of their component parts".

This chapter focusses on perspectives of patients under the care of specialized palliative care services involving the multi-professional team. Thus, it is the strength of palliative care to complement the diagnosis-driven approach of medical cancer care by a person-centred assessment, participatory care plan and patient-directed interventions. Consequently, palliative care approaches patients and their suffering with a bio-psycho-social-spiritual concept. Thus, psychological aspects are integral part of the palliative care model. It is the aim of palliative care to give back as much self-control as possible to the patient and to provide support wherever, whenever and whoever needed. The target of such care is less a cell or an organ, but patient and their carers—or by words of Dame Cicely Saunders—the unit of care. Collaboration within the palliative care team and among all professionals with different backgrounds is a frequent term when discussing and planning patient care. In palliative care the relevance of psycho-oncological aspects is considerable in the understanding of the overall suffering of patients approaching death and their loved ones and in their care and support.

Psycho-oncology is a multidisciplinary subspecialty of oncology concerned with the emotional responses of patients at all stages of disease, their families and staff (Holland 2013).

Therefore, psycho-oncology and palliative care share the view of seeing the patient as a whole and the suffering not only as a medical problem. Both disciplines intervene to empower patients to ameliorate their living with their disease and to increase quality of life in patients without aiming at healing their somatic condition. Both disciplines regard the non-medical aspects as an essential part of suffering but also as a potential source of energy or even healing. In 2003, William Breitbart edited for the first time the journal "Palliative & Supportive Care", "the first international journal of palliative medicine that focuses on the psychiatric, psychosocial, spiritual, existential, ethical, philosophical and humanities aspects of palliative care"(Breitbart 2003). In a personal reflection Breitbart (2006) challenges one of the most significant values in palliative care and in psycho-oncology: time. Time is the main essence—for reflection, creating trust and a relationship, doing "unfinished business", coping, communicating, but also for setting priorities: how would I like to spend my remaining lifetime, with whom and where?

Psycho-oncology and palliative care are both frequently involved in the care of patients with advanced cancer, but there is little evidence about "dosage", best time for involvement and the process of interaction of these two disciplines. There is a substantial overlap of the two definitions of psycho-oncology and palliative care, a fact that explains potential conflicts but also how they complement each other in daily clinical care. There may be side effects of palliative care and psycho-oncology that need to be recognized early if used alone or in combination. One is adding distress to the patient and family by an overdose of support and/or insufficient coordination of care activities. Another is to disregard the patient's own resources even in a clinical situation of weakness and frailty, and to focus—as we do in medicine in general—on deficits rather than strengths and resources. In addition it is of highest importance to distinguish three levels of interaction and reflection: the patient, the patient's surrounding or family and finally the professional team.

This chapter will discuss and highlight recent advances in palliative care with particular focus on psycho-oncological aspects. The authors attempt to focus on data derived from specific studies in the "palliative care" population (which is still difficult to define!): from assessment to interventions and outcomes having in mind a common "credo": professionalism in palliative care and psycho-oncology relies on the capability to continuously evaluate if treatment and care allows and gives back a certain sense of control to the patient and family, of coherence, as Antonovsky defined, even in a "palliative situation"—and provides space and time for essential issues at the end of life defined by patients themselves. A most valuable basis for counselling support and therapy in palliative care is in fact the concept of salutogenesis with its three components comprehensibility, manageability and meaningfulness (Antonovsky 1996). In clinical practice these components may be used as a stepwise approach for reducing distress in patients and family carers: understanding the current situation and reasons for limitations will allow to tailor expectations and to find concrete measures such as self-help strategies for handling the situation, and finally to promote acceptance or even making sense out of the current situation.

2 Assessment

2.1 Timely Identification, Assessment Strategies and Tools in Palliative Care

A or possibly THE major issue in palliative care is late referral. In psycho-oncology and palliative care, access to this kind of support and care is still lacking clearly defined "red flags", thus the recognition of needs remain unsystematic.

Usually the physical and cognitive resources of patients in late stage of a cancer disease are scarce. It therefore is of paramount importance that supportive care is well coordinated and aims are clearly defined and communicated. Patients' and family members' needs must be the leading criteria for the involvement of palliative care or psycho-oncology and potential underlying reasons such as helplessness of professionals should be identified.

Today, recognition or "diagnosis" of important psychosocial and spiritual distress and "palliative care needs" in patients with advanced cancer has been highlighted in several guidelines (e.g. (National Comprehensive Cancer Network (NCCN) 2016b). A recently published systematic review on referral criteria for outpatient palliative cancer care concludes that a significant heterogeneity regarding the timing and process for referral exists. The authors underline the need for standardized referral criteria (Hui et al. 2016). In clinical practice, staffing, scientific recognition and financial reimbursement still pose significant barriers for early integration of palliative care in standard oncology care. A major impediment to a proactive approach of advance care planning may derive from physicians themselves. In a recent report, uncertainty about the right timing of end-of-life (EOL) discussions as well as emotional involvement were reported to hinder a proactive stance (Pfeil et al. 2015). The authors call for educational activities regarding communication skills.

There is growing evidence that early integration of palliative care—several months prior to death—not only reduces distress and improves quality of life, but also decreases health care utilization and lastly costs (Temel et al. 2010, 2011; Zhang et al. 2009). Evidence seems to be sufficient for the American Society for Clinical Oncology (ASCO) to recommend early palliative care as best practice in some cancer diagnoses (Smith et al. 2012). Early integration of palliative care and communicating with patient and family about difficult issues such as the end of life can alleviate distress. There is also evidence that end-of-life (EOL) discussions and place of death (hospital/ICU vs. at home) not only have a positive impact on patient outcomes but also on caregiver bereavement adjustment (Wright et al. 2008, 2010) despite considering that the outcomes of early involvement of palliative care are still unclear, but advance care planning strategies in general seem to have positive impact on compliance with patients' end-of-life wishes and decrease unwanted health care utilization such as emergency hospitalizations (Brinkman-Stoppelenburg et al. 2014; Zambrano et al. 2016). Outcomes such as spiritual aspects, or the social network, for which more comprehensive information is needed, are just as important in palliative care as any disease-modifying treatment option (Gaertner and Becker 2014) since these topics provide meaningful information about the person himself. Early integration of palliative care and communicating with patients and families about difficult issues such as the end of life can alleviate distress. Increased or persisting distress is usually also a criterion for the integration of psycho-oncology. A thorough assessment of patients' needs and the coordinated interplay of the two disciplines are most beneficial for patients and their family.

2.2   Assessment Strategies and Tools

Assessing and documenting complexity is one of the big challenges in palliative and end of life care. This is also true for the organization of tasks and responsibilities in an interprofessional care team, but also for financial/reimbursement issues. Comprehensive cancer care is one of the attempts to organize such tasks and responsibilities through a shared care model. One of the challenges in highly complex situations, as we encounter them in palliative care, can be seen in the fact that medical diagnoses alone may not reflect sufficiently individual problems and suffering.

The MASCC Psychosocial Study Group published a conclusive paper on main psychosocial concerns and needs of cancer patients and families throughout all phases of the disease (Surbone et al. 2010). In this document we find a call for action in terms of systematic assessment, training and even a "new paradigm of supportive care that addresses psychosocial issues from diagnosis through treatment and post-treatment phases, up to end-of-life or long-term survivorship, …".

In palliative care settings, assessment must be tailored to the patients' situation. Burden and length of the assessment must be minimized and the type of assessment must be related to concrete implications. This means that assessment instruments should have a screening tool character and serve as a foundation to support and enable further communication not necessarily linked directly to the patient but to family and team about the components of despair and possible resources of support.

For the purpose of providing a person-centred assessment system in palliative care, with symptom assessment as only one part of it, the "SENS"-framework has been developed (Eychmuller 2012). 'SENS' stands for Symptom management, End- of –life decisions, Network- organization and Support of the family and has been developed by focusing on patients' needs. Thus, the 'SENS' framework helps to assess various aspects of daily life and to create a care plan based as far as possible on self-determination and patients' wishes.

Other multidimensional or rather multiple-symptom-assessment systems in palliative care are commonly used in clinical practice but all rely on the patient's cognitive function which can alter dramatically even within days or hours. Based on NCCN Clinical Practice Guidelines for Palliative Care (National Comprehensive Cancer Network (NCCN) 2016b), the Edmonton Symptom Assessment System (ESAS) or single item tools for various symptoms (Butt et al. 2008) can be used. Most studies on multi-symptom assessment tools are developed and tested mainly in ambulatory patient populations except ESAS. A recent review (Hudson et al. 2016) reported that the ESAS and the Distress Thermometer (DT) were most often used as assessment tool for symptoms or distress in palliative care settings.

3   Assessment in and Involvement to Psycho-Oncological Support Service

Late referral to psycho-oncological services too is a major issue. Increased distress or persisting distress is a criterion for the integration of psycho-oncology as well as the patient or caregivers uttered need for psychological support. Early diagnosis and referral of patients for psychosocial support is especially important with respect to psycho-oncological care, because elevated levels of psychosocial distress not only complicate treatment, but also negatively impact the quality of life of patients and their family members, adversely affect compliance and lead to poorer medical treatment results (Colleoni et al. 2000; Faller et al. 1999; Ganz 2008; Parker et al. 2003).

Psychological disorders like adjustment disorders, anxiety disorders or depression, only represent a portion of the reasons why cancer patients and their family members should be offered psycho-oncological care. The more general term, distress, is more appropriate for describing the psychosocial difficulties—whether they fulfil the criteria for a psychiatric disorder or not—experienced by many patients and their family members. Estimates are high regarding the number of patients and family members who do not fulfil the formal criteria for a psychological disorder according to the ICD or DSM but they do suffer from clinically relevant psychosocial distress (Bultz and Carlson 2005; Herschbach and Heusser 2008; Holland 2006). International guidelines therefore reflect the urgency to quickly and efficiently identify (according to a predefined cut-off) individuals who may require more intense diagnostic and potentially psycho-oncological care (Holland et al. 2007). The standards for care of patients exhibiting psychosocial distress described by the NCCN are of particular importance in this area (National Comprehensive Cancer Network (NCCN) 2016a).

Screening for distress with the DT identifies comorbidities, including depression and anxiety and is therefore a widely used screening tool in the specific field of psycho-oncology. The DT contains one item ("Please circle the number (0–10) that best describes how much distress you have been experiencing in the past week including today") with a vertical visual analogue scale from 0 ("no distress") to 10 ("extreme distress") and a problem list that entails five problem categories (practical problems, family problems, emotional problems, spiritual/religious concerns, physical problems), with a total of 36 potential causes of expressed distress, each of which can be answered with 'yes' or 'no'.

The DT is a reliable and valid screening tool used in many psycho-oncological studies (Dolbeault et al. 2008; Donovan et al. 2014; Hughes et al. 2011; Mitchell 2007). The DT is also validated for relatives (Zwahlen et al. 2008). Distress screening is now an international standard in comprehensive care of cancer patients (Institute of Medicine (IOM) 2008; National Comprehensive Cancer Network (NCCN) 2016a) and, in many countries, its use is a criterion for cancer centre accreditation (Bultz et al. 2014; Pirl et al. 2014).

Screening tools such as the DT must be used to identify patients most in need of supportive care, and must be intended to give patients and their families' access to supportive care services. This is particularly true as resources and energy of patients and families in the palliative situation is scarce.

4 Barriers to Uptake or Acceptance of Psycho-Oncological Support Service

A problem identified in various studies is that the extent of distress correlates only moderately or not at all with the wish for support (Baker-Glenn et al. 2011; Faller et al. 2016a, b; Merckaert et al. 2010; Schaeffeler et al. 2015; Sollner et al. 2004) or actual utilization of the resources offered (Brebach et al. 2016; Carlson and Bultz 2003; Faller et al. 2016a, b; Waller et al. 2013). This might be particularly true for patients in the palliative situation (Azuero et al. 2014; Kadan-Lottick et al. 2005; Mosher et al. 2014). It also remains to be elucidated whether referred palliative patients are those who are most likely to benefit (Ellis et al. 2009).

Several recent studies report why distressed patients do not seek professional support despite a certain level of distress. In their review, Dilworth and colleagues describe the primary patient-reported reason as "no subjective need for psychosocial services" (38.7% of pts) (Dilworth et al. 2014). This patient-related reason includes, e.g. the preference to self-manage symptoms, not feeling distressed enough, the impression that help would not be effective, and receiving enough support from family and friends (Clover et al. 2015; Dilworth et al. 2014; Faller et al. 2016a, b). There seems to be no difference in patients treated with palliative or curative intention (Azuero et al. 2014; Kadan-Lottick et al. 2005; Mosher et al. 2014). Patients' underlying motivations for reporting no need for psychological help are wide-ranging and numerous. Some patients may regard psychosocial care as stigmatizing and therefore are reluctant to seek help. Patients' fear of being considered weak and unable to cope with the disease, or being told what to do by the psycho-oncologist, and the idea that emotional "strength" also means physical "strength" might have considerable influence on patients' behaviour and lead to rejection of psychological support (Baker et al. 2013; Dilworth et al. 2014; Mehnert and Koch 2008; Neumann et al. 2010).

On the side of professionals there are potential barriers to the integration of psycho-oncologists: on the one hand there is the attitude of medical staff that assumes the non-physical suffering and psychological aspect as less important. On the other hand a palliative care team must be trained in recognizing, diagnosing and managing distress in patients and needs an algorithm when to refer to mental health professionals.

5 Screening and Communication

Discussing with patients their level of distress using a screening tool such as DT creates an opportunity for the interprofessional team and patients to effectively communicate about psychosocial issues and psychosocial health needs. Indeed, it was shown that Oncologists used the DT more to initiate communication about distress than as an assessment tool (Tondorf et al. submitted). Mitchell et al. (2012) reported that a screening tool such as the DT positively influenced communications about psychosocial issues and distress, and clinicians believed the screening program improved communication in more than 50% of assessments (Mitchell et al. 2012). Bultz, et al. (2011) emphasize that interaction with patients is the essential element of an effective screening procedure. However, a conversation about psychosocial distress after screening is not as simple as it sounds. When examining patient–clinician communication during a standard distress screening procedure oncologists and patients differed substantially in their recall of communication (Tondorf et al. submitted). The most striking disagreements were over whether the oncologist "provided practical information about psycho-oncological support" (90% versus 21%), and whether the oncologist "recommended attending the psycho-oncology service" (55% versus 26%).

Research and practice in psychotherapy and medical care has shown that effective strategies include communication techniques that establish an atmosphere of cooperation rather than dependence (Doherty et al. 1994; Langewitz 2013; McDaniel and Hepworth 2000). Validating patients' perception, authentic empathic listening, focusing on resources and cooperation are key elements for improving the quality of care in terms of therapeutic relationship, patient participation and treatment process (Doherty et al. 1994; Langewitz 2013; McDaniel and Hepworth 2000).

Going back to our patient example, the main area of distress of Mrs. B. at the beginning of the contact with the palliative care professionals was the loss of control and her fear to burden her daughter. Her distress did not correspond with symptoms of depression or anxiety nor was it solely the pain, which made her suffer most. A sensitive and focused dialogue only could reveal needs and potential sources of support.

6 Depression and Anxiety

In a meta-analysis of studies performed with patients in palliative cancer care Mitchell et al. (Mitchell et al. 2011) reported interesting data. Stratified for various classification systems (ICD, DSM) as well as for stage of disease, this review did not support the common clinical assumption of higher percentages of depression in patients with cancer (depression or adjustment disorder 24.7%, all types of mood disorder 29.0%). In addition, the study did not reveal any significant difference between palliative-care and non-palliative-care settings. Surprisingly, adjustment disorders or anxiety seemed to be slightly more common in non- palliative patients. Previous results reported by Lichtenthal and colleagues also showed that the prevalence of depression and anxiety disorders were not increased in patients with advanced cancers. However, patients closer to death exhibited increased existential distress and physical symptom burden (Lichtenthal et al. 2009). This might be explained again by the heterogeneous definition of "palliative situation".

Prevalence of anxiety and its relationship with psychological distress in the "palliative patient" is poorly understood. A recent study in terminally ill cancer patients showed moderately increased symptoms of anxiety in 18.6% and clinically relevant symptoms in 12.4% of all participants. The levels of anxiety did not differ in outpatients versus palliative care inpatients. The Hospital Anxiety and Depression Scale was used to measure symptoms of anxiety and depression, and was administered along with measures of hopelessness and the desire for hastened death (Kolva et al. 2011). Palliative care inpatients reported significantly more symptoms of depression and desire for hastened death. The authors believe that an imminent death may lead to an increase of these symptoms.

Anxiety, however, plays an important if not dominant role in symptom perception and expression, particularly in pain. It is well known from multiple studies in neuropsychology and physiology that uncertainty and pain are directly linked (Brown et al. 2008; Yoshida et al. 2013). Clinicians therefore need to explore in depth patients' fears and beliefs together with standard symptom assessment.

6.1 Demoralization, Hopelessness and Wish for Hastened Death

There are many components of despair at the end of life. While some patients suffer from depression and anxiety, others do not fulfil the criteria for these psychiatric diagnoses but suffer from demoralization and hopelessness or loss of meaning—symptoms and syndromes that cannot be categorized according to psychiatric diagnosis. Kissane et al. (2001) wrote an informative article about the importance of demoralization in palliative care, Nissim et al. (2009) investigated the desire for hastened death and hopelessness and Chochinov and colleagues looked at dignity (2008). To be aware of and to assess demoralization and hopelessness and the wish for hastened death might be crucial to support some patients in the palliative situation.

6.2 Assessing Quality of Life

The WHO defines quality of life as the predominant outcome of palliative care (2002). In clinical practice, however, evaluation of individual quality of life can be difficult. Patients are often too weak and cognitively unstable to provide reliable answers to quality of life assessment tools or questionnaires. In addition, most tools have not been evaluated adequately in this challenging clinical situation (Albers et al. 2010). While acknowledging such limitations, highly individualized quality of life measurement tools such as McGill Quality of Life Questionnaire (Cohen and Mount 2000; Cohen et al. 1997) and more recently the SMiLE—instrument (Fegg et al. 2008) have been specifically developed and tested in patients with far advanced cancer or other diseases. The idea behind both instruments, as an example, is to assess individual domains that may contribute to patient-related quality of life and at the same time to give weight to these domains in regard of actual importance. Results from the studies are encouraging but such an approach seems to be linked to research settings rather than to daily routine.

7 Being Culturally Sensitive

In a society with more and more migrants and people of diverse cultural origin being familiar with their specific care needs and rituals is essential (Hunter and Soom Ammann 2016). Specific assessment tools or concrete questions evaluating the heterogenic needs can be just as helpful as knowledge on their background, listening to their stories and reflecting one's own cultural background.

Intermezzo: Mrs. B.
Mrs. B. may not be "representative" for all patients suffering from advanced cancer. Mrs. B. had a long story of self-effectiveness and a rather high level of need of keeping control of her life. Thus, it is no surprise that during assessing her needs and strengths, it was easy to define her goals and to collaborate actively to give weight and priority to various personal aspects. She was clear in defining worries in regard to her daughter as first priority. She was clear in choosing her preferred place of care (at home) and to assess quantity and quality of her individual care team apart from her daughter. She regained control over her miserable illness in the moment, when medical reasoning was complemented by problem-based assessment and care planning. We might underestimate the effect of activating individual coping mechanisms when switching from medical language and diagnosis to day-to-day problems and related problem-solving skills.

8 Setting up of an Individual Care Plan

8.1 Multi-professional Teamwork

With increased complexity of patients and their family's situation and depending on the amount of emotional distress in the system, specialized palliative care and psycho-oncological interventions are required. Thus, in more complex situations the coordination of interdisciplinary support is essential.

Psycho-oncology and palliative care are both frequently involved in patients with advanced cancer, but there is little evidence about "dosage", best time for involvement and process of interaction of these two domains. "The most successful psycho-oncology, psychosocial and behavioural oncology units have been those able to use this diversity to their advantage by evaluating patients and referring them to the most appropriate resource. They function as truly multidisciplinary organizations, drawing on the knowledge of each to enrich the others, while remaining fully integrated in the patients' total medical care" (Holland 2006). The "team" by itself in consequence may become a healing factor—or if distressed and badly coordinated—a risk factor for the patient and family (Nakazawa et al. 2010).

Intermezzo: Mrs. B
The crucial point in Mrs. B.'s patient journey was the moment of taking over the leadership for her remaining lifetime (Detering et al. 2010). Based on her previous

life experiences this shift back to control was the key: it was up to her to organize continuity of care and "her" network at home; it was up to her to decide and anticipate that her place for dying might NOT be at home but on the palliative care ward whenever possible; it was up to her to make active plans for the limited amount of lifetime; it was up to her to make peace with her limited physical function. And it was finally up to her to discuss with her daughter the need for psychological support including the time of bereavement.

9 Interventions

As recommended by various guidelines (e.g. NCCN) best symptom control, advance care planning and care of the dying should be an integral part of any intervention near the end of life. Education in self-administration of drugs (enteral or subcutaneously) by patient or a family member plays an important role in any crisis intervention (Shipley and Fairweather 2001). Dealing with fatigue and loss of appetite has been reported repetitively to become an important topic in each oncological consultation—not only for the patient, but also for the family (NICE 2011). But palliative care interventions offer more than just "symptomatology", and there might be a danger to over-medicalize "treatment".

Not only medical treatment can be overdosed but psycho-oncological support must also be sensitively tailored to patients and their family's situation and the limitations within the circumstances depending on factors such as time, cognitive functioning and level of energy. Due to limitations and contingent on the risk of acute deterioration, interventions usually should focus on immediate positive effects on despair and acute stressors. As the EAPC paper (European Association for Palliative Care) (Junger and Payne 2011) puts it *"In fact, claims regarding the relevance and effectiveness of psychological support provided to dying patients and their relatives should be made with caution. When defining their own professional role, tasks and responsibilities, psychologists should reflect critically upon the real benefits of their contribution. They should avoid a 'pathologisation' or 'psychologisation' of the normal intrapersonal and interpersonal challenges in the context of physical and existential suffering near the end of life". (p. 238).*

The EAPC suggest distinguishing between four levels of psycho-oncological interventions in the palliative situation: (1) Compassionate communications and general psychological support; (2) Psychological techniques, such as problem solving; (3) Counselling and specific psychological interventions, such as anxiety management and (4) Specialist psychological interventions, such as psychotherapy.

Foundation of psycho-oncological support and essential for most terminally ill patients and their families is a sustainable and trustful relationship. The importance of the relationship in the palliative situation should not be underestimated as most patients have a sense of loss of control and vulnerability. The circumstances often lead to a rapidly intensified relationship between patient and psycho-oncologist as well as the awareness of time limits and approaching death might lead to personal developments that can be supported by general psychological support. These aspects demonstrate how difficult it is to measure how and why patients and families might benefit from psycho-oncological support at the end of life. One major difficulty in psychosocial research at the end-of-life, however, is defining patient relevant outcomes.

Nonetheless, there is evidence for specialist psycho-oncological interventions with particular tailoring to terminally ill patients as Breitbart (2010, 2012) showed in a meaning-centred group setting. One other promising approach is dignity therapy (Chochinov et al. 2011). These first results for a specific population demonstrate both, feasibility and clinical benefit, and can be considered as promising strategies for the future.

Spiritual care interventions, such as being based on the MATCH guideline (Mercy, Austerity, Truthfulness, Cleanliness and Holy name (Sankhe et al. 2016) offered to patients and families could have additional positive effects not only on the spiritual well-being but also on a general feeling of wellness. Guidelines for the interprofessional team might support.

10 Recent Advances to Improve Patients Overall Well-Being

- Patient
  New approaches to minimize distress in patients are currently tested. One example of improving well-being and quality of life in patients with advanced cancer is the opportunity to engage in an eight-session meaning-centred group psychotherapy (Breitbart et al. 2010, 2015) aiming at supporting the patients in finding a sense of meaning in their lives. This intervention demonstrated to improve their quality of life as well as reducing psychological symptoms.
- Family
  Applebaum and Breitbart (2013) reviewed several interventions to support informal cancer caregivers. Caregivers benefited the most from goal-oriented, structured and time-limited integrative psychotherapeutic interventions. Supporting family members who take care of the dying at home is important to lessen distress even throughout the bereavement period. Hudson et al. (2015) reduced psychological distress of family caregivers of home-based palliative care patients by a short psychoeducational intervention by a designated family caregiver support nurse.

10.1 Outcomes and Expectations

However, one of the major sources for distress—for patients, but also partners/family and professional carers—can be found in overoptimistic or unrealistic expectations in any intervention in our world of "doing" and "everything is feasible". Calman (1984) introduced a new concept in regard to discussing and tailoring patients' (and carers') expectations as a central strategy to avoid additional distress. These early results have been studied repetitively, among others by Hagerty et al. (2005) in palliative and psycho-oncological care. The Calman gap concept remains one of the pragmatic approaches for physician/psychologist-patient interaction and highlights the importance of the concept of expectations (Broderick et al. 2011). Physical activity frequently cannot be altered or improved which may be difficult to accept especially for sportive people as in our case report. Therefore, physical activity should be "replaced" or complemented by psychological, social and/or spiritual activity—a strategy that sometimes may patients feel helpless and lost in a to date unknown world. Thus, for any intervention we offer to a severely ill person with low level of energy and short timely prognosis, we should consider potential harm in terms of unrealistic expectations and/or lack of individual coping strategies.

11 Summary

Mrs. B. was not able to tell her family and the professional team any details about her experiences in the very last days of her life. But she could tell her family and the professional carers how important these last weeks at home surrounded by her family were to her. The family on the other hand told the professional team that the joint care planning, its discussion and finally all interventions responded not only to their mother's needs and wishes, but also integrated at its best the family—and helped to reduce family distress at least to a manageable amount.

Providing space and security for essential things to happen, and to give back a sense of control even in a situation of weakness and fatigue—such elements seem to be mandatory for the final months of life. In times of cost-effectiveness and evidence-based objective measurements this therapeutic approach may be primarily considered as non-scientific, but evidence from neuropsychology, physiology and from (randomized) controlled trials in assessment and interventions in psychosocial and even spiritual care increasingly support such strategies. The stress-model and recent advances in brain research may add additional evidence and build the bridge to a more scientific acceptance of a humanistic approach. The whole story seems to be about stress reduction and even "healing" in an otherwise desperate life situation, with "healing" being applied not only to the patient, but also to family carers and professionals (Mount and Kearney 2003). Research may finally turn out to support historic findings as formulated earlier by Paracelsus (1493–1541): "Die beste Arznei für den Menschen ist der Mensch. Der höchste Grad dieser Arznei ist die Liebe". Or: the best drug for humans is another human being. The highest degree of this drug is love".

References

Albers G, Echteld MA, de Vet HC, Onwuteaka-Philipsen BD, van der Linden MH, Deliens L (2010) Evaluation of quality-of-life measures for use in palliative care: a systematic review. Palliat Med 24(1):17–37. doi:10.1177/0269216309346593

Antonovsky A (1996) The salutogenic model as a theory to guide health promotion. Health Promot Int 11(1):11–18

Applebaum AJ, Breitbart W (2013) Care for the cancer caregiver: a systematic review. Palliative & supportive care, 11(3), 231–252. doi:10.1017/S1478951512000594

Azuero C, Allen RS, Kvale E, Azuero A, Parmelee P (2014) Determinants of psychology service utilization in a palliative care outpatient population. Psychooncology 23(6):650–657. doi:10.1002/pon.3454

Baker P, Beesley H, Dinwoodie R, Fletcher I, Ablett J, Holcombe C, Salmon P (2013) 'You're putting thoughts into my head': a qualitative study of the readiness of patients with breast, lung or prostate cancer to address emotional needs through the first 18 months after diagnosis. Psychooncology 22(6):1402–1410. doi:10.1002/pon.3156

Baker-Glenn EA, Park B, Granger L, Symonds P, Mitchell AJ (2011) Desire for psychological support in cancer patients with depression or distress: validation of a simple help question. Psychooncology 20(5):525–531. doi:10.1002/pon.1759

Brebach R, Sharpe L, Costa DS, Rhodes P, Butow P (2016) Psychological intervention targeting distress for cancer patients: a meta-analytic study investigating uptake and adherence. Psychooncology 25(8):882–890. doi:10.1002/pon.4099

Breitbart W (2003) Palliative and supportive care: introducing a new international journal; the "Care" journal of palliative medicine. Palliat Support Care 1(1):1–2

Breitbart W (2006) Waiting. Palliat Support Care 4(3):313–314

Breitbart W, Rosenfeld B, Gibson C, Pessin H, Poppito S, Nelson C, Olden M (2010) Meaning-centered group psychotherapy for patients with advanced cancer: a pilot randomized controlled trial. Psychooncology 19(1):21–28. doi:10.1002/pon.1556

Breitbart W, Poppito S, Rosenfeld B, Vickers AJ, Li Y, Abbey J, Cassileth BR (2012) Pilot randomized controlled trial of individual meaning-centered psychotherapy for patients with advanced cancer. J Clin Oncol 30(12):1304–1309. doi:10.1200/JCO.2011.36.2517

Breitbart W, Rosenfeld B, Pessin H, Applebaum A, Kulikowski J, Lichtenthal WG (2015) Meaning-centered group psychotherapy: an effective intervention for improving psychological well-being in patients with advanced cancer. J Clin Oncol 33(7):749–754. doi:10.1200/JCO.2014.57.2198

Brinkman-Stoppelenburg A, Rietjens JA, van der Heide A (2014) The effects of advance care planning on end-of-life care: a systematic review. Palliat Med 28(8):1000–1025. doi:10.1177/0269216314526272

Broderick JE, Junghaenel DU, Schneider S, Bruckenthal P, Keefe FJ (2011) Treatment expectation for pain coping skills training: relationship to osteoarthritis patients' baseline psychosocial characteristics. Clin J Pain 27(4):315–322. doi:10.1097/AJP.0b013e3182048549

Brown CA, Seymour B, Boyle Y, El-Deredy W, Jones AK (2008) Modulation of pain ratings by expectation and uncertainty: behavioral characteristics and anticipatory neural correlates. Pain 135(3):240–250. doi:10.1016/j.pain.2007.05.022

Bultz BD, Carlson LE (2005) Emotional distress: the sixth vital sign in cancer care. J Clin Oncol 23(26):6440–6441. doi:10.1200/JCO.2005.02.3259

Bultz BD, Groff SL, Fitch M, Blais MC, Howes J, Levy K, Mayer C (2011) Implementing screening for distress, the 6th vital sign: a Canadian strategy for changing practice. Psychooncology 20(5):463–469. doi:10.1002/pon.1932

Bultz BD, Cummings GG, Grassi L, Travado L, Hoekstra-Weebers J, Watson M (2014) 2013 President's plenary international psycho-oncology society: embracing the IPOS standards as a means of enhancing comprehensive cancer care. Psychooncology 23(9):1073–1078. doi:10.1002/pon.3618

Butt Z, Wagner LI, Beaumont JL, Paice JA, Peterman AH, Shevrin D, Cella D (2008) Use of a single-item screening tool to detect clinically significant fatigue, pain, distress, and anorexia in ambulatory cancer practice. J Pain Symptom Manage 35(1):20–30. doi:10.1016/j.jpainsymman.2007.02.040

Calman KC (1984) Quality of life in cancer patients–an hypothesis. J Med Ethics 10(3):124–127

Carlson LE, Bultz BD (2003) Cancer distress screening. Needs, models, and methods. J Psychosom Res 55(5):403–409

Chochinov HM, Hassard T, McClement S, Hack T, Kristjanson LJ, Harlos M, Murray A (2008) The patient dignity inventory: a novel way of measuring dignity-related distress in palliative care. J Pain Symptom Manage 36(6):559–571. doi:10.1016/j.jpainsymman.2007.12.018

Chochinov HM, Kristjanson LJ, Breitbart W, McClement S, Hack TF, Hassard T, Harlos M (2011) Effect of dignity therapy on distress and end-of-life experience in terminally ill patients: a randomised controlled trial. Lancet Oncol 12(8):753–762. doi:10.1016/S1470-2045(11)70153-X

Clover KA, Mitchell AJ, Britton B, Carter G (2015) Why do oncology outpatients who report emotional distress decline help? Psychooncology 24(7):812–818. doi:10.1002/pon.3729

Cohen SR, Mount BM (2000) Living with cancer: "good" days and "bad" days–what produces them? Can the McGill quality of life questionnaire distinguish between them? Cancer 89 (8):1854–1865

Cohen SR, Mount BM, Bruera E, Provost M, Rowe J, Tong K (1997) Validity of the McGill Quality of Life Questionnaire in the palliative care setting: a multi-centre Canadian study demonstrating the importance of the existential domain. Palliat Med 11(1):3–20

Colleoni M, Mandala M, Peruzzotti G, Robertson C, Bredart A, Goldhirsch A (2000) Depression and degree of acceptance of adjuvant cytotoxic drugs. Lancet 356(9238):1326–1327. doi:10.1016/S0140-6736(00)02821-X

Detering KM, Hancock AD, Reade MC, Silvester W (2010) The impact of advance care planning on end of life care in elderly patients: randomised controlled trial. BMJ 340:c1345. doi:10.1136/bmj.c1345

Dilworth S, Higgins I, Parker V, Kelly B, Turner J (2014) Patient and health professional's perceived barriers to the delivery of psychosocial care to adults with cancer: a systematic review. Psychooncology 23(6):601–612. doi:10.1002/pon.3474

Doherty WJ, McDaniel SH, Hepworth J (1994) Medical family therapy: an emerging arena for family therapy. J Family Therapy 16(1):31–46

Dolbeault S, Bredart A, Mignot V, Hardy P, Gauvain-Piquard A, Mandereau L, Medioni J (2008) Screening for psychological distress in two French cancer centers: feasibility and performance of the adapted distress thermometer. Palliat Support Care 6(2):107–117. doi:10.1017/S1478951508000187

Donovan KA, Grassi L, McGinty HL, Jacobsen PB (2014) Validation of the distress thermometer worldwide: state of the science. Psychooncology 23(3):241–250. doi:10.1002/pon.3430

Ellis J, Lin J, Walsh A, Lo C, Shepherd FA, Moore M, Rodin G (2009) Predictors of referral for specialized psychosocial oncology care in patients with metastatic cancer: the contributions of age, distress, and marital status. J Clin Oncol 27(5):699–705. doi:10.1200/JCO.2007.15.4864

Eychmuller S (2012) SENS is making sense—on the way to an innovative approach to structure palliative care problems. Ther Umsch 69(2):87–90. doi:10.1024/0040-5930/a000256

Faller H, Bulzebruck H, Drings P, Lang H (1999) Coping, distress, and survival among patients with lung cancer. Arch Gen Psychiatry 56(8):756–762

Faller H, Weis J, Koch U, Brahler E, Harter M, Keller M, Mehnert A (2016a) Perceived need for psychosocial support depending on emotional distress and mental comorbidity in men and women with cancer. J Psychosom Res 81:24–30. doi:10.1016/j.jpsychores.2015.12.004

Faller H, Weis J, Koch U, Brahler E, Harter M, Keller M, Mehnert A (2016b) Utilization of professional psychological care in a large German sample of cancer patients. Psychooncology. doi:10.1002/pon.4197

Fegg MJ, Kramer M, L'Hoste S, Borasio GD (2008) The Schedule for Meaning in Life Evaluation (SMiLE): validation of a new instrument for meaning-in-life research. J Pain Symptom Manage 35(4):356–364. doi:10.1016/j.jpainsymman.2007.05.007

Fox E (1997) Predominance of the curative model of medical care. A residual problem. JAMA 278 (9):761–763

Gaertner J, Becker G (2014) Patients with advanced disease: the value of patient reported outcomes. Oncol Res Treat 37(1–2):7–8. doi:10.1159/000358498

Ganz PA (2008) Psychological and social aspects of breast cancer. Oncology (Williston Park)22 (6):642–646, 650; discussion 650, 653

Hagerty RG, Butow PN, Ellis PM et al (2005) Communicating with realism and hope: incurable cancer patients' views on the disclosure of prognosis. J Clin Oncol 23(6):1278–1288

Herschbach P, Heusser P (2008) Einführung in die psychoonkologische Behandlungspraxis, 1st edn. Klett-Cotta, Stuttgart

Holland JC (2006) Psycho-oncology: from empirical research to screening program. In: Herschbach P, Heussner P, Sellschopp A (eds) Psycho-Onkologie, Perspektiven heute. Pabst Science Publishers, pp 9–43

Holland JC (2013) Distress screening and the integration of psychosocial care into routine oncologic care. J Natl Compr Canc Netw 11(5 Suppl):687–689

Holland JC, Andersen B, Breitbart WS, Dabrowski M, Dudley MM, Fleishman S, Nccn (2007) Distress management. J Natl Compr Canc Netw 5(1):66–98

Hudson P, Trauer T, Kelly B, O'Connor M, Thomas K, Zordan R, Summers M (2015) Reducing the psychological distress of family caregivers of home based palliative care patients: longer term effects from a randomised controlled trial. Psychooncology 24(1):19–24. doi:10.1002/pon.3610

Hudson P, Collins A, Bostanci A, Willenberg L, Stephanov N, Phillip J (2016) Toward a systematic approach to assessment and care planning in palliative care: a practical review of clinical tools. Palliat Support Care 14(2):161–173

Hughes KL, Sargeant H, Hawkes AL (2011) Acceptability of the distress thermometer and problem list to community-based telephone cancer helpline operators, and to cancer patients and carers. BMC Cancer 11:46. doi:10.1186/1471-2407-11-46

Hui D, Meng YC, Bruera S, Geng Y, Hutchins R, Mori M, Bruera E (2016) Referral criteria for outpatient palliative cancer care: a systematic review. Oncologist 21(7):895–901. doi:10.1634/theoncologist.2016-0006

Hunter A, Soom Ammann E (2016) End-of-life care and rituals in contexts of post-migration diversity in Europe: an introduction. J Intercult Stud 37(2):95–102. doi:10.1080/07256868.2016.1142052

Institute of Medicine (IOM) (2008) Cancer care for the whole patient: meeting psychosocial health needs. The National Academies Press, Washington DC

Junger S, Payne S (2011) Guidance on postgraduate education for psychologists involved in palliative care. Europ J Pall Care 18(5):238–252

Kadan-Lottick NS, Vanderwerker LC, Block SD, Zhang B, Prigerson HG (2005) Psychiatric disorders and mental health service use in patients with advanced cancer: a report from the coping with cancer study. Cancer 104(12):2872–2881. doi:10.1002/cncr.21532

Kissane DW, Clarke DM, Street AF (2001) Demoralization syndrome—a relevant psychiatric diagnosis for palliative care. J Palliat Care 17(1):12–21

Kolva E, Rosenfeld B, Pessin H, Breitbart W, Brescia R (2011) Anxiety in terminally ill cancer patients. J Pain Symptom Manage 42(5):691–701. doi:10.1016/j.jpainsymman.2011.01.013

Langewitz W (2013) Kommunikation im medizinischen Alltag. Ein Leitfaden für die Praxis. Schweizerische Akademie der Medizinischen Wissenschaften, Basel

Lichtenthal WG, Nilsson M, Zhang B, Trice ED, Kissane DW, Breitbart W, Prigerson HG (2009) Do rates of mental disorders and existential distress among advanced stage cancer patients increase as death approaches? Psychooncology 18(1):50–61. doi:10.1002/pon.1371

McDaniel SH, Hepworth J (2000) Kooperation mit Patienten, Ihren Familien und dem Behandlungsteam. Ein neuer Ansatz im Umgang mit Macht und Abhängigkeit. In Kröger F,

Hendrischke A, McDaniel S (eds) Familie, System und Gesundheit. Systemische Konzepte für ein soziales Gesundheitswesen. Carl-Auer-Systeme, Heidelberg

Mehnert A, Koch U (2008) Psychological comorbidity and health-related quality of life and its association with awareness, utilization, and need for psychosocial support in a cancer register-based sample of long-term breast cancer survivors. J Psychosom Res 64(4):383–391. doi:10.1016/j.jpsychores.2007.12.005

Merckaert I, Libert Y, Messin S, Milani M, Slachmuylder JL, Razavi D (2010) Cancer patients' desire for psychological support: prevalence and implications for screening patients' psychological needs. Psychooncology 19(2):141–149. doi:10.1002/pon.1568

Mitchell AJ (2007) Pooled results from 38 analyses of the accuracy of distress thermometer and other ultra-short methods of detecting cancer-related mood disorders. J Clin Oncol 25 (29):4670–4681. doi:10.1200/JCO.2006.10.0438

Mitchell AJ, Chan M, Bhatti H, Halton M, Grassi L, Johansen C, Meader N (2011) Prevalence of depression, anxiety, and adjustment disorder in oncological, haematological, and palliative-care settings: a meta-analysis of 94 interview-based studies. Lancet Oncol 12 (2):160–174. doi:10.1016/S1470-2045(11)70002-X

Mitchell AJ, Lord K, Slattery J, Grainger L, Symonds P (2012) How feasible is implementation of distress screening by cancer clinicians in routine clinical care? Cancer 118(24):6260–6269. doi:10.1002/cncr.27648

Mosher CE, Winger JG, Hanna N, Jalal SI, Fakiris AJ, Einhorn LH, Champion VL (2014) Barriers to mental health service use and preferences for addressing emotional concerns among lung cancer patients. Psychooncology 23(7):812–819. doi:10.1002/pon.3488

Mount B, Kearney M (2003) Healing and palliative care: charting our way forward. Palliat Med 17 (8):657–658

Nakazawa Y, Miyashita M, Morita T, Umeda M, Oyagi Y, Ogasawara T (2010) The palliative care self-reported practices scale and the palliative care difficulties scale: reliability and validity of two scales evaluating self-reported practices and difficulties experienced in palliative care by health professionals. J Palliat Med 13(4):427–437. doi:10.1089/jpm.2009.0289

National Comprehensive Cancer Network (NCCN) (2016a) Distress Management, Version 2

National Comprehensive Cancer Network (NCCN) (2016b) Palliative Care Version 1.2016. J Natl Compr Canc Netw 14:82–113

Neumann M, Galushko M, Karbach U, Goldblatt H, Visser A, Wirtz M, Pfaff H (2010) Barriers to using psycho-oncology services: a qualitative research into the perspectives of users, their relatives, non-users, physicians, and nurses. Support Care Cancer 18(9):1147–1156. doi:10. 1007/s00520-009-0731-2

NICE (2011) The Diagnosis and Treatment of Lung Cancer (Update) (Vol. 212). Cardiff (UK)

Nissim R, Gagliese L, Rodin G (2009) The desire for hastened death in individuals with advanced cancer: a longitudinal qualitative study. Soc Sci Med 69(2):165–171. doi:10.1016/j.socscimed. 2009.04.021

Parker PA, Baile WF, de Moor C, Cohen L (2003) Psychosocial and demographic predictors of quality of life in a large sample of cancer patients. Psychooncology 12(2):183–193. doi:10. 1002/pon.635

Pfeil TA, Laryionava K, Reiter-Theil S, Hiddemann W, Winkler EC (2015) What keeps oncologists from addressing palliative care early on with incurable cancer patients? An active stance seems key. Oncologist 20(1):56–61. doi:10.1634/theoncologist.2014-0031

Pirl WF, Fann JR, Greer JA, Braun I, Deshields T, Fulcher C, Bardwell WA (2014) Recommendations for the implementation of distress screening programs in cancer centers: report from the American Psychosocial Oncology Society (APOS), Association of Oncology Social Work (AOSW), and Oncology Nursing Society (ONS) joint task force. Cancer 120 (19):2946–2954. doi:10.1002/cncr.28750

Sankhe A, Dalal K, Agarwal V, Sarve P (2016) Spiritual care therapy on quality of life in cancer patients and their caregivers: a prospective non-randomized single-cohort study. J Relig Health. doi:10.1007/s10943-016-0324-6

Schaeffeler N, Pfeiffer K, Ringwald J, Brucker S, Wallwiener M, Zipfel S, Teufel M (2015) Assessing the need for psychooncological support: screening instruments in combination with patients' subjective evaluation may define psychooncological pathways. Psychooncology 24 (12):1784–1791. doi:10.1002/pon.3855

Shipley V, Fairweather J (2001) A programme of individualized and self-administration of medicines in a hospice. Int J Palliat Nurs 7(12):581–586. doi:10.12968/ijpn.2001.7.12.9282

Smith TJ, Temin S, Alesi ER, Abernethy AP, Balboni TA, Basch EM, Von Roenn JH (2012) American Society of Clinical Oncology provisional clinical opinion: the integration of palliative care into standard oncology care. J Clin Oncol 30(8):880–887. doi:10.1200/JCO.2011.38.5161

Sollner W, Maislinger S, Konig A, Devries A, Lukas P (2004) Providing psychosocial support for breast cancer patients based on screening for distress within a consultation-liaison service. Psychooncology 13(12):893–897. doi:10.1002/pon.867

Surbone A, Baider L, Weitzman TS, Brames MJ, Rittenberg CN, JohnsonJ, MPS Group (2010) Psychosocial care for patients and their families is integral to supportive care in cancer: MASCC position statement. Support Care Cancer 18(2):255–263. doi:10.1007/s00520-009-0693-4

Temel JS, Greer JA, Muzikansky A, Gallagher ER, Admane S, Jackson VA, Lynch TJ (2010) Early palliative care for patients with metastatic non-small-cell lung cancer. N Engl J Med 363 (8):733–742. doi:10.1056/NEJMoa1000678

Temel JS, Greer JA, Admane S, Gallagher ER, Jackson VA, Lynch TJ, Pirl WF (2011) Longitudinal perceptions of prognosis and goals of therapy in patients with metastatic non-small-cell lung cancer: results of a randomized study of early palliative care. J Clin Oncol 29(17):2319–2326. doi:10.1200/JCO.2010.32.4459

Tondorf T, Rothschild S, Koller MT, Rochlizu C, Kiss A, Zwahlen D (submitted) Talking about psychosocial distress screening: what oncologists and cancer patients recall

Waller A, Williams A, Groff SL, Bultz BD, Carlson LE (2013) Screening for distress, the sixth vital sign: examining self-referral in people with cancer over a one-year period. Psychooncology 22(2):388–395. doi:10.1002/pon.2102

WHO (2002) Definition palliative care. 2013

Wright AA, Zhang B, Ray A, Mack JW, Trice E, Balboni T, Prigerson HG (2008) Associations between end-of-life discussions, patient mental health, medical care near death, and caregiver bereavement adjustment. JAMA 300(14):1665–1673. doi:10.1001/jama.300.14.1665

Wright AA, Keating NL, Balboni TA, Matulonis UA, Block SD, Prigerson HG (2010) Place of death: correlations with quality of life of patients with cancer and predictors of bereaved caregivers' mental health. J Clin Oncol 28(29):4457–4464. doi:10.1200/JCO.2009.26.3863

Yoshida W, Seymour B, Koltzenburg M, Dolan RJ (2013) Uncertainty increases pain: evidence for a novel mechanism of pain modulation involving the periaqueductal gray. J Neurosci 33 (13):5638–5646. doi:10.1523/JNEUROSCI.4984-12.2013

Zambrano SC, Fliedner MC, Eychmuller S (2016) The impact of early palliative care on the quality of care during the last days of life: what does the evidence say? Curr Opin Support Palliat Care 10(4):310–315. doi:10.1097/SPC.0000000000000240

Zhang B, Wright AA, Huskamp HA, Nilsson ME, Maciejewski ML, Earle CC, Prigerson HG (2009) Health care costs in the last week of life: associations with end-of-life conversations. Arch Intern Med 169(5):480–488. doi:10.1001/archinternmed.2008.587

Zwahlen D, Hagenbuch N, Carley MI, Recklitis CJ, Buchi S (2008) Screening cancer patients' families with the distress thermometer (DT): a validation study. Psychooncology 17(10):959–966. doi:10.1002/pon.1320

Family Caregivers to Adults with Cancer: The Consequences of Caring

Anna-leila Williams

Abstract

A person living with cancer will potentially have some degree of physical, cognitive, and/or psychological impairment, periods of unemployment, financial concerns, social isolation, and existential questions, any or all of which can impact the family and friends who surround them. In our current era of health care, patients with cancer receive invasive diagnostic studies and aggressive treatment as outpatients, and then convalesce at home. As such, cancer family caregivers are de facto partners with the healthcare team. The cancer family caregiver role is demanding and may lead to increased morbidity and mortality —in effect, the cancer family caregiver can become a second patient in need of care. This chapter discusses the consequences cancer family caregivers may accrue. The topics covered include caregiver mood disturbance and psychological impairment and some of the mutable factors that contribute to these states (i.e., sleep disturbance, decline in physical health, restriction of activities, and financial concerns), uncertainty, spiritual concerns, and caregiver witnessing. There is a discussion of the factors that influence the caregiving experience (caregiver characteristics, patient characteristics, and social supports). The chapter concludes with comments on intervention studies that have been conducted to ameliorate the burden of caregiving, and the state of caregiver research.

Keywords

Cancer family caregiver · Uncertainty · Witnessing · Spirituality · Religiosity · Social support · Burden · Distress

A. Williams (✉)
Frank H. Netter MD School of Medicine, Quinnipiac University, Hamden, CT, USA
e-mail: anna-leila.williams@quinnipiac.edu

© Springer International Publishing AG 2018
U. Goerling and A. Mehnert (eds.), *Psycho-Oncology*, Recent Results
in Cancer Research 210, https://doi.org/10.1007/978-3-319-64310-6_6

1   Introduction

With more than 14 million people worldwide experiencing a cancer diagnosis in any given year (World Health Organization International Agency for Research on Cancer 2014), the consequences are far-reaching. A person living with cancer will potentially have some degree of physical, cognitive, and/or psychological impairment, periods of unemployment, financial concerns, social isolation, and existential questions, any or all of which can impact, directly and indirectly, the family and friends who surround them.

1.1   Terminology

For the purpose of this discussion, the term *family caregiver* is defined as the primary person upon whom the patient relies for assistance with physical care, symptom management, and psychosocial needs, and who does not receive financial remuneration for caregiving (Seifert et al. 2008). This definition indicates the family caregiver does not need to be a blood or adoptive relative, nor a household member, and thus encompasses friends, neighbors, and relatives (such as adult children) who maintain separate homes.

The attention directed toward cancer family caregivers has led to considerable growth in research over the past two decades. Unfortunately, a single definition of family caregiver has failed to emerge in the published literature. Several studies neglect to define the parameters for the selection of their family caregiver study populations. Of those who provide a definition, a range of parameters have been expressed which encompass the caregiver's relationship to the patient, caregiver's responsibilities, and/or the patient and caregiver sharing a common household. Table 1 lists a subset of the cancer family caregiver definitions published in the research literature from 2006 to 2016. The consequences of not having a single definition for cancer family caregivers are many. Most notably, different study population sampling criteria likely contribute to inconsistent outcomes across studies. Obviously, the responsibilities and consequent burdens experienced by family caregivers who exclusively provide instrumental tasks, such as transportation and grocery shopping, are different than those experienced by family caregivers who address the patient's physical and psychological needs, such as wound care, bathing, medication management, and emotional support. As such, the ability to aggregate study outcomes, and have the cancer family caregiver research mature and progress has been stymied.

Throughout this chapter, the author deliberately avoids using the term "loved one" and instead uses the less emotionally charged terms "patient," "ill family member" and "person living with cancer." Caring for someone with cancer does not require love, nor does the process of caring necessarily engender love. Close interpersonal relations are enveloped in a spectrum of emotions, and the patient–caregiver dyad can be formed and the caregiver role assumed for reasons other than

Table 1 A subset of cancer family caregiver definitions published in the research literature, 2006–2016

Study citation (first author year)	Definitions
Kim (2006)	"...an individual in a family-like relationship who constantly provided help to [the person with cancer]."
Mellon (2006)	"...family [member]/significant other over 18 years who had been through the cancer experience with [the patient] and had been [the patient's] main source of emotional or instrumental support."
Sherwood (2006)	"...someone who provided ongoing support to the care recipient (including financial, emotional, and/or physical support)."
Walsh (2007)	"...the main person who provided unpaid practical and emotional support to the patient on a regular basis and was in contact with the palliative care team."
Seifert (2008)	"...someone who is involved with and helps the patient with his or her care and/or household activities; the caregiver was not necessarily a relative nor did he or she need to be living with the patient."
Hendrix (2009)	"...an individual who lived in the same household as the cancer patient and provided the most 'hands-on' care."
O'Hara (2010)	"... someone close to them [the patients] who was involved with their care..."
Beesley (2011)	"The definition of caregiver was deliberately left for the patient to interpret however, when clarity was sought, a caregiver was described as someone who provided the patient with physical or emotional support. Paid caregivers were excluded."
Guay (2012)	"...the spouse, first-degree relative, or other designated person who provides direct assistance to the patient in his or her activities of daily living."
Kershaw (2015)	"...identified by patients as their primary provider of emotional and/or physical care."
Paiva (2015)	"...individuals significantly involved in the ill individual's treatment and care (most of the week) and could be the individual's child, spouse, parent, sibling, boy/girlfriend, grandparent, uncle, aunt, or first cousin."
Bayen (2016)	"...the family member or friend who was most responsible for decision making and care of the patient."
Ha-Hyun Kim (2016)	"...family members (spouse, son, son-in-law, daughter, daughter-in-law, parent, brother, sister, or other relative who provided direct assistance to the patient)..."
Youngmee Kim (2016)	"...family-like individuals who have provided consistent help during a survivor's cancer experience."
Mosher (2016)	"The person who provided most of their [the patients'] unpaid, informal care."
Hanly (2016)	"...a family member, friend or another person who had been helping take care of them [the patients] since their diagnosis."
Shaffer (2016a)	"...a relative or friend who provided the patient help and would likely accompany the patient to clinic visits."

love, including a sense of obligation, feelings of guilt, or financial concerns. To assume the cancer family caregiver and patient are "loved ones" denies the intensity of the dyad's relationship, and potentially constrains emotional expression from both parties.

1.2 Why Focus on the Cancer Family Caregiver?

Caring for someone who is ill is a ubiquitous behavior, common to our humanity throughout recorded time. So why do family caregivers deserve mention in a textbook of psycho-oncology if they are merely fulfilling a time honored human to human covenant? The answer is twofold. First, in our current era of health care, patients with cancer often receive invasive diagnostic studies and aggressive treatment as outpatients, and then convalesce at home. Cancer family caregivers, who customarily receive little or no training from health professionals, assume responsibility for home care and are de facto partners with the healthcare team. Cancer family caregivers are required to provide complex physical and psychological care, as well as help the patient navigate a complicated healthcare system and maintain the household (Kent et al. 2016). The intricacies of the cancer family caregiver role and responsibilities are demanding, therefore leading us to the second justification for focusing on family caregivers. We now have several decades' worth of data that describe the consequences of fulfilling the role of caregiver. The increased morbidity and mortality incurred by cancer family caregivers, some of which will be mentioned in this chapter, indicate the family caregiver, in effect, can be a second patient in need of care (Northouse et al. 2012).

2 Mood Disturbance and Psychological Impairment

Mood disturbances and psychological impairment are the most commonly explored variables in the cancer family caregiver literature. Researchers have used a variety of instruments to measure conceptual and diagnostic categorizations of psychological impairment, namely: anxiety, depression, stress, tension, strain, emotional well-being, and psychological distress (Williams and McCorkle 2011). The lack of a common metric makes it difficult to precisely assess the extent of psychological impairment among cancer family caregivers, and the subgroup of caregivers who are at greatest risk; however, it is noteworthy that across almost all metrics, caregivers consistently have anxiety, depression, and psychological distress rates two or more times that of the general population (Bayen et al. 2016; Leroy et al. 2016; Rumpold et al. 2016a, b; Williams et al. 2013). The lack of precision in the research literature around caregiver psychological impairment in no way obscures what is undoubtedly a major burden for cancer family caregivers. Several studies which concurrently measured psychological impairment in patients and family caregivers, found the family caregivers had higher rates of impairment than the patients with cancer (Braun et al. 2007; Kershaw et al. 2015; Leroy et al. 2016; Mellon et al. 2006).

The application of multidimensional statistical analyses to family caregiver data has provided greater insight into the interweave among mood disturbance, physical health, ability to cope, and caregiver perceived burden (Bayen et al. 2016; Hanly et al. 2016; Leroy et al. 2016; Perez-Ordóñez et al. 2016; Rumpold et al. 2016b; Shaffer et al. 2016a, b). The literature illuminates the path by which family caregivers can become mired in their role, and offers evidence for supportive measures that can lead to favorable outcomes for caregivers. For example, family caregivers who have their own physical health issues and those who are employed have a high likelihood to endure mood disturbance and perceived burden (Bayen et al. 2016; Hanly et al. 2016). Whereas family caregivers who exercise problem-focused coping strategies seem to effectively mitigate mood disturbance and perceived burden (Perez-Ordóñez et al. 2016).

There also appears to be a "sweet spot" for caregiving in which the healthy and otherwise secure family caregiver may accrue psychological well-being from their caregiving responsibilities. With only a small amount of research in this area, it seems that limiting the amount of time devoted to caregiving to less than 6 h per week may promote the family caregiver's happiness and well-being (Hanly et al. 2016). Unfortunately, cancer family caregivers far exceed this "sweet spot", with estimates ranging from 30 to 58 h per week devoted to caregiving responsibilities (Kim and Schulz 2008; Yabrof et al. 2009).

2.1 Patient–Caregiver Relationship—Bidirectional Influence

Cancer family caregiver mood disturbance and psychological impairment not only contribute to the caregiver's personal suffering, but also impact their relationship with the family member with cancer, and the care they are able to provide that family member. A wealth of data, compiled in two meta-analyses (Hagedoorn et al. 2000; Hodges et al. 2005) shows mutual, bidirectional influences on psychological distress and quality of life among the patient–caregiver dyad. Recent research continues to support the idea of mutual influence, both positive and negative, among the patient–caregiver dyad (Kershaw et al. 2015; Tan et al. 2015).

The patient–caregiver dyad research has progressed to examine the influence of the relationship itself on outcomes for both members of the dyad (Nissen et al. 2016; Reblin et al. 2016). Specifically, the type, quality, and context of the dyadic relationship have been scrutinized and indicate supportive relationships can enhance the quality of life outcomes and be protective against distress and perceived burden. In contrast, patient–caregiver relationships meeting criteria for detached or low-expressive types were subject to diminished mental and physical health (Nissen et al. 2016). While patient–caregiver relationship research is still developing, early studies point to the value of identifying the dyadic relationship type, quality, and context with the intention of intervening with families that are detached or low-expressive. Interventions could focus on building trust and learning to express emotions.

2.2   Mutable Factors that Contribute to Mood Disturbance

Several mutable factors contribute to cancer family caregivers' risk for mood disturbance, including sleep disturbance, physical illness, restriction of activities, and financial concerns. Similar to the general population, the cancer family caregiver population has an increased prevalence of anxiety and depression among those with disturbed sleep (Carter 2003; Carter and Acton 2006; Gibbins et al. 2009; Lee et al. 2015). Cancer family caregivers, especially those who share a household with the ill family member, provide care 24 hours per day. Nighttime duties may include medication administration, toileting assistance, symptom management, and support for treatment side effects, as well as providing emotional support to the patient. As one would expect, disturbed sleep is a common concern for cancer family caregivers, with reports of prevalence rates ranging from 40 to 76% (Gibbins et al. 2009; Lee et al. 2015).

Decline in the cancer family caregiver's physical health has been shown to contribute to an increased risk of depression among cancer family caregivers. Several studies have demonstrated that decline in cancer family caregiver physical health is driven largely by the patient's physical limitations and the caregiver's perception of the caregiving experience, including their sense of burden, social functioning, and abandonment (Bayen et al. 2016; Kim et al. 2015; Shaffer 2016b). Self-efficacy in one's caregiving skills also seems to determine caregiver physical and mental health (Kershaw et al. 2015). As with the general population, lower educational attainment is associated with worse physical and mental health among cancer family caregivers (Shaffer 2016b).

Not surprisingly, as the cancer family caregiver's life becomes curtailed by caregiver responsibilities, there is an increased risk for mood disturbance and psychological impairment (Bayen et al. 2016; Cameron et al. 2002; Williamson et al. 1998). When pleasurable and meaningful activities related to work or leisure are usurped by the daily tasks and stressors of caring for someone with cancer, the cancer family caregiver's identity, coping strategies, self-care efforts, and social network may be disrupted (Goldstein et al. 2004; Mosher et al. 2013a). The loss of pleasurable and meaningful activities can also add to the cancer family caregiver's perceived burden from caring, all of which increase the risk for mood disturbance and psychological impairment (Bayen et al. 2016; Kim et al. 2005).

Families affected by cancer invariably incur financial burden secondary to the illness (Bayen et al. 2016; Hanly et al. 2013; Round et al. 2015; van Houtven et al. 2011). A 2013 Irish study aimed to comprehensively define the economic costs of caring for someone with colon cancer during the diagnosis and treatment phase (Hanly et al. 2013). They collected data "… on specified hospital-related caring activities (including travelling, waiting and visiting time during diagnosis, surgery and/or chemotherapy/radiotherapy), hospital-related out-of-pocket costs (including parking, meals and accommodation), domestic-related caring activities (extra hours spent on housework, activities of daily living (ADL), instrumental activities of daily living (IADL) and cancer-specific care) and domestic-related out-of-pocket costs (including medications, household expenses and cancer-related items such as home help, private nurse and stoma expenses)." The highest contributor to financial burden was the cost of the cancer family caregiver's time, which incurred primarily as lost wages and lost productivity.

A 2015 study modeled estimates for costs of caring for someone with cancer at the end of life (Round et al. 2015). The results, similar to the study of earlier phases of disease (Hanly et al. 2013), found the greatest expense, by far, was the cost of the cancer family caregiver's time. Cancer family caregivers report that in order to fulfill their caregiving responsibilities they have had to shift from full-time to part-time work, switch the time of day during which they work, use personal sick leave, change the nature of their work (ex. stop taking business trips), or take early retirement (Bayen et al. 2016; Williams and Bakitas 2012). The consequences of these work adjustments include decreased household income and potentially long-term derailment of career opportunities.

3   Uncertainty

Uncertainty is a constant companion for patients and family caregivers living with cancer throughout all stages of disease. Diagnosis, staging, treatment decisions, treatment-related side effects, disease and treatment monitoring, survivorship, recurrence, end of life—are all wrought with uncertainty and inflict turmoil on everyday life (Kent et al. 2016; Stajduhar et al. 2008; Temel et al. 2008). Patients and cancer family caregivers who are uncertain as to how the patient will feel or function in the near or distant future, have difficulty planning appointments, meals, work assignments, childcare responsibilities, social engagements, or vacations (Williams and Bakitas 2012). Essentially any activity or responsibility that takes planning requires a contingency because of the uncertainty of the patient's well-being. Managing uncertainty is a formidable trial for many people and cancer family caregivers are no exception. A 2009 qualitative study queried 33 bereaved and current cancer family caregivers of critically ill patients about what they felt was important for them to prepare for death and bereavement. Several factors related to life experience and cognitive, affective, and behavioral dimensions emerged as important to the caregivers. Notably, the participants *unanimously* reported uncertainty (as it relates to medical, psychosocial, religious/spiritual, and pragmatic issues) as their principal challenge; and identified communication as the chief means of managing uncertainty (Hebert et al. 2009).

4   Spiritual Concerns

The crucible of cancer family caregiving is laden with uncertainty, identity disruption, and physical and emotional challenges, and therefore, potentially provides the ideal environment for spiritual and existential questions to arise (Adams et al.

2014; Murray et al. 2010). The literature on cancer family caregiver spirituality is small but burgeoning, and indicates spirituality may have been a potently influential variable that was overlooked in earlier research.

In a large national study, the American Cancer Society's Study of Cancer Survivors and Quality of Life Survey for Caregivers assessed spiritual well-being and its association with several patient and caregiver variables (Kim et al. 2011). Spiritual well-being was defined as the ability to find meaning and peace. Results show a significant association between spiritual well-being and mental health, for both patients and caregivers. Interestingly, when the caregivers in this study reported higher spiritual well-being, their family members with cancer reported better physical health. Determining whether patient physical health contributes to caregiver spirituality or vice versa, or if the relationship is bidirectional, awaits replication in a longitudinal study.

A small epidemiologic study of family caregivers to adults with advanced cancer enrolled in palliative care found *all* of the participants self-identified as "spiritual" and said their spirituality was a major means by which they coped with their family member's illness (Guay et al. 2012). That said, more than half of the participants reported they had "spiritual pain" [defined as "a pain deep in your soul (being) that is not physical" (Mako et al. 2006)]. Participants who identified as having spiritual pain were significantly more likely to have elevated levels of anxiety, depression, denial, behavioral disengagement, and dysfunctional coping strategies than participants who did not identify spiritual pain.

Two studies have considered the influence of patient spirituality on caregiver psychological adjustment and quality of life (Douglas and Daly 2012; Tan et al. 2015). A longitudinal study of patients with stage III or IV lung, gastrointestinal, or gynecological cancers and their family caregivers looked at the relationships among spirituality, health-related quality of life, and physical and psychological functioning. As expected, caregiver depression was inversely related to patient physical quality of life. Of interest, patient spiritual well-being mediated the relationship between patient physical quality of life and caregiver depression (Douglas and Daly 2012). In addition, a study conducted in Singapore showed patients who were able to derive meaning from their cancer experience and who resolved existential concerns related to their cancer diagnosis were associated with family caregivers' well-being and satisfaction with their caregiving role (Tan et al. 2015).

Religiosity is a construct that is related to, but different from, spirituality. Religiosity encompasses the formal practices of religious affiliation, belief, and practice, and has been rarely studied in the cancer family caregiver population. With emerging evidence of the mitigating effect of religion-related variables on depression in other populations, it is an area worthy of attention. A 2015 United States study of cancer family caregivers showed nearly two-thirds of the study population answered affirmatively to the question, "Have you ever prayed for your own health?", which is considerably higher than the percent of general population who responded affirmatively (Williams et al. 2015). These results, while limited to a single study population, raise the possibility that assuming the caregiver role may change one's prayer practices. Knowing that one must be healthy to fulfill caregiver responsibilities, cancer family caregivers may be inclined to pray for one's own health. A qualitative study investigating spirituality and religiosity among cancer family caregivers in Brazil supports the premise that peoples' prayer practices may change once they become caregivers (Paiva et al. 2015). Participants stated their faith in God had increased and they were more reflective about life since becoming a caregiver. In addition, participants stated religiosity gave them strength and helped them cope with their caregiver responsibilities.

5   Caregiver Witnessing

Inherent in the family caregiver role is bearing witness to the plight of the person with cancer (Weitzner et al. 1999). The cancer family caregiver's journey with their ill family member begins with the shock of diagnosis and travels through the exploration of treatment decisions, the stress of managing symptoms and treatment side effects, to the uncertainty of survivorship or the challenge of end of life and death. Beyond their personal experiences at each of the phases of disease, the cancer family caregiver often has the added task of witnessing the ill family member's ordeal of enduring aggressive care and its aftermath. The cancer family caregiver may have an intimate view of the patient's physical pain, emotional anguish, physical deterioration, and delirium. The consequences of witnessing for the family caregiver have not yet been fully explicated. Qualitative studies speak to the brutal reality of what cancer family caregivers witness (Murray et al. 2010; Stetz and Brown 1997; Williams and Bakitas 2012). A few epidemiologic studies have linked cancer family caregiver witnessing to their development of posttraumatic stress disorder and major depressive disorder (Barry et al. 2002; Wright et al. 2010).

The Yale Bereavement Study was the first study to evaluate the bereaved caregiver's perceptions of the patient's suffering during the illness, the violent nature of the death, and their sense of being prepared for the death, and how these factors are associated with major depressive disorder, posttraumatic stress disorder, and prolonged grief disorder (Barry et al. 2002). Earlier research classified deaths as violent based on how the death occurred (i.e., motor vehicle crash, homicide, suicide). The Yale Bereavement Study allowed the bereaved caregiver to classify the death as violent or peaceful, according to how much they perceived the patient to have pain and other physical symptoms. The authors, reporting on 122 bereaved adults who were interviewed at 4 months post-death (baseline) and 9 months post-death (follow-up), found perception of the death as violent led to a 1.5 times increased likelihood of major depressive disorder at baseline. A major limitation of The Yale Bereavement Study is its reliance on retrospective ratings of the bereaved person's perceptions, and the simultaneous evaluation of those ratings and assessment of the psychiatric diagnoses. It is possible individuals with post-death major depressive disorder and prolonged grief disorder are inclined to perceive the circumstances surrounding the death negatively. Similarly, the directionality of the associations between the bereaved caregiver's perceptions and the psychiatric diagnoses is ambiguous. That said, The Yale Bereavement Study was a groundbreaking, ambitious, and creative undertaking that laid the foundation for future research related to caregiver witnessing.

6 Factors that Influence the Caregiving Experience

6.1 Caregiver Characteristics

Much of the cancer family caregiver descriptive research has attempted to discern which factors influence the caregiving experience, either increasing or mitigating one's risk for psychosocial burden. While the assertion is often made that younger caregivers and female caregivers are at increased risk for developing anxiety and depression (Given and Sherwood 2006; Kim and Given 2008; Maguire et al. 2016; Rumpold et al. 2016a; Schrank et al. 2016), there is also a body of literature that refutes these findings (Fenix et al. 2006; Ha-Hyun Kim et al. 2016; Grov et al. 2005; Williams et al. 2013). In all likelihood, the outcomes depend upon which variables the researchers controlled for, such as socioeconomics, education, having other dependents in the household, employment status, length of time as caregiver, number of hours devoted to caregiving, types of caregiving tasks, social connections and supports, personality trait, spirituality, religiosity, coping strategy, and perception of the role. A recent study demonstrated that cancer family caregiver characteristics were inconsequential with the exception of predicting their own health and finances (Maguire et al. 2016). Quite possibly, the experience of caregiving supersedes gender, age, and race/ethnicity, and instead leads the caregiver to draw on core human elements that transcend demographics.

6.2 Patient Characteristics

Patient characteristics have been found to profoundly influence the cancer family caregiving experience. Caregivers caring for patients with greater physical decline, less functional ability, higher number of symptoms, and those who are close to death are at increased risk for distress and burden (Kim and Given 2008; Krug et al. 2016; Maguire et al. 2016).

The National Quality of Life Survey for Caregivers, over an 8-year period, looked at the consequences of caring for someone with cancer in the United States (Kim et al. 2015). Their findings contradict previous studies that found associations between severity of the patient's health status and that of the caregiver. For the first time, The National Quality of Life Survey for Caregivers has documented effect of the caregiver's subjective assessment of stress after 2 years of caregiving on the caregiver's physical health, namely development of arthritis, chronic back pain, and heart diseases. Of note, the 2-year associations further predict caregiver health at 8 years post diagnosis (Youngmee Kim et al. 2016). Those caregivers whose patient had died by the 8-year mark were significantly more likely to report mood disorders and psychological distress than caregivers whose patients were in remission (Youngmee Kim et al. 2016).

6.3 Caregiver Social Supports

There is mounting evidence that the caregiving experience can be a time for personal growth and transformation, an opportunity to prioritize interpersonal relationships, heal old relational wounds, and reflect on and engage in meaningful and purposeful work (Colgrove et al. 2007; Ferrel and Baird 2012; Moore et al. 2011). One factor that contributes to these positive aspects of caregiving may be the caregiver's social support network. It appears that if the caregiver has a supportive network of family and friends who can provide companionship, emotional support, instrumental care (meals, housecleaning, errands), and respite care, the cancer family caregiver can have the space and time necessary to garner perspective on the arduous role of caregiving (Fujinami et al. 2015; Kim et al. 2013; Mosher et al. 2013b).

7 Interventions

Several interventions to ameliorate cancer family caregiver burden have been proposed, however, few intervention studies have shown favorable effect. In 2013, the United States Veterans Administration published a systematic review that included intervention studies targeting family caregivers to adults with cancer and memory-related illness (Griffin et al. 2013). With the intention of testing the hypothesis that interventions which aid the family caregiver ultimately benefit the patient, the systematic review focused on patient outcomes only. The systematic review included a total of 27 unique cancer family caregiver randomized controlled trials which used a variety of methodologies (e.g., telephone or web-based counseling provided to patient and family member separately, adaptations of couples' cognitive behavioral therapy, family-assisted approaches to patient care, family-focused cognitive behavioral therapy interventions that include family coping, and problem solving). Of note, all of the cancer family caregiver studies were found to be of fair or poor methodologic quality with moderate or high risk of bias and evidence ratings of low or insufficient. The systematic review concludes, "Overall, the available data indicated that compared to usual or standard care, family involved interventions did not consistently improve global quality of life; mental, physical, or social functioning; depression/anxiety; or symptom control among patients with cancer." (Griffin et al. 2013)

A 2016 meta-analysis of 36 intervention studies that used at least one aspect of cognitive behavioral therapy for cancer family caregivers found no effect (O'Toole et al. 2016). When one considers the broad evidential support for cognitive behavioral therapy to treat psychological distress, coupled with the high rate of psychological distress among cancer family caregivers, the lack of effect found in the meta-analysis speaks to the complexity of cancer family caregiver needs.

The physical activity literature is robust and provides solid evidence for salubrious effects on physical and psychological well-being. Fourteen physical activity intervention studies for cancer family caregivers were included in a 2016 systematic review (Lambert et al. 2016). The interventions included dancing, brisk walking, yoga, and aerobic exercises with an instructor. None of the studies achieved a high-quality methodologic rating; nine achieved a moderate quality rating. Overall, the physical activity interventions improved cancer family caregiver well-being, quality of life, sleep quality, and self-efficacy for caregiving.

The cancer family caregiver intervention research continues to grow, however, the methodologic quality remains circumspect with many studies hampered by small sample sizes, high attrition, and cryptic or incomplete reporting.

8 State of the Research

Over the past 20 years, a sizable descriptive psychosocial assessment of cancer family caregivers has accrued. Several major problems with the literature are evident, namely: failure to set sampling parameters based on caregiver and patient characteristics; focus on psychosocial issues of family caregivers in isolation, rather than assessing the interrelationship between psychosocial, physical, and spiritual/existential needs; inattention to the dynamic nature of the caregiving role over time; and inconsistent use of measurement tools.

In an effort to improve assessment of cancer family caregiver burden, Shilling et al. (2016) conducted a systematic review to identify, psychometrically evaluate, and appraise research instruments that measure the impact of caregiving. For the preponderance of instruments, the authors were unable to find evidence of psychometric performance with cancer family caregivers. They also identified several domains that have been largely ignored by caregiver researchers, namely: impact on paid employment and career planning, sexual activity, impact on other family members, and functioning of the family unit.

Clearly, there is a need to standardize definitions and outcome measures used in cancer family caregiver research. The time is ripe for new measures to be developed that accurately and reliably assess the broad spectrum of domains that are affected by cancer family caregiving (Williams and Bakitas 2012; Shilling et al. 2016). The use of multiple measurement tools presents a major barrier to any type of comparative or aggregate analysis across studies, which is an essential next step in a field where most studies are comprised of small samples.

9 Conclusion

Cancer family caregivers are in the unenviable position of being essential members of the healthcare team and having their own considerable healthcare needs. Popular belief holds that by supporting the cancer family caregiver, we in turn support the patient who invariably receives higher quality, more conscientious care at home. Unfortunately, there is at present, no scientific evidence to endorse the claim that supporting the caregiver positively effects patient outcomes. Regardless, cancer family caregivers provide a valuable service to their patient, the healthcare system, and society as a whole—while accruing considerable personal costs. Cancer family caregivers deserve quality research, and appropriate preventive, supportive, and acute care.

References

Adams RN, Mosher CE, Cannady RS, Lucette A, Kim Y (2014) Caregiving experiences predict changes in spiritual well-being among family caregivers of cancer patients. Psycho-Oncology 23:1178–1184

Barry LC, Kasl SV, Prigerson HG (2002) Psychiatric disorders among bereaved persons: the role of perceived circumstances of death and preparedness for death. Am J Geriatr Psychiatry 10:447–457

Bayen E, Laigle-Donadey F, Proute M (2016) The multidimensional burden of informal caregivers in primary malignant brain tumor. Support Care Cancer. doi:10.1007/s00520-016-3397-6

Beesley VL, Price MA, Webb PM (2011) Loss of lifestyle: health behaviour and weight changes after becoming a caregiver of a family member diagnosed with ovarian cancer. Support Care Cancer 19:1949–1956

Braun M, Mikulincer M, Rydall A, Walsh A, Rodin G (2007) Hidden morbidity in cancer: spouse caregivers. J Clin Oncol 25:4829–4834

Cameron J, Franche R, Cheung A, Stewart D (2002) Lifestyle interference and emotional distress in family caregivers of advanced cancer patients. Cancer 94:521–527

Carter P (2003) Family caregivers' sleep loss and depression over time. Cancer Nurs 26:253–259

Carter P, Acton GJ (2006) Personality and coping: predictors of depression and sleep problems among caregivers of individuals who have cancer. J Gerontological Nurs 32:45–53

Colgrove LA, Kim Y, Thompson N (2007) The effect of spirituality and gender on the quality of life of spousal caregivers of cancer survivors. Ann Behav Med 33:90–98

Douglas S, Daly BJ (2012) The impact of patient quality of life and spirituality upon caregiver depression for those with advanced cancer. Palliat Support Care 11:389–396

Fenix JB, Cherlin EJ, Prigerson HG, Johnson-Hurzeler R, Kasl SV, Bradley EH (2006) Religiousness and major depression among bereaved family caregivers: a 13-month follow-up study. J Palliat Care 22:286–292

Ferrel BR, Baird P (2012) Deriving meaning and faith in caregiving. Semin Oncol Nurs 28:256–261

Fujinami RS, Virginia S, Finley Z, Uman G, Grant M, Ferrell B (2015) Family caregivers' distress levels related to quality of life, burden, and preparedness. Psycho-Oncology 24:54–62

Gibbins J, McCoubrie R, Kendrick AH, Senior-Smith G, Davies AN, Hanks GW (2009) Sleep-wake disturbances in patients with advanced cancer and their family carers. J Pain Symptom Manage 38:860–870

Given B, Sherwood PR (2006) Family care for the older person with cancer. Semin Oncol Nurs 22:43–50

Goldstein M, Concato J, Fried T, Kasl S, Johnson-Hurzeler R, Bradley E (2004) Factors associated with caregiver burden among caregivers of terminally ill patients with cancer. J Palliat Care 20:38–43

Griffin JM, Meis L, Greer N, Jensen A, MacDonald R, Rutks I, Carlyle M, Wilt TJ (2013) Effectiveness of family and caregiver interventions on patient outcomes among adults with cancer or memory-related disorders: a systematic review. VA-ESP Project #09-009, p 38

Grov E, Dahl A, Moum T, Fossa S (2005) Anxiety, depression, and quality of life in caregivers of patients with cancer in late palliative phase. Annals Oncol 16:1185–1191

Guay M, Parsons HA, Hui D, De la Cruz MG, Thorney S, Bruera E (2012) Spirituality, religiosity, and spiritual pain among caregivers of patients with advanced cancer. Am J Hosp Palliat Care 30:455–461

Hagedoorn M, Buunk BP, Kuijer RG, Wobbes T, Sanderman R (2000) Couples dealing with cancer: role and gender differences regarding psychological distress and quality of life. Psycho-Oncology 9:232–242

Hanly P, Ó Céilleachair A, Skally M, O'Leary E, Kapur K, FitzpatrickP, Staines A, Sharp L (2013) How much does it cost to care for survivors of colorectal cancer? Caregiver's time, travel and out-of-pocket costs. Support Care Cancer 21:2583–2592

Hanly P, Maguire R, Balfe M, Hyland P, Timmons A, O'Sullivan E, Butow P, Sharp L (2016) Burden and happiness in head and neck cancer carers: the role of supportive care needs. Support Care Cancer 24:4283–4291

Hebert RS, Schulz R, Copeland VC, Arnold RM (2009) Preparing family caregivers for death and bereavement: insights from caregivers of terminally ill patients. J Pain Symptom Manage 37:3–12

Hendrix CC, Abernethy A, Sloane R, Misuraca J, Moore J (2009) A pilot study on the influence of an individualized and experiential training on cancer caregiver's self-efficacy in home care and symptom management. Home Health Nurse 27:271–278

Hodges J, Humphries G, MacFarlane G (2005) A meta-analytic investigation of the relationship between the psychological distress of cancer patients and their carers. Soc Sci Med 60:1–12

Kent E, Rowland J, Northouse L, Litzelman K, Chou W, Shelburne N, Timura C, O'Mara A, Hus K (2016) Caring for caregivers and patients: research and clinical priorities for informal cancer caregiving. Cancer. doi:10.1002/cncr.29939

Kershaw T, Ellis KR, Yoon H, Schafenacker A, Katapodi M, Northouse L (2015) The interdependence of advanced cancer patients' and their family caregivers' mental health, physical health, and self-efficacy over time. Ann Behav Med 49:901–911

Kim Y, Given BA (2008) Quality of life of family caregivers of cancer survivors: across the trajectory of the illness. Cancer 112(11 Suppl):2556–2568

Kim Y, Schulz R (2008) Family caregivers' strains: comparative analysis of cancer caregiving with dementia, diabetes, and frail elderly caregiving. J Aging Health 20:483–503

Kim Y, Duberstin PR, Sorensen S (2005) Levels of depressive symptoms in spouses of people with lung cancer: effects of personality, social support, and caregiving burden. Psychosomatics 46:123–130

Kim Y, Baker F, Spillers RL, Wellisch DK (2006) Psychological adjustment of cancer caregivers with multiple roles. Psycho-Oncology 15:795–804

Kim Y, Carver CS, Spillers RL, Crammer C, Zhou ES (2011) Individual and dyadic relations between spiritual well-being and quality of life among cancer survivors and their spousal caregivers. Psycho-Oncology 20:762–770

Kim Y, Carver CS, Rocha-Lima C, Shaffer KM (2013) Depressive symptoms among caregivers of colorectal cancer patients during the first year since diagnosis: a longitudinal investigation. Psycho-Oncology 22:362–367

Kim Y, Carver CS, Shaffer KM, Gansler T, Cannady RS (2015) Cancer caregiving predicts physical impairments: roles of earlier caregiving stress and being a spousal caregiver. Cancer 121:302–310

Kim HH, Kim SY, Kim JM, Kim SW, Shin IS, Shim HJ, Hwang JE, Chung IJ, Yoon JS (2016) Influence of caregiver personality on the burden of family caregivers of terminally ill cancer patients. Palliat Support Care 14:5–12

Kim Y, Shaffer KM, Carver CS, Cannady RS (2016) Quality of life of family caregivers 8 years after a relative's cancer diagnosis: follow-up of the national quality of life survey for caregivers. Psycho-Oncology 25:266–274

Krug K, Miksch A, Peters-Klimm F, Engeser P, Szecsenyi J (2016) Correlation between patient quality of life in palliative care and burden of their family caregivers: a prospective observational cohort study. BMC Palliat Care. doi:10.1186/s12904-016-0082-y

Lambert SD, Duncan LR, Kapellas S, Bruson AM, Myrand M, Santa Mina D, Culos-Reed N, Lambrou A (2016) A descriptive systematic review of physical activity interventions for caregivers: effects on caregivers' and care recipients' psychosocial outcomes, physical activity levels, and physical health. Ann Behav Med 50:907–919

Lee KC, Yin JJ, Lin PC, Lu SH (2015) Sleep disturbances and related factors among family caregivers of patients with advanced cancer. Psycho-Oncology 24:1632–1638

Leroy T, Fournier E, Penel N, Christophe V (2016) Crossed views of burden and emotional distress of cancer patients and family caregivers during palliative care. Psycho-Oncology 25:1278–1285

Maguire R, Hanly P, Hyland P, Sharp L (2016) Understanding burden in caregivers of colorectal cancer survivors: what role do patient and caregiver factors play? Eur J Cancer Care. doi:10.1111/ecc.12527

Mako C, Gale K, Poppito SR (2006) Spiritual pain among patients with advanced cancer in palliative care. J Palliat Med 9:1106–1113

Mellon S, Northouse LL, Weiss LK (2006) A population-based study of the quality of life of cancer survivors and their family caregivers. Cancer Nurs 29:120–131

Moore AM, Gamblin TC, Geller DA, Youssef MN, Hoffman KE, Gemmell L, Likumahuwa SM, Bovbjerg DH, Marsland A, Steel JL (2011) A prospective study of posttraumatic growth as assessed by self-report and family caregiver in the context of advanced cancer. Psycho-Oncology 20:479–487

Mosher CE, Champion VL, Azzoloi CG (2013a) Economic and social changes among distressed family caregivers of lung cancer patients. Support Care Cancer 21:819–826

Mosher CE, Jaynes HA, Hanna N, Ostroff JS (2013b) Distressed family caregivers of lung cancer patients: an examination of psychosocial and practical challenges. Support Care Cancer 21:431–437

Mosher CE, Winger JG, Hanna N, Jalal SI, Einhorn LH, Birdas TJ, Ceppa DP, Kesler KA, Schmitt J, Kashy DA, Champion VL (2016) Randomized pilot trial of a telephone symptom management intervention for symptomatic lung cancer patients and their family caregivers. J Pain Symptom Manage 52:469–482

Murray SA, Kendall M, Boyd K, Grant L, Highet G, Sheikh A (2010) Archetypal trajectories of social, psychological, and spiritual well-being and distress in family care givers of patients with lung cancer. BMJ 304:c2581

Nissen KG, Trevino K, Lange T, Prigerson HG (2016) Family relationships and psychosocial dysfunction among family caregivers of patients with advanced cancer. J Pain Symptom Manage 52:841–849

Northouse L, Williams AL, Given B, McCorkle R (2012) Psychosocial care for family caregivers of patients with cancer. J Clin Oncol 30:1227–1234

O'Hara RE, Hull JG, Lyons KD, Bakitas M, Hegel MT, Li Z, Ahles TA (2010) Impact on caregiver burden of a patient-focused palliative care intervention for patients with advanced cancer. Palliat Support Care 8:395–404

O'Toole MS, Zachariae R, Renna ME, Mennin DS, Applebaum A (2016) Cognitive behavioral therapies for informal caregivers of patients with cancer and cancer survivors: a systematic review and meta-analysis. Psycho-Oncology. doi:10.1002/pon.4144

Paiva BSR, Carvalho AL (2015) "Oh, yeah, I'm getting closer to god": spirituality and religiousness of family caregivers of cancer patients undergoing palliative care. Support Care Cancer 23:2383–2389

Perez-Ordóñez F, Frías-Osuna A, Romero-Rodríguez Y, Del-Pino-Casado R (2016) Coping strategies and anxiety in caregivers of palliative cancer patients. Eur J Cancer Care 25:600–607

Reblin M, Donaldson G, Ellington L, Mooney K, Caserta M, Lund D (2016) Spouse cancer caregivers' burden and distress at entry to home hospice: the role of relationship quality. J Soc Pers Relat 33:666–686

Round J, Jones L, Morris S (2015) Estimating the cost of caring for people with cancer at the end of life: a modelling study. Palliat Med 29:899–907

Rumpold T, Schur S, Amering M, Kirchheiner K, Masel EK, Watzke H, Schrank B (2016a) Informal caregivers of advanced-stage cancer patients: every second is at risk for psychiatric morbidity. Support Care Cancer 24:1975–1982

Rumpold T, Schur S, Amering M, Ebert-Vogel A, Kirchheiner K, Masel E, Watzke H, Schrank B (2016b) Hope as determinant for psychiatric morbidity in family caregivers of advanced cancer patients. Psycho-Oncology. doi:10.1002/pon.4205

Schrank B, Ebert-Vogel A, Amering M, Masel EK, Neubauer M, Watzke H, Zehetmayer S, Schur S (2016) Gender differences in caregiver burden and its determinants in family members of terminally ill cancer patients. Psycho-Oncology 25:808–814

Seifert ML, Williams AL, Dowd MF, Chappel-Aiken L, McCorkle R (2008) The caregiving experience in a racially diverse sample of cancer family caregivers. Cancer Nurs 31:399–407

Shaffer KM, Jacobs JM, Nipp RD, Carr A, Jackson VA, Park ER, Pirl WF, El-Jawahri A, Gallagher ER, Greer JA, Temel JS (2016a) Mental and physical health correlates among family caregivers of patients with newly-diagnosed incurable cancer: a hierarchical linear regression analysis. Support Care Cancer. doi:10.1007/s00520-016-3488-4

Shaffer KM, Kim Y, Carver CS (2016b) Physical and mental health trajectories of cancer patients and caregivers across the year post-diagnosis: a dyadic investigation. Psychol Health 31:655–674

Sherwood PR, Given BA, Given CW, Schiffman RF, Murman DL, Lovely M, von Eye A, Rogers LR, Remer S (2006) Predictors of distress in caregivers of persons with a primary malignant brain tumor. Res Nurs Health 29:105–120

Shilling V, Matthews L, Jenkins V, Fallowfield L (2016) Patient-reported outcome measures for cancer caregivers: a systematic review. Qual Life Res 25:1859–1876

Stajduhar KI, Martin WL, Barwich D, Fyles G (2008) Factors influencing family caregivers' ability to cope with providing end-of-life cancer care at home. Cancer Nurs 31:77–85

Stetz KM, Brown MA (1997) Taking care: caregiving to persons with cancer and AIDS. Cancer Nurs 20:12–22

Tan JY, Lim HA, Kuek NM, Kua EH, Mahendran R (2015) Caring for the caregiver while caring for the patient: exploring the dyadic relationship between patient spirituality and caregiver quality of life. Support Care Cancer 23:3403–3406

Temel JS, McCannon J, Greer JA, Jackson VA, Ostler P, Pirl WF, Lynch TJ, Billings JA (2008) Aggressiveness of care in a prospective cohort of patients with advanced NSCLC. Cancer 113:826–833

Van Houtven CH, Ramsey SD, Hornbrook MC, Atienza AA, van Ryn M (2011) Economic burden for informal caregivers of lung and colorectal cancer patients. Oncologist 15:883–893

Walsh K, Jones L, Tookman A, Mason C, McLoughlin J, Blizard R (2007) Reducing emotional distress in people caring for patients receiving specialist palliative care. Br J Psychiatr 190:142–147

Weitzner MA, McMillan SC, Jacobsen PB (1999) Family caregiver quality of life: differences between curative and palliative cancer treatment settings. J Pain Symptom Manage 17:418–428

Williams AL, Bakitas M (2012) Cancer family caregivers: a new direction for interventions. J Palliat Med 15:775–783

Williams AL, McCorkle R (2011) Cancer family caregivers during the palliative, hospice, and bereavement phases: a review of the descriptive psychosocial literature. Palliat Support Care 9:315–325

Williams AL, Holmes-Tisch AJ, Dixon J, McCorkle R (2013) Factors associated with depressive symptoms in cancer family caregivers of patients receiving chemotherapy. Support Care Cancer 21:2387–2394

Williams AL, Dixon J, Feinn R, McCorkle R (2015) Cancer family caregiver depression: are religion-related variables important? Psycho-Oncology 24:825–831

Williamson G, Shaffer D, Schulz R (1998) Activity restriction and prior relationship history as contributors to mental health outcomes among middle-aged and older spousal caregivers. Health Psychol 17:152–162

World Health Organization International Agency for Research on Cancer, Stewart BW, Wild CP (eds) World Cancer Report 2014, p 16

Wright AA, Keating NL, Balboni TA, Matulonis UA, Block SD, Prigerson HG (2010) Place of death: correlations with quality of life of patients with cancer and predictors of bereaved caregivers' mental health. J Clin Oncol 28:4457–4464

Yabroff KR, Kim Y (2009) Time costs associated with informal caregiving for cancer survivors. Cancer 115(18 Suppl):4362–4373

Rehabilitation for Cancer Patients

Joachim Weis and Jürgen M. Giesler

Abstract

Rehabilitation for cancer patients aims at reducing the impact of disabling and limiting conditions resulting from cancer and its treatment in order to enable patients to regain social integration and participation. Given current trends in cancer incidence and survival along with progress in medical treatment, cancer rehabilitation is becoming increasingly important in contemporary health care. Although not without limitations, the International Classification of Functioning, Disability and Health (ICF) provides a valuable perspective for cancer rehabilitation in understanding impairments in functioning and activity as the result of an interaction between a health condition and contextual factors. The structure of cancer rehabilitation varies across countries as a function of their healthcare systems and social security legislations, although there is a broad consensus with respect to its principal goals. Cancer rehabilitation requires a careful assessment of the individual patient's rehabilitation needs and a multidisciplinary team of health professionals. A variety of rehabilitation interventions exist, including psycho-oncological and psycho-educational approaches. Research on the effectiveness of cancer rehabilitation provides

J. Weis (✉)
Universitätsklinikum Freiburg Medizinische Fakultät, Klinik Für Onkologische Rehabilitation UKF Reha GGmbH, Albert-Ludwigs-Universität Freiburg, Breisacher Str. 117, Freiburg 79106, Deutschland, Germany
e-mail: joachim.weis@ukf-reha.de

J.M. Giesler
Sektion Versorgungsforschung und Rehabilitationsforschung, Universitätsklinikum Freiburg, Medizinische Fakultät, Albert-Ludwigs-Universität Freiburg, Hugstetter Str. 49, Freiburg 79106, Deutschland, Germany
e-mail: juergen.giesler@uniklinik-freiburg.de

© Springer International Publishing AG 2018
U. Goerling and A. Mehnert (eds.), *Psycho-Oncology*, Recent Results
in Cancer Research 210, https://doi.org/10.1007/978-3-319-64310-6_7

evidence of improvements in relevant outcome parameters, but faces some methodological challenges as well.

Keywords

Psychosocial distress · Rehabilitation · Coping · Psychosocial interventions · Assessment

1 Increasing Relevance of Rehabilitation in Cancer

As has been well documented (Bray et al. 2012), cancer incidence continues to rise worldwide as does the number of cancer survivors. For the year 2012, e.g., the International Agency for Research on Cancer (IARC) estimates that about 14 million people have been diagnosed with cancer all over the world (Cancer Research UK 2014; Ervik et al. 2016; Ferlay et al. 2015). For the same year, the 5-year prevalence of cancer worldwide has been estimated with approximately 32 million persons (Cancer Research UK 2014). By the year 2030 the number of persons newly diagnosed with cancer annually is expected to rise to about 24 million (Cancer Research UK 2014). Irrespective of considerable variation between different countries in these parameters, these trends reflect the effects of various factors. Among these, advances in medical treatment and early detection of cancer during the past three decades as well as the increasingly higher life expectancy of the population play a significant role. In addition, changes in lifestyle associated with the development of modern industrialized societies have to be taken into account here. As a consequence of these trends, an increasing number of persons will require medical treatment for cancer, long-term surveillance, and eventually palliative care in the future. Thus, cancer has turned into a life-threatening chronic condition for a large proportion of patients that pose new challenges for comprehensive cancer care. These include, among others, a change in patient role toward more active participation in treatment decisions and treatment itself depending on the individual patients' needs and expectations.

Oncologic treatment typically includes surgery, chemotherapy, and/or radiation which in general have become increasingly more complex, long lasting as well as more invasive. That is, treatment may produce significant toxicities which cause substantial short- and long-term side effects, functional loss in various behavioral and life domains (physical, cognitive, emotional, social, and vocational) as well as psychosocial distress. Quality of life and functional status for a considerable proportion of patients will thus be substantially reduced. Against this background, cancer rehabilitation may generally be defined as the coordinated efforts of healthcare professionals to help patients overcome, minimize, or compensate the functional impairments and activity limitations brought about by the disease and its treatment. Due to the different developments described above, the importance of cancer rehabilitation has steadily increased during the last decades. Thus, rehabilitation has become an increasingly essential part of comprehensive cancer care covering the entire continuum of early detection, diagnosis, primary and adjuvant treatment, survivorship, and aftercare to end-of-life phases.

2 Focus and Basic Concepts of Cancer Rehabilitation

If one follows the WHO's definition of rehabilitation in general (WHO 1981), cancer rehabilitation may be understood as the "use of all means at reducing the impact of disabling and handicapping conditions" associated with cancer and its treatment with the aim of enabling patients to regain physical, social, psychological, and work-related functionality and "to achieve optimal social integration" (see also Gerber 2001; Gerber et al. 2005; Meyer et al. 2011). This process starts already during or immediately after the end of the primary treatment in terms of secondary and tertiary prevention.

Basic to this understanding of cancer rehabilitation is a concept of functional health that the International Classification of Functioning, Disability and Health (ICF) of the WHO (2001; German version: German Institute of Medical Documentation and Information 2005) builds upon. From this perspective, a person would be considered functionally healthy if his/her body functions are in accordance with accepted norms, if he/she can do what a person without a health condition would be expected to be able to do, and if he/she could live his/her life in personally important life domains in a way as it would be expected of a person without functional impairments and restrictions to activities and participation.

As can be seen from Fig. 1, the ICF distinguishes between health conditions and contextual factors. Thus, it provides a new perspective on disability and functional impairment which are now explicitly viewed as outcomes of an *interaction* between these health conditions and contextual factors. This perspective integrates a social and a biomedical model of disability into a biopsychosocial one. In addition, Fig. 1 shows that the ICF distinguishes between body functions and structures, activities, and participation in order to describe levels of restricted functioning. *Body functions* refer to physiological functions of body systems (including psychological functions), whereas *body structures* comprise anatomical parts of the body such as organs, limbs, and their components. Problems at this level may take the form of significant deviation or loss and are termed *impairments*. On the next level, *activity* means the execution of a task or an action by an individual and difficulties in executing tasks are termed *activity limitations*. Finally, *participation* refers to a person's involvement in a life situation and problems experienced by the individual in this respect are referred to as *participation restrictions*. *Environmental factors* (comprising a person's physical, social, and attitudinal environment) and personal factors (e.g., a person's optimism) may moderate how a given health condition impacts on the three levels of functioning and activity and thus on the manifestation of disability. As an example in the field of cancer, one might consider the case of a

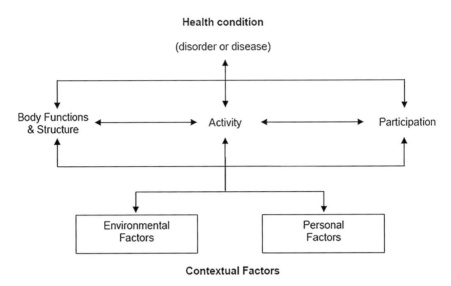

Fig. 1 Model of disability underlying the ICF (WHO 2001)

patient with peripheral neuropathy and ankle weakness resulting from chemotherapy (Gilchrist et al. 2009). This might lead to a limitation in this patient's ability to walk. However, whether or not this would result in a participation restriction in the vocational domain as well would of cause depend on the person's vocation (e.g., if he were a fire fighter as opposed to a computer programmer).

Intended as a complement to the International Classification of Diseases (ICD), the ICF provides an extensive set of categories by which a person's functional impairments, activity restrictions, and limitations deriving from a health condition may be described in detail with additional reference to contextual factors. To be clinically useful, however, subsets of this extensive list have to be built which refer to specific health conditions and represent so-called ICF core sets. In the field of cancer, core sets for breast as well as for head and neck cancer have been developed and are currently undergoing validation (Becker et al. 2010; Brach et al. 2004; Glaessel et al. 2011; Leib et al. 2012; Tschiesner et al. 2010, 2011). This research lends support to the content validity of the respective core set categories on the one hand, but on the other also identifies the need for further amendments (Khan et al. 2012; Kirschneck et al. 2014). Thus, there still is a need for additional development and further validation. Although the general perspective provided by ICF has been positively evaluated so far, it remains to be seen, then, whether core sets covering impairments and limitations associated with other tumor diagnoses will emerge. Furthermore, reservations concerning the applicability and practicability of ICF categories in the field of cancer rehabilitation (e.g., Bornbaum et al. 2013) will have to be resolved.

3 Structure of Rehabilitation Care

Considering the continuum of cancer care, cancer rehabilitation has its place at the interface of acute and follow-up or aftercare. How rehabilitation services are delivered varies greatly from country to country as a function of the social security system into which it is embedded. In most European countries and in the United States of America, rehabilitation services are mostly based in outpatient settings, whereas in Germany one finds a unique system in which rehabilitation services are provided predominantly through inpatient settings although outpatient rehabilitation services have partially gained importance in recent years, too.

Hellbom et al. (2011) have provided a brief overview of the structures of cancer rehabilitation and the state of rehabilitation research in Nordic and European countries. As they point out, cancer rehabilitation there ranges from primarily outpatient programs as in Sweden, Norway and the Netherlands over 1-week courses as in Finland, Denmark, Iceland and, again, Sweden and Norway to (predominantly inpatient) 3-week programs in Germany (for Germany see also Koch and Morfeld 2004; Koch et al. 2000). Extending this perspective, Stubblefield et al. (2013) focus on commonalities and differences in the structure of rehabilitation services between Europe and the United States of America.

One of many interesting characteristics of the German rehabilitation system is that rehabilitation costs are primarily covered by the German statutory pension insurance or the patient's health insurance—depending on whether or not the patient still is in the labor force. Different from patients with other health conditions, however, cancer patients in Germany generally are entitled to apply for rehabilitation measures. Rehabilitation of cancer patients not yet retired is guided by the aim of restoring their earning capacity (as a prerequisite of social participation) which is well captured by the official slogan "rehabilitation rather than pension". Another specific feature of rehabilitation in Germany is a special form of rehabilitation that is termed "post-acute rehabilitation". This refers formally to rehabilitation services that are about to begin not later than 2 weeks after discharge from the acute care hospital. This type of rehabilitation measures represented about 35% of all rehabilitation measures in 2014 (German Statutory Pension Insurance 2015).

In 2014, the German statutory pension insurance provided a total of 152,260 in- and outpatient cancer rehabilitation measures (German Statutory Pension Insurance 2015). These represent 16% of all its rehabilitation measures for adults in that year. 83% of all rehabilitation measures in 2014 were inpatient measures and 14% were outpatient measures (both for adults). The latter represents an increase of 11 percentage points compared to the year 2000. This mainly reflects the effort that has been taken during that time in order to develop outpatient services in Germany as well in order to tailor services more specifically to the needs of some subgroups of the patient population. However, compared to the total of inpatient rehabilitation measures provided in 2014 the proportions of women and men with cancer receiving inpatient rehabilitation amounted to 20 and 15%, respectively, while the proportion of patients with cancer receiving outpatient rehabilitation was 2% in both women and men, respectively, in comparison to the total of outpatient rehabilitation measures.

In the United States of America, the form of delivering cancer rehabilitation has undergone some notable changes during the last decades according to observations by Alfano et al. (2012). These authors note a shift in rehabilitation service delivery away from tertiary cancers centers to community centers coupled with a fragmentation of cancer care in community settings. In combination these trends limit the potential of cancer rehabilitation. In order to improve this unsatisfactory situation, Alfano et al. (2012) suggest to revitalize the link between primary treatment and rehabilitation services and to also consider the possibility to integrate some elements of the European forms of rehabilitation into the US system of health care. It remains to be seen how this will translate into practice. Nevertheless, these recommendations fit well with initiatives by the Institute of Medicine to establish the concept of a cancer survivorship plan that describes the tasks for survivorship care of any individual patient (Oeffinger and McCabe 2006; Salz et al. 2012, Stout et al. 2012; Stubblefield et al. 2013).

The structure of delivering cancer rehabilitation not only varies widely across countries, but also is undergoing dynamic processes of change in response to changes in medical care and society in general. Despite the marked variation in the delivery of cancer rehabilitation services across different countries, however, there appears to be a general consensus that cancer rehabilitation is a multidisciplinary task (for details see Section "Cancer Rehabilitation: A Multidisciplinary Task").

4   Rehabilitation Needs and Assessment

Physical and psychosocial sequelae of cancer and its treatment differ widely between patients and the stages of the cancer trajectory. Problems during the initial phase immediately after treatment are different from those that may arise in later phases, e.g., after a recurrence or at the end of life (Gerber 2001). More specifically, the spectrum of sequelae may include fear of recurrence, anxiety, depression, cognitive dysfunction, fatigue, pain syndromes, peripheral neuropathy, sexual dysfunction, problems with body image, balance and gait problems, various mobility issues, lymphedema, problems with bladder and bowel functioning, stoma care, problems with swallowing, and speech and communication difficulties (Alfano et al. 2012; Fialka-Moser et al. 2003; Stubblefield and O'Dell 2009). Given this broad range of potential impairments in combination with the wide variability between patients, each cancer patient requesting rehabilitation has to be assessed individually with respect to his/her rehabilitation needs (Gamble et al. 2011; Ruppert et al. 2010). This assessment will take place routinely at admission in terms of a medical examination and interview. It may be complemented by a short psychological assessment by a psychologist or on the basis of a standard distress screening procedure. Determining a patient's rehabilitation needs could be improved using standardized instruments designed to measure the quality of life. These may be either generic or may focus on the specific problems and distress of cancer patients. Aside from assisting in the assessment of rehabilitation needs before or at admission, these instruments may be used efficiently in evaluating the effects of rehabilitation programs at discharge or follow-up examinations as well. Schag et al. (1991) and Ganz et al. (1992) were among the first to develop a comprehensive instrument for assessing rehabilitation needs in cancer patients.

Table 1 Illustrative selection of instruments and domains available to assessment in cancer rehabilitation

Domain, instrument, and reference[a]	
Quality of life: **Cancer specific**	
EORTC QLQ C30	European Organization for Research and Treatment of Cancer: Quality of Life Questionnaire C-30 (Aaronson et al. 1993)
FACIT	Functional Assessment of Chronic Illness Therapy (Webster et al. 2003)
Quality of life: **Generic**	
NHP	Nottingham Health Profile (Hunt et al. 1981; Kohlmann et al. 1997)
SF-36	Short Form 36 (Ware et al. 1994; Morfeld et al. 2011)
Health-related cognitions	
IPQ-R	Illness Perception Questionnaire Revised (Moss-Morris et al. 2002)
MHLC	Multidimensional Health Locus of Control scales (Wallston et al. 1978)
SOC	Sense of Coherence Questionnaire (Antonovsky 1993; Eriksson and Lindström 2006)
Coping with cancer	
CBI	Cancer Behavior Inventory (Merluzzi et al. 2001)
COPE	COPE Inventory (Carver et al. 1989)
FKV[b]	Freiburger Fragebogen zur Krankheitsverarbeitung (Muthny 1989)
TSK[b]	Trierer Skalen zur Krankheitsverarbeitung (Klauer and Filipp 1993)
WCCL	Ways of Coping Check List (Folkman 2013)
Social support	
ISSS	Index of Sojourner Social Support Scale (Ong and Ward 2005)
SSUK[b]	Skalen zur sozialen Unterstützung bei Krankheit (Ullrich and Mehnert 2010)
Pain	
(WHY)MPI	Multidimensional Pain Inventory (Kerns et al. 1985)
PDI	Pain disability Index (Tait et al. 1987)
Distress/Comorbidity	
BDI-II	Beck Depression Inventory II (Beck et al. 1996)
DT	Distress Thermometer (Holland et al. 2007; Mitchell 2007)
BSI	Brief Symptom Inventory (Derogatis and Melisaratos 1983; Derogatis and Savitz 1999)
GHQ	General Health Questionnaire (Lundin et al. 2016)
HADS	Hospital Anxiety and Depression Scale (Zigmond and Snaith 1983; Bjelland et al. 2002)

Note [a]In the case of some instruments, the reader is referred to more recent publications providing reviews of research on the respective instrument. [b]Available only in German

Overviews of instruments may be obtained from a variety of sources (e.g., Bengel et al. 2008; Mpofu and Oakland 2010). Table 1 illustrates some of the more frequently used instruments that are generally available to assessments in cancer rehabilitation settings.

5 Goals and Interventions

Given the multifaceted impairments and sequelae due to cancer and its treatment, cancer rehabilitation usually addresses a variety of goals. On a general level, cancer rehabilitation aims at restoring the patient's physical, emotional, social, role, and cognitive functioning. This may also include reintegration into work–life. Besides helping the patient regain functional autonomy, preventing further impairment of functioning may frequently represent another important task for rehabilitation of cancer patients. Following a suggestion by Bergelt and Koch (2002) rehabilitation goals may be classified as biomedical/treatment-related, psychosocial, educational, or vocational. Table 2 presents an illustrative list of rehabilitation goals covering these categories.

Specifying rehabilitation goals for the individual patient will take his/her individual needs into account as well as the results of all other assessments. In addition, the goals to be specified should be attainable within a reasonable amount of time. Based on this principle and the previous assessments, an individual rehabilitation plan will be developed in close cooperation with the patient. Also, patients and— wherever possible and indicated—their family will be encouraged to actively participate as partners in the rehabilitation process and thus contribute to attain their goals. In the end, the rehabilitation plan will combine a variety of medical and psychosocial interventions considered necessary to achieve the specified objectives. As an illustration, Table 3 presents an overview of the treatment options typically available in cancer rehabilitation programs.

In general, rehabilitation interventions for cancer patients include exercise (Baumann 2013), diet counseling (Reichel et al. 2013), neuropsychological training (Ercoli et al. 2015), and psychological interventions (Faller et al. 2013). Medical counseling and treatment are tailored to the various physical health problems resulting from cancer and its treatment. In addition, specialized programs have been developed that address issues and sequelae of patients from a given diagnostic or treatment subgroup (e.g., patients with breast or prostate cancer or patients having undergone stem cell transplantation). Thus, rehabilitation programs designed specifically for women with breast cancer may, e.g., focus on comprehensive management of lymphedema, postoperative management of breast reconstruction, psychological counseling or psychotherapy, and art- or dance therapy in order to address problems with body image and self-esteem. Similarly, patients suffering

Table 2 Types of intervention goals in cancer rehabilitation (slightly modified after Bergelt & Koch 2002)

Biomedical/treatment-related goals
To continue therapies as recommended after primary treatment
To identify and treat sequelae of cancer and its treatment (e.g., pain, fatigue, lack of endurance, peripheral neuropathy, sleep disorders)
To improve physical condition and performance status focusing on strength, endurance, and mobility
Psychosocial goals
To support the process of coping with the disease and the accompanying physical changes
To restore and improve social, emotional, and cognitive functioning
To enhance self-help strategies, competencies, and resources for disease management
To facilitate adaptation to irreversible limitations and help the patient develop compensatory skills and abilities
To help the patient stabilize with respect to his/her personal, familial, social, and vocational situation
Educational goals
To provide information on cancer, its treatment, and forms of psychosocial support
To provide information on risk factors and to initiate modification in health-related behaviors like dietary habits, exercise, smoking, or alcohol consumption
Vocational goals
To help the patient achieve vocational reintegration, resume previous occupation, or retrain in order to attain a position appropriate under given circumstances

Table 3 Interventions in cancer rehabilitation

Medical treatment including pain management and complementary medicine
Physical therapy and exercise programs
Diet consultation
Smoking cessation education
Psychological counseling/individual psychotherapy
Psycho-education
Art therapy/Occupational Therapy
Neuropsychological training

from severe fatigue and decreased physical performance for a prolonged period of recovery after having received stem cell transplantation may also profit from a specialized program that might combine elements of physical exercise and psycho-educational interventions (Du et al. 2015).

Table 4 Elements of psycho-educational programs in cancer rehabilitation

Information about cancer and its treatment
Social and emotional support, sharing of experience
Stress management
Cognitive behavioral self-instruction and self-control techniques
Relaxation, guided imagery

6 Psycho-oncology in Rehabilitation

Psycho-oncological interventions are an essential part of a comprehensive cancer rehabilitation program. They address the cognitive, behavioral, and emotional facets of the patients' (and their families') response to cancer and its treatment, especially the most common mental and social issues (psychosocial distress, depression and anxiety, fear of recurrence). During the last decades, numerous psycho-oncological interventions based on individual or group therapy approaches have been developed (Newell et al. 2002; Holland et al. 2015), which are carried out also in rehabilitation centers (Reese et al. 2016). As meta-analyses and systematic reviews have shown, evidence of the effectiveness of these interventions is available at the high ranking EBM levels I or II (Faller et al. 2013; Edwards et al. 2008). In a rehabilitation setting, psycho-educational interventions address the psychosocial distress, support the patients' coping and help them find their individual way of living with the cancer experience and a new life perspective. In addition, group interventions give participants the opportunity to share their experiences and find a solution to their problems. These interventions are frequently based on a cognitive–behavioral approach and include various elements as summarized in Table 4. They typically encompass 4–12 sessions with a maximum of 10–12 patients each. These interventions are operated on the basis of a structured agenda that focuses on the most prevalent issues of cancer patients and aim at initiating an active coping behavior.

7 Cancer Rehabilitation: A Multidisciplinary Task

Due to the multifaceted nature of cancer and its treatment, cancer rehabilitation requires a multidisciplinary team of healthcare professionals (Alfano et al. 2012; Hellbom et al. 2011; Ruppert et al. 2010). The interventions provided by these professionals in accordance with an individual patient's rehabilitation plan have to be coordinated by a member of the team who in most cases will be the rehabilitation physician. The multidisciplinary cancer rehabilitation team may thus include members from the following professions: oncology, psychology, nursing, nutritional counseling, physiotherapy and physical therapy, occupational therapy, art therapy (including music therapy, dance therapy, etc.), social work/vocational counseling as well as spiritual care. As a team, these professionals work together very closely, thus requiring a regularly based professional interchange in terms of multidisciplinary case conferences across the course of rehabilitation. In addition, external supervision will support the work of the multidisciplinary cancer rehabilitation team as a well-established instrument of quality assurance.

8 Evaluation of Cancer Rehabilitation

Cost-effectiveness has become a major issue in healthcare and rehabilitation services over the past years. As a consequence, evaluating the effectiveness and efficiency of rehabilitation in general and cancer rehabilitation in particular has also become a major field of research over the last three decades wherever healthcare systems are providing rehabilitation services. Efforts at addressing the effectiveness of rehabilitation services empirically may also be useful in providing a basis for attempts at implementing programs for quality assurance in rehabilitation settings.

Evaluation of cancer rehabilitation may be carried out at the level of single intervention module of which a rehabilitation program is made up and at the level of multicomponent programs as a whole. Thus, evaluation of cancer rehabilitation covers the whole spectrum from randomized controlled studies of specific interventions to health services research addressing the effects of established programs at more complex levels. However, while randomization may be easily performed when evaluating single interventions, randomization may be difficult to perform at the level of evaluation a program as a whole.

For the majority of the countries focused upon by Hellbom et al. (2011), studies on the effectiveness of rehabilitation interventions for cancer patients are available. However, these authors also support the assumption that the level of available evidence of the effectiveness of single interventions in rehabilitation settings varies —with largely positive results for interventions like relaxation training or psychosocial counseling, whereas evidence levels are lower for effects of interventions like, e.g., lymph drainage or art therapy (Weis and Domann 2006). Similarly, higher levels of evidence appear to be available for interventions targeting fatigue and physical exercise (Mishra et al. 2012; Puetz et al. 2012; Spelten et al. 2003; Spence et al. 2007; van Weert et al. 2005, 2006, 2010). With respect to the rehabilitation of patients with prostate cancer, however, Hergert et al. (2009) report rather limited evidence of the effectiveness of the majority of the interventions investigated by the studies they reviewed. As a consequence, these authors suggest additional and methodologically stronger research in this field of rehabilitation.

In Germany, efforts at establishing quality assurance and research programs in rehabilitation settings started in the 1980s. As a result, various means of quality assurance have been implemented (expert visitations of rehabilitation centers, expert reviews of discharge records and recommendations, and patient surveys) and are considered to be working successfully. In addition, these efforts will profit from the recent publication of clinical and practice guidelines for psychosocial cancer care (German Statutory Pension Insurance 2016; Guideline Program Oncology 2014; Reese et al. 2016).

Regarding the effectiveness of cancer rehabilitation at the program level earlier as well as more recent research in Germany provides evidence of patients improving with respect to health-related quality of life, subjective well-being, and physical functioning or symptoms (Bartsch et al. 2003; Heim et al. 2001; Krüger et al. 2009; Teichmann 2002; Weis and Domann 2006). In general, rehabilitation effects found for patients with cancer or other chronic conditions in Germany have been interpreted as clinically meaningful (Haaf 2005). That rehabilitation measures are cost-effective as well may probably also be assumed insofar as it can be shown that the costs for rehabilitation reach the break-even point if a person's retirement may be postponed for at least 4 months (German Statutory Pension Insurance Scheme 2015).

As a comparative study by Weis et al. (2006) showed, patients with non-metastatic breast cancer receiving rehabilitation differed from a group of comparable patients not planning to have rehabilitation by lower emotional functioning, higher psychosocial distress, and more disease-specific impairments. This was taken to indicate that processes of (adequate) referral by health professionals and self-selection by patients themselves were in operation as might have been expected in light of the objectives of rehabilitation. In addition, controlling for the influence of prior chemotherapy, Weis et al. (2006) found improvements in their patients with respect to health-related quality of life, anxiety, and depression as measured by the HADS, and in specific symptoms. When compared to the patients not attending cancer rehabilitation, effects of the factor "treatment/time of assessment" were mainly found to be of moderate size and higher for patients having received rehabilitation.

Although the available evidence thus suggests positive effects of cancer rehabilitation, there still are some unresolved issues and challenges to be addressed by future research (see also Stubblefield et al. 2013). One of these issues concerns the question whether the improvements reported for various outcome parameters during rehabilitation are sufficiently stable beyond discharge. In fact, some studies have reported a decrease in health-related quality of life or well-being after discharge and initial improvements—in some cases to even lower levels than those observed at admission (e.g., Weis et al. 2006). Consequently, further research is needed in order to clarify whether improvement or deterioration across time varies as a function of the demands of the rehabilitation program, the transfer of newly acquired skills to daily life, the disease, socio-demographic characteristics, and the patient's social and psychological status. Another issue, of course, is the fact that the majority of studies to date do not employ a randomized controlled design that alone would allow causal inferences. Therefore, setting up valid designs whenever randomized control is not feasible will continue to present a major challenge for researchers in the field of cancer rehabilitation who are interested in causal inferences. In addition, setting up a valid design in rehabilitation research implies the need to carefully select the variables of interest and operationalize them appropriately. These may be sampled from various domains of patient reported outcomes in terms of, e.g., quality of life and subjective well-being, or from biomedical or socioeconomic domains covering outcomes such as frequency of rehospitalization, survival, health behavior, healthcare costs, return to work, or others.

9 Summary and Outlook

This chapter presented a brief overview of some major features of cancer rehabilitation. The model of functional health as provided by the ICF served as a background for conceptualizing cancer rehabilitation as a system of coordinated efforts to overcome the functional impairments and activity limitations that have resulted from cancer and its treatment with the aim of restoring functional independence and participation of a patient at the highest possible level. Although countries obviously differ with respect to the way they organize cancer rehabilitation services, they widely share a consensus with respect to the goals of these services. Epidemiologic trends in cancer incidence and prevalence that have contributed to an increase in the importance of cancer rehabilitation thus far were described. It was further pointed out that cancer rehabilitation requires careful individual assessment and in the light of the multifaceted sequelae of cancer and its treatment is probably best provided by a multidisciplinary team. Next, a variety of interventions available to cancer rehabilitation were introduced. Finally, results from evaluation research on the effectiveness of cancer rehabilitation at the level of either single interventions or a rehabilitation program as a whole were discussed. This research suggests meaningful improvements of relevant outcome parameters like quality of life and functional status during the course of rehabilitation and there is also some evidence of cost-effectiveness. However, methodological challenges exist as well, e.g., with respect to the stability of improvements in the patients' quality of life, subjective well-being, and psychological status beyond rehabilitation and with respect to the feasibility of randomization. Nevertheless, future research in cancer rehabilitation will be able to effectively address issues like these and thus will continue to help refine and optimize cancer rehabilitation services. Furthermore, cancer rehabilitation will gain additional importance given the persistence of the epidemiologic trends illustrated in this chapter. Insofar as the utility of cancer rehabilitation programs could further be supported by empirical studies this would once more highlight that cancer rehabilitation serves both the individual patient and society as a whole.

References

Aaronson NK, Ahmedzai S, Bergman B, Bullinger M, Cull A, Duez NJ, Filiberti A, Flechtner H, Fleishman SB, de Haes JCJM, Kaasa S, Klee MC, Osoba D, Razavi D, Rofe PB, Schraub S, Sneeuw KCA, Sullivan M, Takeda F (1993) The European Organisation for Research and

Treatment of Cancer QLQ-C30: a quality-of-life instrument for use in international clinical trials in oncology. J Natl Cancer Inst 85:365–376

Alfano CM, Ganz PA, Rowland JH, Hahn EE (2012) Cancer survivorship and cancer rehabilitation: revitalizing the link. J Clin Oncol 30:904–906. doi:10.1200/JCO.2011.37. 1674

Antonovsky A (1993) The structure and properties of the sense of coherence scale. Soc Sci Med 36:725–733

Bartsch HH, Weis J, Moser M (2003) Cancer-related fatigue in patients attending oncological rehabilitation programs: prevalence, patterns and predictors. Onkologie 26:51–57

Baumann FT (2013) Physical exercise programs following cancer treatment. Eur Rev Aging Phys Act 10(1):57–59. doi:10.1007/s11556-012-0111-7

Beck AT, Steer RA, Ball R, Ranieri W (1996) Comparison of Beck Depression Inventories -IA and -II in psychiatric outpatients. J Pers Assess 67(3):588–597

Becker S, Kirchberger I, Cieza A, Berghaus A, Harréus U, Reichel O, Tschiesner U (2010) Content validation of the comprehensive ICF core set for head and neck cancer (HNC): the perspective of psychologists. Psychooncology 19:594–605. doi:10.1002/pon.1608

Bengel J, Wirtz M, Zwingmann C (2008) Diagnostische Verfahren in der Rehabilitation. (Diagnostik für Klinik und Praxis – Band 5). Hogrefe, Göttingen

Bergelt C, Koch U (2002) Rehabilitation bei Tumorpatienten In Schwarzer R, Jerusalem M, Weber H Gesundheitspsychologie von A – Z. Hogrefe, Göttingen, pp 455–458

Bjelland I, Dahl AA, Haug TT, Neckelmann D (2002) The validity of the Hospital anxiety and depression scale. an updated literature review. J Psychosom Res 52(2):69–77

Bornbaum CC, Doyle PC, Skarakis-Doyle E, Theurer JA (2013) A critical exploration of the international classification of functioning, disability, and health (ICF) framework from the perspective of oncology: recommendations for revision. J Multidiscip Healthc 6:75–686. doi:10.2147/JMDH.S40020

Brach M, Cieza A, Stucki G, Füßl M, Cole A, Ellerin B, Fialka-Moser V, Kostanjsek N, Melvin J (2004) ICF core sets for breast cancer. J. Rehabil Med Suppl. 44:121–127

Bray F, Jemal A, Grey N, Ferlay J, Forman D (2012) Global cancer transitions according to the Human Development Index (2008–2030): a population-based study. Lancet Oncol 13:790–801. doi:10.1016/S1470-2045(12)70211-5

Cancer Research UK (2014) World Cancer fact sheet. World Cancer burden (2012). http://publications.cancerresearchuk.org/downloads/Product/CS_REPORT_WORLD.pdf. Accessed Jan 21 2017)

Carver CS, Scheier MF, Weintraub JK (1989) Assessing coping strategies: a theoretically based approach. J Pers Soc Psychol 56:267–283

Derogatis LR, Melisaratos N (1983) The brief symptom inventory: an introductory report. Psychol Med 13(3):595–605

Derogatis LR, Savitz KL (1999) The SCL-90-R, brief symptom inventory, and matching clinical rating scales. In Maruish ME (ed) The use of psychological testing for treatment planning and outcome assessment, 2nd edn. Erlbaum, Mahwah, pp 679–724

Du S, Hu L, Dong J, Xu G, Jin S, Zhang H, Yin H (2015) Patient education programs for cancer-related fatigue: a systematic review. Patient Educ Couns 98(11):1308–1319

Edwards AG, Hulbert-Williams N, Neal RD (2008) Psychological interventions for women with metastatic breast cancer. Cochrane Database Syst Rev 16: CD004253. doi:10.1002/14651858. CD004253.pub3

Ercoli LM, Petersen L, Hunter AM (2015) Cognitive rehabilitation group intervention for breast cancer survivors: results of a randomized clinical trial. Psycho-Oncology 24:1360–1367. doi:10.1002/pon.3769

Eriksson M, Lindström B (2006) Antonovsky's sense of coherence scale and the relation with health: a systematic review. J Epidemiol Community Health 60(5):376–381

Ervik M, Lam F, Ferlay J, Mery L, Soerjomataram I, Bray F (2016) Cancer today. Lyon, France: International Agency for Research on Cancer. Cancer Today. Available from http://gco.iarc.fr/today. Accessed Jan 21 2017

Faller H, Schuler M, Richard M, Heckl U, Weis J, Küffner R (2013) Effects of psycho-oncologic interventions on emotional distress and quality of life in adult patients with cancer: systematic review and meta-analysis. J Clin Oncol 31(6):782–793. doi:10.1200/JCO.2011.40.8922

Ferlay J, Soerjomataram I, Dikshit R, Eser S, Mathers C, Rebelo M, Parkin DM, Forman D, Bray F (2015) Cancer incidence and mortality worldwide: sources, methods and major patterns in GLOBOCAN 2012. Int J Cancer 136(5):E359–E386. doi:10.1002/ijc.29210

Fialka-Moser V, Crevenna R, Korpan M, Quittan M (2003) Cancer rehabilitation. Particularly with aspects on physical impairment. J Rehabil Med 35:153–162

Folkman S (2013) Ways of coping checklist (WCCL). In: Gellman MD, Turner JR (eds) Encyclopedia of behavioral medicine. Springer, New York, p 2041–2042

Gamble GL, Gerber LH, Spill GR, Paul KL (2011) The future of cancer rehabilitation: emerging subspecialty. Am J Phys Med Rehabil 90(5 Suppl 1):S76–S87. doi:10.1097/PHM. 0b013e31820be0d1

Ganz PA, Schag CA, Lee JJ, Sim MS (1992) The CARES: a generic measure of health-related quality of life for patients with cancer. Qual Life Res 1:19–29

Gerber L (2001) Cancer rehabilitation in the future. Cancer 92, 4 (Suppl.):975–979

Gerber L, Vargo M, Smith R (2005) Rehabilitation of the cancer patient. In: DeVita V et al (eds) Cancer: principles and practice of oncology, 7th edn. Lippincott William Philadelphia, pp 3089–3110

German Institute of Medical Documentation and Information (2005) Internationale Klassifikation der Funktionsfähigkeit. Behinderung und Gesundheit, WHO, Geneva

German Statutory Pension Insurance (2015) Reha-Bericht 2015. Die medizinische und berufliche Rehabilitation der Rentenversicherung im Licht der Statistik. DRV Bund, Berlin

German Statutory Pension Insurance (2016) Reha-Therapiestandards Brustkrebs. DRV Bund, Berlin

Gilchrist LS, Galantino ML, Wampler M, Marchese VG, Morris GS, Ness KK (2009) A framework for assessment in oncology rehabilitation. Phys Ther 89:286–306. doi:10.2522/ptj. 20070309

Glaessel A, Kirchberger I, Stucki G, Cieza A (2011) Does the comprehensive international classification of functioning, disability and health (ICF) core set for breast cancer capture the problems in functioning treated by physiotherapists in women with breast cancer? Physiotherapy 97:33–46. doi:10.1016/j.physio.2010.08.010

Guideline Program Oncology (German Cancer Society. German Cancer Aid, Association of the Scientific Medical Societies in Germany) (2014) Psychoonkologische Diagnostik, Beratung und Behandlung von erwachsenen Krebspatienten, Langversion 1.1, 2014, AWMF-Registernummer: 032/051OL. http://leitlinienprogramm-onkologie.de/Leitlinien.7.0. html. Accessed 21 Jan 2017

Haaf HG (2005) Ergebnisse zur Wirksamkeit der Rehabilitation. Rehabilitation 44:259–276 (English abstract)

Heim ME, Kunert S, Ozkan I (2001) Effects of inpatient rehabilitation on health-related quality of life in breast cancer patients. Onkologie 24:268–272

Hellbom M, Bergelt C, Bergenmar M, Gijsen B, Loge JH, Rautalahti M, Smaradottir A, Johansen C (2011) Cancer rehabilitation: a Nordic and European perspective. Acta Oncol 50:179–186. doi:10.3109/0284186X.2010.533194

Hergert A, Hofreuter K, Melchior H, Morfeld M, Schulz H, Watzke B, Koch U, Bergelt C (2009) Effektivität von Interventionen in der Rehabilitation bei Prostatakarzinompatienten – Ein systematischer Literaturüberblick. Phys Med Rehab Kuror 19:311–325

Holland JC, Bultz BD, National comprehensive Cancer Network (NCCN) (2007) The NCCN guideline for distress management: a case for making distress the sixth vital sign. J Natl Compr Canc Netw 5(1):3-7

Holland JC, Breitbart WS, Jacobson PB, Loscalzo MJ, McCorkle R, Butow PN (eds) (2015) Psycho-oncology, 3rd edn. Oxford University Press, New York

Hunt SM, McKenna SP, McEwen J, Williams J, Papp E (1981) The Nottingham health profile: subjective health status and medical consultations. Soc Sci Med A 15(3 Pt 1):221–229

Kerns RD, Turk DC, Rudy TE (1985) The West Haven-Yale multidimensional pain inventory (WHYMPI). Pain 23(4):345–356

Khan F, Amatya B, Ng L, Demetrios M, Pallant JF (2012) Relevance and completeness of the international classification of functioning, disability and health (ICF) comprehensive breast cancer core set: the patient perspective in an Australian community cohort. J Rehabil Med 44 (7):570–580. doi:10.2340/16501977-0972

Kirschneck M, Sabariego C, Singer S, Tschiesner U (2014) Assessment of functional outcomes in patients with head and neck cancer according to the international classification of functioning, disability and health core sets from the perspective of the multi-professional team: results of 4 Delphi surveys. Head Neck 36(7):954–968. doi:10.1002/hed.23399

Klauer T, Filipp SH (1993) Trierer Skalen zur Krankheitsbewältigung, 1st edn. Göttingen, Hogrefe

Koch U, Morfeld M (2004) Weiterentwicklungsmöglichkeiten der ambulanten Rehabilitation in Deutschland. Rehabiitation 43(5):284–95. (English abstract)

Koch U, Gundelach C, Tiemann F, Mehnert A (2000) Teilstationaere onkologische Rehabilitation – Ergebnisse eines Modellprojektes. Rehabilitation 39:363–372 (English abstract)

Kohlmann T, Bullinger M, Kirchberger-Blumstein I (1997) German version of the Nottingham Health Profile (NHP): translation and psychometric validation. Soz Präventivmed 42:175–185. doi:10.1007/BF01300568

Krüger A, Leibbrand B, Barth J, Berger D, Lehmann C, Koch U, Mehnert A (2009) Verlauf der psychosozialen Belastung und gesundheitsbezogenen Lebensqualität bei Patienten verschiedener Altersgruppen in der onkologischen Rehabilitation. Z Psychosom Med Psychother 55:141–161 (English abstract)

Leib A, Cieza A, Tschiesner U (2012) Perspective of physicians within a multidisciplinary team: content validation of the comprehensive ICF core set for head and neck cancer. Head Neck 34:956–966. doi:10.1002/hed.21844

Lundin A, Hallgren M, Theobald H, Hellgren C, Torgén M (2016) Validity of the 12-item version of the General Health Questionnaire in detecting depression in the general population. Public Health 136:66–74. doi:10.1016/j.puhe.2016.03.005

Merluzzi TV, Nairn RC, Hegde K, Martinez Sanchez MA, Dunn L (2001) Self-efficacy for coping with cancer: revision of the cancer behavior inventory (version 2.0). Psychooncology 10 (3):206–217

Meyer T, Gutenbrunner C, Bickenbach J, Cieza A, Melvin J, Stucki G (2011) Towards a conceptual description of rehabilitation as a health strategy. J Rehabil Med 43:765–769. doi:10. 2340/16501977-0865

Mishra SI, Scherer RW, Geigle PM, Berlanstein DR, Topaloglu O, Gotay CC, Snyder C (2012) Exercise interventions on health-related quality of life for cancer survivors. Cochrane Database Syst Rev 8: CD007566. doi:10.1002/14651858.CD007566.pub2

Mitchell AJ (2007) Pooled results from 38 analyses of the accuracy of distress thermometer and other ultra-short methods of detecting cancer-related mood disorders. J Clin Oncol 25:4670–4681

Morfeld M, Kirchberger I, Bullinger M (2011) SF-36. Fragebogen zum Gesundheitszustand. 2., ergänzte und überarbeitete Auflage 2011. Hogrefe, Göttingen

Moss-Morris R, Weinman J, Petrie KJ, Horne R, Cameron LD, Buick D (2002) The revised illness perception questionnaire (IPQ-R). Psychol Health 17:1–16

Mpofu E, Oakland T (eds) (2010) Rehabilitation and health assessment: applying ICF guidelines. Springer, New York

Muthny FA (1989) Freiburger Fragebogen zur Krankheitsverarbeitung, 1st edn. Weinheim, Beltz

Newell SA, Sanson-Fisher RW, Savolainen NJ (2002) Systematic review of psychological therapies for cancer patients: overview and recommendation for future research. J Natl Cancer Inst 94:558–584

Oeffinger KC, McCabe MS (2006) Models for delivering survivorship care. J Clin Oncol 24:5117–5124

Ong ASJ, Ward C (2005) The construction and validation of a social support measure for sojourners: the Index of Sojourner Social Support (ISSS) scale. J Cross Cult Psychol 36:637–661

Puetz TW, Herring MP (2012) Differential effects of exercise on cancer-related fatigue during and following treatment: a meta-analysis. Am J Prev Med 43:e1–e24. doi:10.1016/j.amepre.2012.04.027

Reese C, Weis J, Schmucker D, Mittag O (2016) Development of practice guidelines for psychological interventions in the rehabilitation of patients with oncological disease (breast, prostate, or colorectal cancer): Methods and results. Psychooncology. doi:10.1002/pon.4322. [Epub ahead of print]

Reichel C, Oehler, G, Burghardt W (2013) Ernährungsmedizin in der Gastroenterologie. In Ernährungsmedizin in der Rehabilitation, Deutsche Rentenversicherung Bund, Abteilung Rehabilitation, ed. (Berlin): 1–217

Ruppert LM Stubblefield MD Stiles J Passik SD (2010) Rehabilitation medicine in Oncology. In: Holland JC Breitbart WS, Jacobson PB, Lederberg MS, Loscalzo MJ, McCorkle R (eds) Psycho-oncology, 2nd edn. Oxford University Press, New York, pp 460–463

Salz T, Oeffinger KC, McCabe MS, Layne TM, Bach PB (2012) Survivorship care plans in research and practice. CA Cancer J Clin. doi:10.3322/caac.20142

Schag CA, Ganz PA, Heinrich RL (1991) Cancer rehabilitation evaluation system–short form (CARES-SF). A cancer specific rehabilitation and quality of life instrument. Cancer 68:1406–1413

Spelten ER, Verbeek JH, Uitterhoeve AL, Ansink AC, van der Lelie J, de Reijke TM, Kammeijer M, de Haes JC, Sprangers MA (2003) Cancer, fatigue and the return of patients to work-a prospective cohort study. Eur J Cancer 39:1562–1567

Spence RR, Heesch KC, Eakin EG, Brown WJ (2007) Randomised controlled trial of a supervised exercise rehabilitation program for colorectal cancer survivors immediately after chemotherapy: study protocol. BMC Cancer 7:154

Stout NL, Binkley JM, Schmitz KH, Andrews K, Hayes SC, Campbell KL, McNeely ML, Soballe PW, Berger AM, Cheville AL, Fabian C, Gerber LH, Harris SR, Johansson K, Pusic AL, Prosnitz RG, Smith RA (2012) A prospective surveillance model for rehabilitation for women with breast cancer. Cancer 118:2191–2200. doi:10.1002/cncr.27476

Stubblefield MD, O'Dell MW (eds) (2009) Cancer rehabilitation: principles and practice. Demos Medical Publishing, New York

Stubblefield MD, Hubbard G, Cheville A, Koch U, Schmitz KH, Dalton SO (2013) Current perspectives and emerging issues on cancer rehabilitation. Cancer 119(Suppl 11):2170–2178. doi:10.1002/cncr.28059

Tait RC, Pollard CA, Margolis RB, Duckro PN, Krause SJ (1987) The pain disability index: psychometric and validity data. Arch Phys Med Rehabil 68(7):438–441

Teichmann JV (2002) Onkologische Rehabilitation: Evaluation der Effektivität stationärer onkologischer Reha-Maßnahmen. Die Rehabilitation 41:48–52 (English abstract)

Tschiesner U, Rogers S, Dietz A, Yueh B, Cieza A (2010) Development of ICF core sets for head and neck cancer. Head Neck 32:210–220. doi:10.1002/hed.21172

Tschiesner U, Oberhauser C, Cieza A (2011) ICF Core Set for head and neck cancer: do the categories discriminate among clinically relevant subgroups of patients? Int J Rehabil Res 34 (2):121–130. doi:10.1097/MRR.0b013e328343d4bc

Ullrich A, Mehnert A (2010) Psychometrische Evaluation und Validierung einer 8-Item-Kurzversion der Skalen zur Sozialen Unterstützung bei Krankheit (SSUK) bei Krebspatienten. Klin Diagn Eval 3(4):259–381 van Weert E, Hoekstra-Weebers J, Grol B, Otter R, Arendzen HJ, Postema K, Sanderman R, van der Schans C (2005) A multidimensional cancer rehabilitation program for cancer survivors: effectiveness on health-related quality of life. J Psychosom Res 58(6):485–496

van Weert E, Hoekstra-Weebers J, Otter R, Postema K, Sanderman R, van der Schans C (2006) Cancer-related fatigue: predictors and effects of rehabilitation. Oncologist 11:184–196

van Weert E, May AM, Korstjens I, Post WJ, van der Schans CP, van den Borne B, Mesters I, Ros WJ, Hoekstra-Weebers JE (2010) Cancer-related fatigue and rehabilitation: a randomized controlled multicenter trial comparing physical training combined with cognitive-behavioral therapy with physical training only and with no intervention. Phys Ther 90(10):1413–1425. doi:10.2522/ptj.20090212. Epub 2010 Jul 22. Erratum in: Phys Ther. 2010 Dec; 90(12):1906

Wallston KA, Wallston BS, DeVellis R (1978) Development of the multidimensional health locus of control (MHLC) scales. Health Education Monographs 6:160–170

Ware JE, Kosinski M, Keller SK (1994) SF-36 physical and mental health summary scales: a user's manual. The Health Institute, Boston

Webster K, Cella D, Yost K (2003) The functional assessment of chronic illness therapy (FACIT) measurement system: properties, applications, and interpretation. Health Qual Life Outcomes 1:79

Weis J, Domann U (2006) Interventionen in der Rehabilitation von Mammakarzinompatientinnen: Eine methodenkritische Uebersicht zum Forschungsstand. Rehabilitation 45:129–142 (English abstract)

Weis J, Moser MT, Bartsch HH (2006) Goal-oriented evaluation of inpatient rehabilitation programs for women with breast cancer (*ZESOR* –Study). In: Jäckel W, Bengel J, Herdt J (eds) Research in rehabilitation: results of a research network in Southwest Germany. Schattauer Verlag, Stuttgart, pp 162–171

WHO (1981) Disability prevention and rehabilitation. Report of the WHO expert committee on disability prevention and rehabilitation. Technical report series 668. WHO, Geneva

WHO (2001) International classification of functioning, disability and health. WHO, Geneva

Zigmond AS, Snaith RP (1983) The hospital anxiety and depression scale. Acta Psychiatr Scand 67(6):361–370. doi:10.1111/j.1600-0447.1983.tb09716.x

Cancer Survivorship in Adults

Cecilie E. Kiserud, Alv A. Dahl and Sophie D. Fosså

Abstract

With the favorable trend regarding survival of cancer in the Western world, there is an increasing focus among patients, clinicians, researchers, and politicians regarding cancer survivors' health and well-being. The number of survivors grows rapidly, and more than 3% of the adult populations in Western countries have survived cancer for 5 years or more. Cancer survivors are at increased risk for a variety of late effects after treatment, some life-threatening such as secondary cancer and cardiac diseases, while others mainly have negative impact on daily functioning and health-related quality of life (HRQOL). The latter factors include fatigue, anxiety disorders, sexual problems, insomnia, and reduced work ability, while depression does not seem to be more common among survivors than in the general population. Life style factors are highly relevant for cancer survivors concerning risk of relapse and somatic comorbidity. The field of cancer survivorship research has grown rapidly. How to best integrate the knowledge of the field into clinical practice with adequate follow-up of cancer survivors at risk for developing late effects, is still an unresolved question, although several models are under consideration.

Keywords

Cancer survivorship · Adults · Somatic late effects · Psychosocial late effects

C.E. Kiserud · A.A. Dahl · S.D. Fosså (✉)
National Advisory Unit for Late Effects After Cancer Treatment, Oslo University Hospital, The Norwegian Radium Hospital, Postbox 4953, 0424 Nydalen, Oslo, Norway
e-mail: s.d.fossa@medisin.uio.no; sdf@ous-hf.no

C.E. Kiserud
e-mail: CKK@ous-hf.no

A.A. Dahl
e-mail: a.a.dahl@ibv.uio.no

© Springer International Publishing AG 2018
U. Goerling and A. Mehnert (eds.), *Psycho-Oncology*, Recent Results in Cancer Research 210, https://doi.org/10.1007/978-3-319-64310-6_8

1 General Aspects

The number of cancer survivors has been steadily increasing in the Western world during the past decades due to increasing cancer incidence, better diagnostic procedures, and more effective treatment modalities. Today the relative 5-year survival is 60–65% for patients diagnosed with cancer (American Cancer Society 2015). In Norway cancer survivors who are alive ≥ 5 years from diagnosis represent about 3% of the total population (The Cancer Registry of Norway 2015). For some cancer types such as testicular cancer, breast cancer, and Hodgkin's lymphoma, the 5-year relative survival exceeds 90%. According to cancer types, the most common survivor groups concern female breast, prostate, colorectal, and gynecologic cancer (American Cancer Society 2015).

Cancer survivorship is defined differently according to time since diagnosis and state of the tumor, but for this chapter we define cancer survivors as persons who have lived at least 5 year beyond diagnosis and are regarded as tumor free.

The favorable development of survival after cancer diagnoses has been followed by a growing clinical and scientific interest concerning health and HRQOL among cancer survivors.

Chemotherapy, radiotherapy, surgery, and hormone therapies are the mainstay of cancer treatments, and they are often combined as various multimodal treatments. Adverse effects may occur during these treatments, and eventually they continue for a long time after treatment or become permanent. Other adverse effects have their onset some time after the treatment has been terminated, but then continue for a long time. Thus, cancer survivors are at increased risk of various medical and psychosocial complications (Fossa et al. 2008, Fosså et al. 2008). Some late effects might be life-threatening, such as second cancer or cardiovascular disorders, while others such as hypogonadism, infertility, sexual dysfunctions, or chronic fatigue might have negative impact of the survivors' daily function and HRQOL, but do not threaten their lives.

A challenge related to studies of late adverse effects is that some of them like second cancer and cardiovascular diseases, typically emerge many years after the termination of treatment. Results of such studies might not completely reflect the risk experienced by patients diagnosed today, since the therapies of today have been modified compared to those used 10–20 years ago. Therefore, the studies of late effects by its nature most often lag behind the treatments currently given. Concerning new and improved treatments, we will have to wait 10–30 years in order to identify their late adverse effects.

Many of the conditions described as late effects like sexual dysfunctions, cardiovascular diseases and chronic fatigue, are also prevalent in the general population. The prevalence of these conditions increase with older age anyhow. Since two-third of cancers is diagnosed after 60 years of age, it is important to study if the prevalence among cancer survivors is significantly higher than in the general population.

The goals of survivorship care are twofold: (1) To reduce the risk of cancer recurrence, second cancer, comorbid severe diseases and adverse effects. (2) To alleviate existing and expected physical and psychological adverse effects. These goals have several challenging implications: (1) To what extent shall cured cancer patients be informed of risks far in the future? (2) How often and how intensively shall survivors be screened for possibly upcoming severe adverse effects? (3) Considering the rapidly growing number of cancer survivors, how shall their health care be organized? To our knowledge, there are no countries yet that have found the definite answers to these challenges.

In this chapter we will give an overview of the field of cancer survivorship, including the most important somatic, psychological, and psychosocial late effects and aspects regarding follow-care of cancer survivors and challenges for research in survivorship issues.

2 Somatic Late Effects

Approximately 15% of cancer survivors will be bothered with treatment-related somatic late effects.

2.1 Second Cancer

Cancer survivors have an increased risk for development of a second cancer, which might be related to an iatrogenic effect of the cancer therapy and/or a genetic predisposition (Curtis et al. 2006). Treatment-related solid second cancers are usually diagnosed at a latency of 10–30 years after radiotherapy, and their development is related to the radiation dose within the target field, but also to scattered irradiation beyond the field borders. A typical example is development of breast cancer after mediastinal irradiation/mantle field irradiation for Hodgkin's lymphoma (Swerdlow et al. 2000), esophageal cancer after thoracic radiotherapy in women with breast cancer (Morton et al. 2014) and pancreatic cancer after radiotherapy for testicular cancer (Hauptman et al. 2016).

During the past two decades increasing documentation has emerged that cytotoxic drugs in a dose-dependent manner are carcinogenic leading to an increased risk of leukemia (Travis et al. 1999; Kollmannsberger et al. 1998), but also of solid tumors (Swerdlow et al. 2001; Fung et al. 2013; Kier et al. 2016).

The association between second cancer and cytotoxic treatment (radiotherapy, cytostatics) has been one of the strongest arguments for the development of risk-adapted strategies in order to reduce the treatment burden and adverse health outcomes as much as possible, while maintaining the highest possible cure rate.

2.2 Cardiotoxicity

Dependent of their previous treatment, long-term cancer survivors may develop asymptomatic or symptomatic left ventricular dysfunction, heart failure, premature coronary atherosclerosis, arrhythmia and/or sudden cardiac death, most often due to myocardial infarction (Lenihan et al. 2013; Zamorano et al. 2016). Mediastinal radiotherapy and treatment with certain cytotoxic drugs (antracyclines, trastuzumab) represent well-known cardiotoxic risk factors, with clear dose-effect associations to cardiac dysfunction.

Age below 15 years at primary treatment also increases the risk of cardiac morbidity. Increased risk of late cardiotoxicity (after 5–30 years) has also been reported in breast cancer survivors who have undergone adjuvant cytotoxic treatment (thoracic radiotherapy, systemic cytostatics) (Darby et al. 2013). The European Society of Medical Oncology and the European Society of Cardiology have recently published recommendations regarding cardiovascular toxicity of cancer treatments (Curigliano et al. 2012; Zamorano et al. 2016). However, currently there is no international consensus about the optimal procedure for early detection or follow-up of increased risk of cardiotoxicity among cancer survivors.

In addition to direct cardiac injury due to cytotoxic treatment, the development of metabolic syndrome (overweight, hyperlipidemia, hypertension, hyperglucosuria) represents a risk for heart disease. This syndrome has been described in long-term testicular (Haugnes et al. 2010) and among ovarian cancer survivors after cisplatin-based chemotherapy (Liavaag et al. 2009). Metabolic syndrome is also responsible for the increased risk of cardiac mortality in prostate cancer survivors, in particular after long-term androgen deprivation therapy (Kenney et al. 2012). Survivors at risk should, therefore, be educated about the importance of a healthy life style (physical activity, healthy diet, no smoking, and moderate use of alcohol) (see also below).

2.3 Gonadal Dysfunction and Infertility

Both surgery, radiotherapy, chemotherapy, and long-term hormone treatment can lead to primary or secondary hypogonadism dependent on whether the damage primarily affects the testicles/ovaries or the pituitary gland/hypothalamus (Lee et al. 2006). In addition, the transport of the ova or the sperm cells may be impeded by fibrosis or stenosis of the ducts because of surgery or radiotherapy.

There are important sex-related differences as to development, prevention, and possible therapy of treatment-related hypogonadism in cancer survivors. After low or intermediate doses of most cytotoxic drugs or after testicular irradiation of less than 2 Gy, the sperm cell production can recover as long as spermatogonial stem cells are preserved. The testosterone producing Leydig cells are relatively resistant to chemotherapy and radiotherapy. Severe endocrine hypogonadism is, therefore, rare after cancer treatment in males. However, clinicians should keep in mind that long-term cancer survivors' testosterone production appears to decrease faster than observed during the physiological aging of the general male population.

The recovery of gonadal function is different in female survivors. At birth the ovaries contain approximately 10 million follicles. This number decreases with aging up to menopause without replacement of the follicles lost each month. After radiotherapy and chemotherapy the loss of follicles is accelerated. As no recovery is possible, female survivors are at risk of premature ovarian failure (menopause before the age of 40).

Treatment of endocrine gonadal failure is based on the application of testosterone or estrogens, however, with important contraindications in survivors after prostate- and breast cancer. Prevention is the best way to limit infertility problems in cancer survivors. Updated guidelines are published constantly (Kenney et al. 2012; Metzger et al. 2013). Pre-treatment sperm cell cryopreservation has been used for many years in adult male cancer patients, but is problematic in pre-pubertal boys. Pre-treatment ovarian or testicular tissue cryo-conservation is still experimental, but reimplantation of thawed ovarian tissue has been followed by pregnancies in a few cancer survivors.

Compared to the general population overall pregnancy rates after adult-onset cancer are decreased by 26% in male and by 39% in female cancer survivors. After implementation of risk-adapted cancer therapy, this discrepancy has been reduced for selected cancer types during the past three decades (e.g., in testicular cancer survivors and male survivors after Hodgkin's lymphoma) (Stensheim et al. 2011).

2.4 Peripheral Neuropathy

One of the most common late effects (20–30%) is peripheral neuropathy caused by chemotherapy containing vinca alkaloids, cisplatin, or taxanes (Windebank and Grisold 2008; Hershman et al. 2014). For some survivors the complaints are limited to numbness of the soles of the feet, whereas others suffer from pain in their legs that might cause severe sleeping problems. In addition cisplatin is ototoxic and can lead to tinnitus and hearing loss (Brydøy et al. 2009; Oldenburg et al. 2007). Though the latter toxicity most often is restricted to decibel frequencies of >4000 Hz, severe ototoxicity might have negative impact on survivors' social and professional life.

2.5 Muscular and Skeletal Effects

As proliferating cells are particularly sensitive to any cytotoxic treatment, radiotherapy to the skeleton and muscles in young adults can be followed by severe muscle atrophy and retarded growth of bones. The negative impact of the target dose is increased by chemotherapy with radiosensitizing drugs (Actionmycin D, Antracyclines, Cisplatin) often applied as a part of multimodal therapy.

In breast cancer survivors reduced function of the ipsilateral arm/shoulder, pain and/or lymphoedema have represented frequent complaints, but the incidence of these late effects has been reduced after the introduction of breast conserving surgery and improved radiotherapy techniques (Nesvold et al. 2011).

Osteoporosis related to male and female endocrine hypogonadism may become a problem in all cancer survivors (Lustberg et al. 2012). Prostate cancer and breast cancer survivors are at particular high risk of developing this late effect, as complete intermittent or permanent hypogonadism is an important part of their treatment. Today several drugs are available which together with Vitamin D, calcium application, and physical activity reduce the risk of osteoporosis by nonhormonal mechanisms (Zolendronic acid, Denusomab).

3 Fatigue

Fatigue is defined as a subjective experience of tiredness, exhaustion and lack of energy (Radbruch et al. 2008). Formal diagnostic criteria for "cancer-related fatigue" as a syndrome was proposed in 1998, but has attracted relatively little attention in the scientific community (Donovan et al. 2013). In this context fatigue is regarded as a symptom.

For most cancer survivors, fatigue is experienced as an adverse effect during treatment and resolves by recovery from therapy, which can be conceptualized as *acute fatigue*. However, for many survivors, fatigue may persist for years after completed cancer therapy and without any signs of active disease. The term *chronic fatigue*, defined as fatigue lasting for 6 months or more or after the triggering stimulus has ended, differentiates between acute fatigue as part of everyday strains (such as acute infections) psychosocial strains, and the feeling of being chronically exhausted. That distinction is supported by the fact that chronic fatigue is reported by 12% of the general population, and the prevalence increases with older age (Loge et al. 1998).

The prevalence of fatigue among cancer survivors vary by assessment method, cancer type and definitions, but most prevalence figures vary between 19 and 38% (Stone and Minton 2008). Survivors of Hodgkin lymphoma and breast cancer are mostly studied. Chronic fatigue is also common among long-term survivors of childhood and adolescence cancers (Hamre et al. 2013). Fatigue is, therefore, probably the most common late effect across all cancer survivors. A study of long-term survivors of testicular cancer showed a positive association between increased time since primary treatment and increased prevalence of chronic fatigue (Sprauten et al. 2015).

The present knowledge about the etiology and pathogenetic mechanisms of fatigue among disease-free cancer survivors is limited (La Voy et al. 2016). That any single mechanism could be identified is unlikely, since fatigue is multifactorial in origin involving both physical and psychological factors. Psychological distress, pain, sleep disturbance, depression, anxiety, physical inactivity, late medical effects, inflammation, and anemia have all been associated with chronic fatigue. Except for anemia, all these etiological factors are relevant in relation to chronic fatigue among cancer survivors.

Interventions to improve chronic fatigue among cancer survivors broadly fall into three categories; drugs, physical exercise, and/or psychosocial interventions (Stone and Minton 2008). An update of a 2008 Cochrane review on drug therapy concluded that psychostimulants are promising, but large scaled randomized controlled trials (RCTs) are warranted (Minton et al. 2010). However, many of the reviewed studies included cancer patients with active disease, and the administration of psychostimulants to disease-free cancer survivors has negative ethical and legal aspects. Exercise interventions, mostly consisting of graded aerobic physical exercises, have slight to moderate positive effects on chronic fatigue among cancer patients in general (Cramp and Daniel 2008). The strongest effects have been observed among cancer survivors, but optimal type, amount and timing of interventions need to be identified.

Psychosocial interventions include education, coping strategy training, behavioral therapy, cognitive therapy, and supportive therapy. These interventions have slight to moderate effects (Pachman et al. 2012). Education about fatigue, teaching self-care, energy conservation, and activity management are easily applicable in ordinary clinical contexts. Combination of sleep regulation focusing on nighttime sleep, rest without sleeping during daytime, and graded physical exercise, are the best documented interventions that are applicable in ordinary clinical practice.

4 Depression and Anxiety

4.1 Depression

Longitudinal studies of depression and anxiety after cancer diagnosis suggest that the high intial prevalence falls slowly over time. A systematic review showed that the prevalence of depression in long-term cancer survivors was similar to that of healthy controls. Interestingly, the prevalence of depressed spouses of cancer survivors was similar to that of survivors (Mitchell et al. 2013a, b). Insomnia is regularly associated with depression and a review reported that these two symptoms were associated with increased mortality risk of cancer (Irwin 2013). Although depression in cancer survivors can be treated with antidepressants and various brief psychotherapies, a review and meta-analysis also supported mindfulness-based therapy (Piet et al. 2012). In fact, exercise under supervision away from home and with a duration of at least 30 min per day, had a significant effect on cancer survivors in a randomized controlled trial (Craft et al. 2012).

4.2 Anxiety

In contrast, the risk of anxiety disorders is significantly higher among cancer survivors than among healthy controls. Anxiety is reported to be as common in their
spouses as in cancer survivors (Mitchell et al. 2013a). Within the time frame of
10 years since diagnosis, anxiety shows a more persistent pattern than depression.
The distribution of anxiety disorders among cancer survivors did not differ from
that of the general population (Greer et al 2011). In general, presence of anxiety has
a negative effect on HRQOL. The common factor may be distressed (type D)
personality, which is the conjoint effect of negative affectivity and social inhibition.
The prevalence of type D personality among cancer survivors (19%) is similar to
the general population (13–24%), but such survivors are at increased risk for
impaired HRQOL and mental health problems (Mols et al. 2012).

4.3 Fear of Recurrence

Recently, more empirical studies have addressed fear of recurrence among cancer
survivors. Although defined in various ways, increasingly consensus focuses on a
fear that cancer could return or progress in the same place or in another part of the
body (Simonelli et al. 2016). Various definitions have lead to multiple self-report
measures for assessment of fear of recurrence without any international recommendations so far (Thewes et al. 2012). This situation may also explain the wide
range of prevalences reported. According to the review of Simard et al. (2013)
based on 130 papers, across cancer sites, 39–97% of cancer survivors reported fear
of recurrence, 22–87% reported moderate to high degree, and 0–15% high degree
of such fear. Fear of recurrence seems to remain stable over time, even if the
objective risk of recurrence decreases as time goes on. This finding points to the
element of irrationality in fear of recurrence that is common to all kinds of
pathological anxiety.

The most consistent predictor of elevated fear of recurrence is younger age.
There is also strong evidence for an association between physical symptoms and
such fear. Additional factors moderately associated with increased fear of recurrence include treatment type, low optimism, family stressors, and fewer significant
others. For socio-demographic factors inconsistent evidence was observed (Crist
and Grunfeld 2013).

Fear of recurrence seems to be a problem even in long-term cancer survivors
among whom the risk of recurrence is minimal. Lower level of education and lower
level of optimism were found to be associated with higher levels of fear of recurrence. Significant negative associations were reported between fear of recurrence
and HRQOL as well as psychosocial well-being (Koch et al. 2013).

4.4 Posttraumatic Stress Disorder (PTSD)

PTSD is a mental disorder caused by exposure to a life-threatening event either personally or as a bystander. Since 1994 the American DSM-IV classification of mental disorders, "being diagnosed with a life-threatening illness" has been defined as such a potentially traumatic event (American Psychiatric Association 1994), and studies of PTSD among cancer patients have flourished since then. However, in 2013 the DSM-5 omitted "being diagnosed with a life-threatening illness" as such an event (American Psychiatric Association 2013). Neither does the World Health Organization's ICD-10 classification include life-threatening disease as a potentially traumatic event (World Health Organization 1993). Therefore, both DSM-5 and ICD-10 preclude getting cancer as a sufficient trauma for the development of PTSD. Some of these problems are discussed by Dahl et al. (2016b).

However, independent of psychiatric diagnostic criteria, survivors of cancer regularly show PTSD symptoms. The PTSD symptoms are quite specific with intrusion in the mind of negative experiences of cancer diagnosis and treatment, and avoidance and hypervigilance in relation to all associations with cancer. The level of PTSD symptoms is regularly high during diagnosis and treatment and then the level gradually tapers off.

In a review of 11 studies PTSD, diagnosed according to the DSM-IV criteria, PTSD was more common in survivors of cancer than it is in the general population (odds ratio 1.66, 95% confidence interval 1.09-2.53). Higher estimates of PTSD in cancer survivors depended upon type of cancer, type of treatment, prior traumas, age, and time since diagnosis (Swartzman et al. 2016).

5 Cognitive Problems

Subjective cognitive problems cover cancer patients' complaints concerning memory, concentration, word finding, planning, and doing multiple tasks. A considerable proportion of patients describe such problems when treated with chemotherapy. However, usually these complaints follow the course of anxiety and depression with gradual reduction over time. A minority gets permanent subjective problems. In an American population study, 14% of cancer patients (brain tumors excluded) reported subjective cognitive complaints versus 8% among cancer-free controls (Jean Pierre et al. 2011).

Objective evidence for cognitive problems can be documented with neuropsychological tests. Koppelmanns et al. (2012) reported considerable neuropsychological deficits in long-term breast cancer survivors compared to cancer-free controls. This result has been replicated in several studies with repeated measurements showing long-term neuropsychological deficits particularly after chemotherapy. Functional brain imaging can visualize reduced metabolism in relevant brain areas during neuropsychological testing. For example, de Ruiter et al. (2011) showed that long-term breast cancer survivors treated with high-dose chemotherapy 10 years previously, showed significantly less metabolic activation under testing compared to controls.

One problem within this field is the lack of correspondence between subjective complaints and objective findings, which should not be hold against the patient. Another problem is that cognitive reduction is multifactorial, which makes it difficult to tease out the specific effect of chemotherapy among other factors. For the clinician, it is important to keep in mind that cognitive reduction can be a long-term adverse effect after cancer therapy, and that this effect may reduce work ability in particular.

A recent Cochrane analysis supported cognitive training in cancer survivors although with limited evidence (Treanor et al. 2016; Zeng et al. 2016). However, cognitive training program like https://www.lumosity.com/ or http://www. neuronation.com/ are easily accessible on the internet for cancer survivors with such problems.

6 Sexual Problems

Many studies of sexual problems in cancer survivors have only used the physiological sexual response model. Recently, this model was supplemented with psychological and social aspects, implying a more comprehensive integrated model of sexual experiences for both sexes (Basson 2015; Katz and Dizon 2016).

New self-report instruments like the *Natsal-3 Sexual Function* questionnaire covers both the physiological, psychological, relational, and social aspects of sexuality as well as help-seeking, and such instruments should be considered for future studies of cancer survivors (Mitchell et al. 2012; Jones et al. 2015).

Concerning sexuality clinicians should be aware of two facts: (1) Various sexual problems are common in the general adult population, and information about pre-cancer function is important in order to understand to what extent pre-existing problems later on are attributed to cancer (Mitchell et al. 2013b). (2) After cancer treatment the optimal aim is to regain the pre-treatment level of sexual function. Cancer hardly improves sexual function, although more openness and emotionality between partners eventually can improve intimacy. Inclusion of the partner in sexual rehabilitation has also become more common (Li et al. 2016; Carroll et al. 2016).

A useful distinction is to separate sexual function in younger and older cancer survivors. *Younger survivors* are more sexual active, and fertility (see separate section) is still an important issue. Younger survivors concerns mainly survivors of breast and gynecological cancer, lymphomas and other hematological cancers, sarcomas, and testicular cancer. Among younger survivors the issue of sexual function in long-term testicular cancer survivors has been debated, but the controlled study with the largest sample, hardly observed significant differences from population-based controls (Dahl et al. 2007). In contrast, long-term male survivors of lymphomas had significantly poorer sexual function than such controls (Kiserud et al. 2009). Young female breast cancer patients often experience long-term lack of sexual interest. The attitude of their partners toward their body and femininity is very important for their sexual well-being. Premature menopause and hormone therapy also is of considerable importance, but less so for long-term survivors.

Most of the same issues are relevant for older breast cancer survivors. In gynecological cancer survivors lack of interest, vaginal dryness, and pains during intercourse are common complaints and can be managed in various ways (Krychman and Millheiser 2013; Dizon et al. 2014). Radical prostatectomy and radiotherapy for prostate cancer as well as adjuvant hormone treatment is frequently followed by severe long-term erectile dysfunction, and full sexual recovery is seldom achieved (Dahl et al. 2016a).

There are few studies of sexuality in long-term survivors.

Finally, a general complaint is the lack of communication about sexuality between survivors and both clinicians and general practitioners.

7 Insomnia

Insomnia is a common sleep disorder in the general population defined by difficulty initiating or maintaining sleep, or early morning awakenings with inability to return to sleep more than three times a week for more than three months. Chronic insomnia is a risk factor for early mortality, sick leaves, and disability pension (Sivertsen et al. 2014). Insomnia is very common during diagnosis and primary treatment of cancer, but the prevalence is gradually reduced during the cancer trajectory (Irwin 2013).

In a mixed sample of cancer patients insomnia was observed in 31%, 22% used hypnotic drugs and a majority also had daytime naps (Davidson et al. 2002). In cancer survivors insomnia has a significant positive association with pain, fatigue, depression, anxiety, and vasomotor symptoms, depending on stage of disease, treatment, and comorbidities (Davis and Goforth 2014).

Prescription of hypnotics for cancer survivors complaining of insomnia is tempting, but the documentation of positive effects is weak (Thedki et al. 2015). In contrast, the effects of cognitive behavior therapy for insomnia are well documented in cancer survivors (Johnson et al. 2016).

8 Lifestyle Factors

Lifestyle factors are important for cancer survivors since they represent risk factors for relapse of the primary cancer and development of secondary cancer (Park et al. 2016), as well as development of comorbid diseases, like diabetes or cardiovascular diseases, which represent additional reduction of HRQOL of the survivors. The lifestyle factors are well known: smoking, unhealthy diet, low physical activity, and high alcohol consumption. Although the severe consequences of unhealthy lifestyle are well known, permanent lifestyle changes have proved difficult to implement by health campaigns or other types of mass influence. Getting cancer has been considered a "teachable moment" for life style changes, but even rather intensive long-term interventions report only moderate success regarding permanent positive changes.

Obesity increases the risk of cancer recurrence and mortality, particularly in survivors of breast and prostate cancers (Ligibel 2012). However, weight gain in the survivorship period does not represent a significantly increased risk for these outcomes, and weight loss does not seem to reduce the risk. Weight loss is important for physical function and reduces the risk for lifestyle diseases like obesity, diabetes, or hypertension. Only a few randomized controlled studies of weight reduction all of them concerning breast cancer survivors, have been published. However, mainly moderate reduction on a nonpermanent basis has been achieved (Demark-Wahnefried et al. 2015).

These authors also described 11 RCTs of *physical activity* mainly in survivors of breast and prostate cancer with improved physical capacity and condition as results. However, any definite effects on cancer relapse or cancer-specific mortality have not been documented. Sedentary cancer survivors have demonstrated effects of structured exercises (Bourke et al. 2014).

Although regular *alcohol intake* is associated with increased risk for many types of cancer, the relation of such a habit with cancer recurrence and morbidity is unclear. The risk for development of additional comorbid somatic diseases is considerable. Alas, the survivorship literature hardly includes any RCTs of alcohol reduction. The same lack of studies concerns interventions against further *sun exposure* in survivors of malignant melanomas.

Smoking cessation was most successful when timed in relation to primary cancer treatment, and both pharmacological treatment and counseling/psychotherapy were effective in RCTs (Nayan et al. 2013).

Many intervention studies of cancer survivors have improvement of multiple factors life style factors as their aim. If multi-target interventions have better results than single target ones, seem unclear (Demark-Wahnefried et al. 2015).

Multiple types of media are now tried out for life style interventions in cancer survivors, thereby improving access and adherence to such programs. Therefore, the future development within this field is promising (Goode et al. 2015).

9   Work Issues

Work ability as a concept covers a person's ability to take part in ordinary work life and has three components: physical, mental, and social ability (van den Berg et al. 2009). Cancer most often infers a weakening of the physical work ability that can be temporary or permanent. However, cancer can also affect the mental and social work ability. Mehnert et al. (2013) review the work challenges of cancer survivors.

In the Nordic countries over 80% of men and women are active in work life, the big difference being that most of the men, but only half of the women hold full-time work. In many other countries the proportion of women at work is significantly lower. Regulations of the work market, unemployment rates, and regulations of social support for those not working are factors affecting the work situation of cancer survivors as well as the population in general.

For those at work, when they get their cancer diagnosis, *return to work* is a most important issue. Many factors have positive influences on return to work: younger age, higher education, single status, high income, positive social support from family and friends; early stage of cancer, good physical fitness level, low level of exhaustion/fatigue/tiredness, absence of pain, no comorbidities present, and good self-rated health; no chemo- or hormone therapy, no pain, lymphedema, or restricted movements; low level of depression, worry, frustration, feelings of guilt, anxiety, and cognitive problems; and finally nonphysical type of work, flexibility of work tasks, and support from colleagues and closest leaders. Factors like manual work, stressful job, lack of support from colleagues, long working hours, and decreased wages, all discourage patients to reenter their jobs (Islam et al. 2014; Kiasuwa Mbengi et al. 2016).

Interventions helping cancer patients return to work, have had moderate success according to a recent Cochrane review (deBoer et al. 2015).

These findings point not only to return to work, but also to the problem of *staying at work* for cancer survivors. Several studies have examined the *problems of cancer survivors at the workplace*. Most studies concern women with breast cancer who report that cognitive problems, hot flashes, and arm–shoulder morbidity reduced their work productivity. Pain in general and fatigue were common problems for survivors of both sexes. In survivors treated with surgery for prostate cancer, physical tasks like lifting and stooping, can be associated with incapacitating urinary leakage, but cognitive problems at work were also common in survivors of prostate cancer. A recent review showed that in spite of physical and/or mental problems, cancer survivors had more presenteism at their jobs than controls, perhaps since they feel that they have something to prove (Soejima and Kamibeppu 2016). Follow-up studies concerning *stability in work life over time* are uncommon so far.

When work ability is grossly and permanently reduced, persons have to leave the work force and go on to disability pension. Compared to matched controls without cancer, survivors have a significantly higher rate of disability pension (Carlsen et al. 2008; Hauglann et al. 2012). Compared to being at work, disability pension implies an income reduction, and several studies have shown that cancer survivors have permanently lower income compared to matched controls without cancer.

Cancer survivors as a group display a reduction in working hours and >10% decline in overall earnings. There are differences across diagnoses with survivors of lymphomas, lung, brain, bone, colorectal, and head-and neck cancer being mostly affected by decline in earnings (Hauglann et al. 2014). Other factors negatively effecting upon earnings are low level of education, lower social support, chemotherapy, self-employment, shorter tenure in the job, and part-time work (Mehnert 2011).

10 Follow-Up Care Organization

Follow-up practices for long-term cancer survivors are probably suboptimal in most countries both regarding content and organization. Specialized late-effects clinics have been established in some countries, and most of them provide care for survivors of childhood cancers. However, the evidence base for the effects of different models is weak at present (Earle and Ganz 2012; Shah et al. 2015; Cheville et al. 2012). For providers, the challenge is to develop and institute care models that address the needs of the fast growing number of survivors. To our knowledge, the only European national initiative has been launched in Great Britain as the National Cancer Survivorship Initiative (http://www.ncsi.org.uk/). In the United States, both the American Cancer Society and the National Cancer Institute are engaged in developing cancer survivorship care. Due to differences in cultures, resources, and organization of the healthcare systems, models found to be effective in one country might not be optimal in other national settings.

Follow-up of cancer survivors includes three distinct parties: (1) The oncologists with expertise in cancer treatment and risk for late effects; (2) The regular primary care physicians with specific knowledge of their patients but often not updated on their risks for late effects after cancer; and (3) The patients with their level of knowledge, attitudes and behavior.

Follow-up care might theoretically be delivered by the oncologists, the regular care physicians, or combinations (shared care). Another option is to give the survivors the full personal responsibility only involving the health care system when the survivors demand it.

Follow-up by oncologists for all cancer survivors is not feasible due to lack of manpower and resources in general. Further, not all survivors are in need of such specialized follow-up care. The National Cancer Survivorship Initiative has estimated that approximately 75% of all survivors can manage their health themselves with support from the primary health care system (http://www.ncsi.org.uk/). On this background, the concept of risk-based care has been launched and includes development of a systematic plan for prevention and surveillance based on risks associated with the cancer therapy, genetic predispositions, the survivors' lifestyle and comorbidities (Oeffinger and McCab 2006).

For cancer survivors to make the optimal decisions regarding their present and future health, they need information regarding the long-term health risks they face and how best to handle them. The literature indicates that today's cancer survivors are not aware of their risks for later adverse health events (Kadan-Lottick et al. 2002; Hess et al. 2011). These findings might not only relate to lacking information per se, but indicate cancer survivors have an ambivalent attitude concerning information about future health risks.

Survivorship care plans have been proposed as a means to operationalize the recommendations regarding follow-up care. Their idea is that a comprehensive care summary and follow-up plan is written by the principal provider of the oncology care. However, a randomized trial could not demonstrate positive effects of such plans among survivors of breast cancer (Grunfeld et al. 2011).

Thus, the present status is that organization and content of follow-up care is still under development. As stated by Earle and Ganz (2012), in this setting it is timely not to let the perfect be the enemy of the good.

11 Cancer Survivorship Research

With the shift from cancer having a poor prognosis to becoming curable diseases, research questions assessing late effects, the particular risk of developing them, how they best can be prevented and managed, and how having had cancer impact HRQOL of survivors, has become increasingly relevant as the number of survivors rapidly increased (Rowland et al. 2013).

At the start of cancer survivorship research in the 1970s, cancer survivors who had recently become curable, who were hit early in life, and survivors with a long life expectancy after cure such as childhood cancers, testicular cancers and Hodgkin's lymphoma, first attracted the researchers' attention. The research field has later rapidly expanded, however, and by year 2011 nearly 17,500 citations related to cancer survivorship science were identified (Rowland et al. 2013). The rapid expansion includes studies of new groups of survivors and broadening of the research field to include not only quantity of life but also the survivors' quality of life. Noteworthy is the finding that late medical effects continue to emerge decades after termination of treatment making continuous surveillance and research on their mechanisms, prevention and treatment even more relevant now than 40 years ago. In conjunction with the expansion of molecular biology, research on the mechanisms of late effects has greatly advanced from year 2000 onward. During the same period, models for providing health care to the survivors and their cost-effectiveness have emerged as a new field of great relevance for the survivors themselves, but also for health administrators and health authorities.

Representative national or regional cancer registries are not available in all countries, but when they are, they provide unique opportunities for studying unselected cohorts of survivors. Some research groups have studied survivors previously included in clinical trials. As opposed to registry data, clinical trials usually provide a broad range of variables for characterization of the exposure—i.e., the disease and treatment, and the host at start of treatment. A limitation of using participants form previous clinical trials is the very low rate of cancer patients being included in trials, which infers that the study subjects are highly selected and the findings will have limited external validity. Observational studies by mailed questionnaires are probably the most frequently used design. Such instruments specifically developed for cancer survivors, have been developed and tested (Pearce et al. 2008). Generic questionnaires, disease-specific questionnaires or questionnaires specifically developed for cancer survivors have been applied. The generic questionnaires allow for comparisons with cancer-free controls including cancer-free members of the general population. The cancer-specific questionnaires often include content of particular relevance for patients receiving treatment, but their content might be less relevant during survivorship. Cancer survivorship-specific questionnaires such as the Impact of Cancer (IOC) scale (Zebrack et al. 2006) addresses important aspects of survivorship such as personal growth, but has limitations regarding comparisons with populations not affected by cancer.

Some important challenges of particular relevance for cancer survivorship research should be pointed out. One is to define who is a cancer survivor? Another is to identify survivors 10–30 years after end of treatment. Legislations, the structure of the health care system, and social mobility all have an effect upon the opportunity to identify cancer survivors. For example, in Norway due to a unique personal identity number, a national uniform healthcare system and relatively low social mobility, we have been able to identify nearly all survivors of specific cancers more than 25–30 years after end of treatment. A third important challenge is how to control for age-related health effects when for example studying adult survivors in their 50s and 60s who were treated as children. Choosing an optimal control group is therefore critical and needs careful consideration. A fourth challenge is to have access to data that allows for detailed description of the exposure and the patient at time of exposure. Most studies till now have been cross-sectional and data on the exposure and the host at time of exposure are often not available or very limited. Cross-sectionals designs limit the possibility to draw inferences about causality. Fifthly, funding of research is a challenge in many countries exaggerated by the present financial crisis. Finally, the diversity of end-points, especially patient-reported, hinders comparisons of findings across studies.

References

American Cancer Society (2015) Cancer Treatment and Survivorship Facts and Figures 2014–2015

American Psychiatric Association (1994) Diagnostic and statistical manual of mental disorders, 4th edn. American Psychiatric Association, Washington DC

American Psychiatric Association (2013) Diagnostic and statistical manual of mental disorders, 5th edn. American Psychiatric Association, Washington DC

Basson H (2015) Human sexual response. In: Vodusek DB, Boller F (eds) Neurology of sexual and bladder disorders. Handbook of Clinical Neurology 2015, vol 130. Elsevier, Amsterdam

Bourke L, Homer KE, Thaha MA et al (2014) Interventions to improve exercise behaviour in sedentary people living with and beyond cancer: a systematic review. Br J Cancer 110:831–841. doi:10.1038/bjc.2013.750

Brydøy M, Oldenburg J, Klepp O et al (2009) Observational study of prevalence of long-term Raynaud-like phenomena and neurological side effects in testicular cancer survivors. J Natl Cancer Inst 101:1682–1695

Carlsen K, Dalton SO, Frederiksen K et al (2008) Cancer and the risk for taking early retirement pension. Scand J Publ Health 36:117–125

Carroll AJ, Baron SR, Carroll RA (2016) Couple-based treatment for sexual problems following breast cancer: A review and synthesis of the literature. Support Care Cancer 24:3651–3659. doi:10.1007/s00520-016-3218-y

Cheville AL, Nyman JA, Pruthi S, Basford JR (2012) Cost considerations regarding the prospective surveillance model for breast cancer survivors. Cancer. Apr 15. 118(8 Suppl):2325–2330. doi:10.1002/cncr.27473

Craft LL, Vaniterson EH, Helenowski IB et al (2012) Exercise effects on depressive symptoms in cancer survivors: a systematic review and meta-analysis. Cancer Epidemiol Biomarkers Prev 21:3–19. doi:10.1158/1055-9965.EPI-11-0634

Cramp F, Daniel J (2008) Exercise for the management of cancer-related fatigue in adults. Cochrane Database of Systematic Reviews 2: CD006145. doi:10.1002/14651858.CD006145. pub2

Crist JV, Grunfeld EA (2013) Factors reported to influence fear of recurrence in cancer patients: a systematic review. Psycho-Oncol 22:978–986. doi:10.1002/pon.3114

Curigliano G, Cardinale D, Suter T et al (2012) Cardiovascular toxicity induced by chemotherapy, targeted agents and radiotherapy: ESMO clinical practice guidelines. Ann Oncol 23:155–1662

Curtis RE, Freedman DM, RonE et al (eds) (2006) New malignancies among cancer survivors: SEER registries: 1973-, National cancer Institute, NHI publNo. 05-5302. Bethesda

Dahl AA, Bremnes R, Dahl O, Klepp et al (2007) Is the sexual function compromised in long-term testicular cancer survivors? Eur Urol 52:1438–1447

Dahl AA, Nilsson R, Axcrona K, Fosså SD (2016a) Addressing erectile dysfunction in prostate cancer survivors after radical prostatectomy. Expert Rev Quality Life Cancer Care 1:403–420. doi:10.1080/23809000.2016.1236660

Dahl AA, Østby-Deglum M, Oldenburg J et al (2016b) Aspects of posttraumatic stress disorder in long-term testicular cancer survivors: cross-sectional and longitudinal findings. J Cancer Surviv 10:842–849

Darby SC, Ewertz M, McGale P et al (2013) Risk of ischemic heart disease in women after radiotherapy for breast cancer. N Engl J Med 368:987–998

Davidson JR, MacLean AW, Brundage MD et al (2002) Sleep disturbances in cancer patients. Soc Sci Med 54:1309–1321

Davis MP, Goforth HW (2014) Long-term and short-term effects of insomnia in cancer and effective interventions. Cancer J 20:330–344. doi:10.1097/PPO.0000000000000071

de Boer AG, Taskila TK, Tamminga SJ, et al (2015) Interventions to enhance return-to-work for cancer patients. Cochrane Database Syst Rev CD007569. doi:10.1002/14651858.CD007569. pub3

de Ruiter MB, Reneman L, Boogerd W et al (2011) Cerebral hyporesponsiveness and cognitive impairment 10 years after chemotherapy for breast cancer. Hum Brain Map 32:1209–1216

Demark-Wahnefried W, Rogers LQ, Alfano CM et al (2015) Practical clinical interventions for diet, physical activity and weight control in cancer survivors. CA Cancer J Clin 65(165):189

Dizon DS, Suzin D, McIlvenna S (2014) Sexual health as a survivorship issue for female cancer survivors. Oncologist 19:202–210. doi:10.1634/theoncologist.2013-0302

Donovan KA, McGinty HL, Jacobsen PB (2013) A systematic review of research using the diagnostic criteria for cancer-related fatigue. Psycho-Oncol 22:737–744

Earle CC, Ganz PA (2012) Cancer survivorship care: don't let the perfect be the enemy of the good. J Clin Oncol 30:3764–3768

Fossa SD, Loge JH, Dahl AA (2008) Long-term survivorship after cancer: how far have we come? Ann Oncol S5:25–29

Fosså S, Vassilopoulou-Sellin R, Dahl A (2008) Long term physical sequelae after adult-onset cancer. J Canc Survivorship 2:3–11

Fung C, Fossa SD, Milano MT et al (2013) Solid tumors after chemotherapy or surgery for testicular nonseminoma: a population-based study. J Clin Oncol 2013(31):3807–3814. doi:10. 1200/JCO.2013.50.3409

Goode AD, Lawler SP, Brakenridge CL et al (2015) Telephone, print, and Web-based interventions for physical activity, diet, and weight control among cancer survivors: a systematic review. J Cancer Surviv 9:660–682. doi:10.1007/s11764-015-0442-2

Greer JA, Solis JM, Temel JS et al (2011) Anxiety disorders in long-term survivors of adult cancers. Psychosom 52:417–423

Grunfeld E, Julian JA, Pond G et al (2011) Evaluating survivorship care plans: results of a randomized, clinical trial of patients with breast cancer. J Clin Oncol 29:4755–4762

Hamre H, Zeller B, Kanellopoulos A et al (2013) High prevalence of chronic fatigue in adult long-term survivors of acute lymphoblastic leukemia and lymphoma during childhood and adolescence. J Adolescent Young Adult Oncol 2:2–9

Hauglann B, Benth JS, Fosså SD et al (2012) A cohort study of permanently reduced work ability in breast cancer patients. J Cancer Surviv 6:345–356

Hauglann B, Benth JS, Fosså SD et al (2014) A controlled cohort study of long-term income in colorectal cancer patients. Support Care Cancer 22:2821–2830. doi:10.1007/s00520-014-2258-4

Haugnes HS, Wethal T, Aass N et al (2010) Cardiovascular risk factors and morbidity in long-term survivors of testicular cancer: a 20-year follow-up study. J Clin Oncol 28:4649–4657

Hauptmann M, Johannesen TB, Gilbert ES, Fosså SD et al (2016) Increased pancreatic cancer risk following radiotherapy for testicular cancer. Br J Cancer 115:901–908

Hershman DL, Lacchetti C, Dworkin RH, Lavoie Smith EM et al (2014) Prevention and management of chemotherapy-induced peripheral neuropathy in survivors of adult cancers: American Society of Clinical Oncology clinical practice guideline. J Clin Oncol 32(18):1941–1967. doi:10.1200/JCO.2013.54.0914

Hess SL, Johannsdottir IM, Hamre H et al (2011) Adult survivors of childhood malignant lymphoma are not aware of their risk of late effects. Acta Oncol 50:653–659

Irwin MR (2013) Depression and insomnia in cancer: prevalence, risk factors, and effects on cancer outcomes. Curr Psychiatry Rep 15:404. doi:10.1007/s11920-013-0404-1

Islam T, Dahlui M, Abd Majid H et al (2014) Factors associated with return to work of breast cancer survivors: a systematic review. BMC Public Health 14(suppl 3):S8

Jean Pierre P, Winters PC, Ahles TA et al (2011) Prevalence of self-reported memory problems in adult cancer survivors: a national cross-sectional study. J Oncol Pract 8:30–34

Johnson JA, Rash JA, Campbell TS et al (2016) A systematic review and meta-analysis of randomized controlled trials of cognitive behavior therapy for insomnia (CBT-I) in cancer survivors. SleepMed Rev 27:20–28. doi:10.1016/j.smrv.2015.07.001

Jones KG, Mitchell KR, Ploubidis GB et al (2015) The Natsal-SF measure of sexual function: comparison of three scoring methods. J Sex Res 52:640–646. doi:10.1080/00224499.2014.985813

Kadan-Lottick NS, Robison LL, Gurney JG et al (2002) Childhood cancer survivors' knowledge about their past diagnosis and treatment: childhood cancer survivor study. JAMA 287:1832–1839

Katz A, Dizon DS (2016) Sexuality after cancer: a model for male survivors. J Sex Med 13:70–78. doi:10.1016/j.jsxm.2015.11.006

Kenney LB, Cohen LE, Shnorhavorian M et al (2012) Male reproductive health after childhood, adolescent, and young adult cancers: a report from the Children's Oncology Group. J Clin Oncol 30:3408–3416

Kiasuwa Mbengi R, Otter R, Mortelmans K et al (2016) Barriers and opportunities for return-to-work of cancer survivors: time for action—rapid review and expert consultation. Syst Rev 5:35. doi:10.1186/s13643-016-0210-z

Kier MG, Hansen MK, Lauritsen J, Mortensen MS, Bandak M et al (2016) Second malignant neoplasms and cause of death in patients with germ cell cancer: a Danish Nationwide Cohort Study. JAMA Oncol 2(12):1624–1627

Kiserud CE, Schover LR, Dahl AA et al (2009) Do male lymphoma survivors have impaired sexual function? J Clin Oncol 27:6019–6026

Koch L, Jansen L, Brenner H et al (2013) Fear of recurrence and disease progression in long-term (≥ 5 years) cancer survivors—a systematic review of quantitative studies. Psycho-Oncology 22:1–11. doi:10.1002/pon.3022

Kollmannsberger C, Beyer J, Droz JP et al (1998) Secondary leukemia following high cumulative doses of etoposide in patients treated for advanced germ cell tumors. J Clin Oncol 16:3386–3391

Koppelmanns V, de Ruiter MB, van der Lijn F et al (2012) Global and focal brain volume in long-term breast cancer survivors exposed to adjuvant chemotherapy. Breast Cancer Res Treat 132:1099–1106

Krychman M, Millheiser LS (2013) Sexual health issues in women with cancer. J Sex Med 10 (Suppl 1):5–15. doi:10.1111/jsm.12034

LaVoy EC, Fagundes CP, Dantzer R (2016) Exercise, inflammation, and fatigue in cancer survivors. Exerc Immunol Rev 22:82–93

Lee SJ, Schover LR, Partridge AH, Patrizio P et al (2006) American Society of Clinical Oncology recommendations on fertility preservation in cancer patients. J Clin Oncol 24(18):2917–2931. Erratum in: J Clin Oncol. 2006 24(36):5790

Lenihan D, Oliva S, Chow EJ et al (2013) Cardiac toxicity in cancer survivors. Cancer 119:2131–2142

Li H, Gao T, Wang R (2016) The role of the sexual partner in managing erectile dysfunction. Nature Rev Urol 13:168–177. doi:10.1038/nrurol.2015.315

Liavaag AH, Tonstad S, Pripp AH et al (2009) Prevalence and determinants of metabolic syndrome and elevated Framingham risk score in epithelial ovarian cancer survivors: a controlled observational study. Int J Gynecol Cancer 19:634–640

Ligibel J (2012) Lifestyle factors in cancer survivorship. J Clin Oncol 30:3697–3704

Loge JH, Ekeberg Ø, Kaasa S (1998) Fatigue in the general Norwegian population—normative data and associations. J Psychosom Res 45:53–65

Lustberg MB, Reinbolt RE, Shapiro CL (2012) Bone health in adult cancer survivorship. J Clin Oncol 30:3665–3674

Mehnert A (2011) Employment and work-related issues in cancer survivors. Critical Rev Oncol/Hematol 77:109–130

Mehnert A, de Boer A, Feuerstein M (2013) Employment challenges for cancer survivors. Cancer 119(Suppl 11):2151–2159. doi:10.1002/cncr.28067

Metzger ML, Meacham LR, Patterson B et al (2013) Female reproductive health after childhood, adolescent, and young adult cancers: guidelines for the assessment and management of female reproductive complications. J Clin Oncol 31:1239–1247

Minton O, Richardson A, Sharpe M et al (2010) Drug therapy for the management of cancer-related fatigue. Cochrane Database Syst Rev.7;7:CD006704

Mitchell KR, Ploubidis GB, Datta J et al (2012) The Natsal-SF: a validated measure of sexual function for use in community surveys. Eur J Epidemiol 27:409–418. doi:10.1007/s10654-012-9697-3

Mitchell AJ, Ferguson DW, Paul J et al (2013a) Depression and anxiety in long-term cancer survivors compared with spouses and healthy controls. Lancet Oncol. doi:10.1016/S1470-2045 (13)70244-4

Mitchell KR, Mercer CH, Ploubidis GB et al (2013b) Sexual function in Britain: findings from the third National Survey of Sexual Attitudes and Lifestyles (Natsal 3). Lancet 382:1817–1829

Mols F, Thong MSY, van de Poll-Franse L et al (2012) Type D (distressed) personality is associated with poor quality of life and mental health among 3080 cancer survivors. J Affect Dis 136:26–34

Morton LM, Gilbert ES, Stovall M et al (2014) Risk of esophageal cancer following radiotherapy for Hodgkin lymphoma. Hematologica 99:193–196

Nayan S, Gupta MK, Strychowsky JE et al (2013) Smoking cessation interventions and cessation rates in the oncology population: an updated systematic review and meta-analysis. Otolaryng Head Neck Surgery 149:200–211

Nesvold IL, Reinertsen KV, Fosså SD et al (2011) The relation between arm/shoulder problems and quality of life in breast cancer survivors: a cross-sectional and longitudinal study. J Canc Surviv 5:62–72

Oeffinger KC, McCab MS (2006) Models for delivering survivorship care. J Clin Oncol 24:5117–5124

Oldenburg J, Kraggerud SM, Cvancarova M et al (2007) Cisplatin-induced long-term hearing impairment is associated with specific glutathione s-transferase genotypes in testicular cancer survivors. J Clin Oncol 25:708–714

Pachman DR, Barton DL, Swetz KM et al (2012) Troublesome symptoms in cancer survivors: fatigue, insomnia, neuropathy, and pain. J Clin Oncol 30:3687–3696

Park SM, Yun YH, Kim YA, Jo M, Won YJ, Back JH, Lee ES (2016) Prediagnosis body mass index and risk of secondary primary cancer in male cancer survivors: a large cohort study. J Clin Oncol 34(34):4116–4124

Pearce NJ, Sanson-Fisher R, Campbell HS (2008) Measuring quality of life in cancer survivors: a methodological review of existing scales. Psychooncology 17:629–640

Piet J, Würtzen H, Zachariae R (2012) The effect of mindfulness-based therapy on symptoms of anxiety and depression in adult cancerpatients and survivors: a systematic review and meta-analysis. J Consult Clin Psychol 80:1007–1020. doi:10.1037/a0028329

Radbruch L, Strasser F, Elsner F et al (2008) Fatigue in palliative care patients-an EAPC approach. Palliat Med 22:13–32

Rowland JH, Kent EE, Forsythe LP et al (2013) Cancer survivorship research in Europe and the United States: Where have we been, where are we going, and what can we learn from each other? Cancer 119(S11):2094–2108

Shah M, Denlinger CS, Oncology (Williston Park) (2015) Optimal post-treatment surveillance in cancer survivors: is more really better? 29(4):230–240

Simard S, Thewes B, Humphris G et al (2013) Fear of cancer recurrence in adult cancer survivors. J Cancer Surviv 7:300–22. doi:10.1007/s11764-013-0272-z

Simonelli LE, Siegel SD, Duffy NM (2016) Fear of cancer recurrence: a theoretical review and its relevance for clinical presentation and management. Psycho-Oncol. doi:10.1002/pon.4168. [Epub ahead of print]

Sivertsen B, Lallukka T, Salo P et al (2014) Insomina as a risk factor for ill health: results from the large population-based HUNT study in Norway. J Sleep Res 23:124–132

Soejima T, Kamibeppu K (2016) Are cancer survivors well-performing workers? A systematic review. Asia Pac J Clin Oncol 12:e383–e397. doi:10.1111/ajco.12515

Sprauten M, Haugnes HS, Brydøy M, et al (2015) Chronic fatigue in 812 testicular cancer survivors during long-term follow-up: increasing prevalence and risk factors. Ann Oncol 26:2133–2140. doi:10.1093/annonc/mdv328

Stensheim H, Cvancarova M, Møller B et al (2011) Pregnancy after adolescent and adult cancer: a population-based matched cohort study. Int J Cancer 129:1225–1236

Stone PC, Minton O (2008) Cancer-related fatigue. Eur J Canc 44:1097–1104

Swartzman S, Booth JN, Munro A et al (2016) Posttraumatic stress disorder after cancer diagnosis in adults: a meta-analysis. Depress Anxiety. doi:10.1002/da.22542. [Epub ahead of print]

Swerdlow AJ, Barber JA, Hudson GV et al (2000) Risk of second malignancy after Hodgkin's disease in a collaborative British cohort: the relation to age at treatment. J Clin Oncol 18:498–509

Swerdlow AJ, Schoemaker MJ, Allerton R et al (2001) Lung cancer after Hodgkin's disease: a nested case-control study of the relation to treatment. J Clin Oncol 19:1610–1618 The Cancer Registry of Norway (2015) Cancer in Norway 2015

Thedki SM, Trinidad A, Roth A (2015) Psychopharmacology in cancer. Curr Psychiatry Rep 17:529

Thewes B, Butow P, Zachariae R et al (2012) Fear of cancer recurrence: a systematic literature review of self-report measures. Psycho-Oncol 21:571–587

Travis LB, Holowaty EJ, Bergfeldt K et al (1999) Risk of leukemia after platinum-based chemotherapy for ovarian cancer. N Engl J Med 340:351–357

Treanor CJ, McMenamin UC, O'Neill RF et al (2016) Non-pharmacological interventions for cognitive impairment due to systemic cancer treatment. Cochrane Database Syst Rev CD011325. doi:10.1002/14651858

van den Berg TIJ, Elders LAM, de Zwart BCH et al (2009) The effects of work-related factors on the Work Ability Index: a systematic review. Occup Environ Med 66:211–220

Windebank AJ, Grisold W (2008) Chemotherapy-induced neuropathy. J Peripher Nerv Syst 13:27–46

World Health Organization (1993) The ICD-10 Classification of Mental and Behavioural Disorders. Diagnostic Criteria for Research. Geneva: World Health Organization

Zamorano JL, Lancellotti P, Muñoz DR, Aboyans V et al (2016) 2016 ESC Position Paper on cancer treatments and cardiovascular toxicity developed under the auspices of the ESC Committee for Practice Guidelines]

Zebrack BJ, Ganz PA, Bernaards CA et al (2006) Assessing the impact of cancer: development of a new instrument for long-term survivors. Psychooncology 15:407–421

Zeng Y, Cheng AS, Chan CC (2016) Meta-analysis of the effects of neuropsychological interventions on cognitive function in non-central nervous system cancer survivors. Integr Cancer Ther 15:424–434

Psychotherapy in the Oncology Setting

Mirjam de Vries and Friedrich Stiefel

Abstract

A person who faces the diagnosis of cancer is subjected to changes within his body, but also with regard to his view of himself and his social relationships. Cancer related psychological distress occurs frequently and has a different prevalence according to—among other factors—cancer type and stage of disease. The main psychiatric disturbances observed in patients with cancer are adjustment disorders and affective disorders (anxiety and depression), which in the majority of patients are due to stressors related to the occurrence and threat of the disease and pre-existing psychological vulnerabilities; however, they might also be a direct consequence of biological causes either resulting from bodily modifications induced by the cancer or from treatment side effects. This chapter provides theoretical and practical information on the main psychotherapeutic approaches for cancer patients, complemented by some reflections on their clinical and scientific evidence.

Keywords

Cancer · Psycho-oncology · Psychotherapy

M. de Vries (✉) · F. Stiefel
Service de Psychiatrie de Liaision, Département de Psychiatrie,
Centre hospitalier universitaire vaudois, Rue du Bugnon 21,
1011 Lausanne, Switzerland
e-mail: Mirjam.de-vries@chuv.ch

F. Stiefel
e-mail: Frederic.stiefel@chuv.ch

F. Stiefel
Faculté de Biologie et Médecine, Université de Lausanne,
Rue du Bugnon 44, 1011 Lausanne, Switzerland

© Springer International Publishing AG 2018
U. Goerling and A. Mehnert (eds.), *Psycho-Oncology*, Recent Results
in Cancer Research 210, https://doi.org/10.1007/978-3-319-64310-6_9

1 Introduction

A person who faces cancer is subjected to changes within his body, but also with regard to his view of himself and his social relationships. Since each individual reacts differently to such a life-threatening event, the psychological responses should not be considered as "adequate" or "inadequate" but rather as adaptive or an expression of psychological distress. A patient might, for example, be considered somehow agitated, increasing his usual activities, but feeling rather good and denying part of the existential threat; this state can be considered as an adaptive response. If the same patient shows signs of fatigue and emerging symptoms of anxiety, his adaptive resources might have become limited and he should be considered as suffering from distress. Cancer related psychological distress occurs frequently: for example, prevalence of major depression in mixed cancer populations is estimated to occur in 10–25% and depressive symptoms in 21–58% (Massie 2004; Mitchell et al. 2011; Pirl 2004), and 14% suffer from pathological demoralization (Kissane et al. 2004a). Furthermore, anxiety disorders were reported in 15–28% of cancer patients (Kerrihard et al. 1999), and a recent meta-analysis showed that almost 40% of them suffered from any type of emotional disorders (Mitchel et al. 2011), a finding which has already been observed in a large prevalence study which identified one third to suffer from distress at a clinical level (Zabora et al. 2001). Psychological distress has been reported to have different prevalence according to cancer site: it was found to be highest in pancreatic (56.7%), lung (43.4%) and brain (CNS) cancer (42.7%), and lower in colon (31.6%), prostate (30.5%), and gynecological cancer (29.6%) (Zabora et al. 2001). Patients with advanced stages may also be more vulnerable to psychological distress, especially when taking into account acute confusional states (Massie 2004; Razavi and Stiefel 1994); however some research, for example in breast cancer, suggests that stage of cancer does not always influence prevalence of psychological distress and other factors such as sociodemographic variables, pre-existing vulnerabilities and life events might explain the variance (Kissane et al. 2004b).

2 Psychological Challenges and Interventions for Patients with Cancer

The main types of psychiatric disturbances observed in patients with cancer are adjustment disorders and affective disorders (anxiety and depression), which in the majority of patients are due to stressors related to the disease and pre-existing psychological vulnerabilities; however, they might also be a direct consequence of biological causes either resulting from bodily modifications induced by the cancer or from treatment side effects (e.g. treatment with interferon or radiation therapy, brain metastases, hypercalcemia, paraneoplastic syndromes, hypothyreosis, treatment with interferon or radiation therapy) (Razavi and Stiefel 1994).

Therefore, treatment of psychological distress calls for a careful evaluation in order to determine the most appropriate intervention, which might be to treat a biological factor or to provide psychological, psycho-pharmalogical or combined treatments. In the following we will only focus on distress for which psychological interventions are appropriate and beneficial.

From the moment of the diagnosis of cancer, the patient will modify his perception of himself, his interpersonal relationships, and his sense of belonging to the (healthy) others: he might reflect on his past and has to adjust to the present and adapt his plans for the future. Pre-existing self-image, quality of interpersonal relationships, and sense of belonging are protective factors or might be a source of increased vulnerability.

Adjustment to cancer is associated with six distinct hurdles, as defined by Faulkner and Maguire (1994): (1) managing uncertainty about the future, (2) searching for meaning, (3) dealing with loss (of control), and (4) having a need for openness, and (5) emotional and (6) medical support. Failing to deal with these hurdles might lead to psychosocial distress. Psychological interventions are conceived to help the patient to cope and adjust to the disease, and have been demonstrated to have a positive effect on distress, anxiety and depression (Devine and Westlake 1995; McLoone et al. 2013; Meyer and Mark 1995; Sheard and Maguire 1999).

While the spectrum of psycho-oncological interventions range from psychopharmacological treatment, relaxation, counselling and support or music-therapy to psychotherapy, we will—after a brief discussion of psycho-education and psychological support—focus on psychotherapy for patients with cancer. Parts of this chapter have been priorly published (De Vries and Stiefel 2014).

2.1 Psycho-education

Psycho-education refers to education offered by a professional to a patient about a mental or physical condition that causes psychological stress. By learning about his condition the patient is thought to feel more in control, which might help to reduce psychological distress. By definition psycho-educational interventions are directed towards specific objectives and therapists take an active role in reaching these goals. For example, psycho-educational interventions in melanoma survivors were shown to increase self-examination, decrease recurrence of melanoma and enhance coping and patient satisfaction. Based on educational concepts, these interventions are thus less oriented to reflect on issues such as intra- or interpersonal conflicts (Mcloone et al. 2013).

2.2 Psychological Support

Psychological support has many definitions and covers various approaches ranging from individual interventions (Hellbom et al. 1998), such as relaxation or structured problem-solving, to community or peer support services. The aims of supportive interventions are also different: e.g. to alleviate worries, to increase the patient's mastering of the situation, to help him to regulate stress or to facilitate his participation in and adherence to treatment. Psychological support is mainly based on non-specific elements, such as the therapist's ability to contain the patient's emotions, his invitation to express thoughts and emotions in an empathic and non-judgmental setting, or the room he provides for testimony of the often traumatizing experience of cancer (Stiefel and Bernard 2008). As an intervention, psychological support might also be offered by non-specialized health personal, since it is generally not subjected to control by training institutes or licensing bodies.

2.3 Psychotherapy

Psychotherapy has been defined by Frank (1988) as the relief of distress or disability in one person by another, based on a particular theory or paradigm, with the requirement that the agent performing the therapy has had training. Franck and Frank (1991) identified four broad dimensions shared by all psycho-therapeutic approaches: (i) a relationship in which the patient considers that the therapist is competent and cares about his state; (ii) a setting which is defined as a place of healing; (iii) a rationale which explains the patient's suffering and how it can be overcome; (iv) a set of procedures, requiring active participation of the patient and the therapist, of which both believe to be means of restoring the patient's health.

Wampold (2001) and Lambert and Ogles (2004) also underline that psychotherapy is a professional activity or service that implies a certain level of skills, which have to be formally recognized by training institutes and licensing bodies, and anchored in a psychological theory; in addition psychotherapeutic treatment should be supported by scientific evidence and provided by mental health specialists, who undergo training, regular supervision and continuous postgraduate education. In many countries, psychotherapeutic treatments can therefore only be provided by certified psychiatrists and psychologists.

In the following, we will first present and discuss the three most widely used psychotherapeutic approaches: psychodynamic, systemic and cognitive behavioural psychotherapy. These approaches have a long history of theoretical and conceptual development and are widely implemented in psychiatric and somatic settings, including oncology. Some of them have gained an important body of evidence confirming their effectiveness and all provide specialized and certified training programs. Finally, specific psychotherapeutic interventions, especially developed for the oncology setting, and the movement of psychotherapy integration will also be discussed.

2.4 Psychodynamic Psychotherapy

Psychodynamic psychotherapies are derived from Freud's work, object relation theory elaborated by Klein and Winnicott and self-psychology based on Sullivan's interpersonal psychotherapy (Lewin 2005). Psychodynamic techniques are intended to develop self-understanding, insight into recurrent problems, maturation, growth and increased autonomy. In the therapeutic process, symptoms and interpersonal difficulties are identified, analysed and interpreted based on the assumption that the subsequent insight and the experiences in the therapeutic relationship can be transferred to "the world outside the therapeutic setting" (Kaplan and Sadock 1998).

Psychodynamic psychotherapies rely on key theoretical concepts, such as (i) the existence of an unconscious, which influences our thoughts, emotions, and behaviours; (ii) the impact of early development, biography and life events on the present state; (iii) the organization of the psyche by the ego, which has the capacity to reason and to anticipate, the id, which is a source of sexual and aggressive drives, and the superego, which contains theses drives by a "guilty conscience"; (iv) the protection of the individual's equilibrium by (unconscious) defence mechanisms, such as rationalization, projection or denial, which are triggered by threatening emotions or thoughts; and (v) the observation that unresolved issues of the patient are re-enacted in the therapeutic setting, where they can be identified, discussed, interpreted and modified.

The different types of psychodynamic psychotherapy reach from insight-oriented psychotherapy, which uncovers repressed thoughts and feelings and aims to enhance patients' autonomy, to supportive psychotherapy, which attempts to suppress anxiety-provoking material and to foster ego functions and adaptive defences (Lewin 2005). Insight-oriented therapy is suitable for less vulnerable patients with intact ego functions, who are motivated to explore their thoughts and feelings in order to enhance reflection and the capacity to analyse adverse events (Rodin and Gillies 2000). Supportive psychotherapy is more often indicated for patients in a palliative phase of their illness, as for most of these patients, the objective is to enhance adaptation, to diminish dysfunctional coping, to decrease psychological distress and to restore psychological well-being (Guex et al. 2000; Krenz et al. 2014; Rodin and Gillies 2000; Ludwig et al. 2011).

A special form of psychodynamic psychotherapy, developed for patients with somatic diseases, is the Psychodynamic Life Narrative (PLN), which can be understood as a way to conceive maladaptive responses to physical illness (Viederman 1983). PLN aims to help the patient to understand their current psychological reactions to illness by linking it to important elements of their life trajectory (Viederman and Perry 1980). This type of therapy is thought to enhance the patient's sense of control and coherence when facing a crisis induced by illness (Viederman 2000).

With regard to the content of psychodynamic interventions it has been observed that the occurrence of cancer is not the sole focus but other issues, such as the specific reaction of the patient towards disease or the modification of his relationships by the disease, are also addressed (Krenz et al. 2014). In addition, a given psychological symptom is not just a target to suppress, since psychodynamic therapies aim to understand its underlying meaning: for example, it would be important for a psychodynamic-oriented therapist to understand whether the depressed mood of a women with breast cancer is due to the fact that she feels pressured by an increased difficulty to fulfill her duties (loss of pre-existing capacities), to a modification of her self-image (loss of her breast) of to an alteration of her relationship with her husband (perceived or imagined withdrawal of investment by others). Depending on the source of the depressive symptoms, the therapeutic approach would be different, focusing on superego pressure, (pre-existing) difficulties with self-esteem or fragile construction and hidden meaning of relationships.

While there are—compared to the body of evidence in the psychiatry setting— only few trials evaluating the effectiveness of psychodynamic therapies in the physically ill and in the cancer setting (Ando et al. 2007; Ludwig et al. 2014; Lurati et al. 2012), many single cases studies have been published (for example Lacy and Higgings 2005; Redding 2005; Tepper et al. 2006).

2.5 Systemic Psychotherapy

Systemic psychotherapy is based on general systems theory, which conceives a system, such as the family, as organized by different elements, which have attributes and functions which can be identified and interrelations which can be understood. Therefore, systemic psychotherapy views social coexistence of people as a complex and integrated whole, which is different than the sum of its parts (Minuchin 1988; Sameroff 1983). Interactions are seen as powerful catalysers or brakes of change. Family therapists utilize special techniques and focus on variables, such as cohesion and hierarchy of the family, as well as attributed roles and implicit and explicit rules (Bressoud et al. 2007). Family members are considered to be helpful resources to patients, who can assist him in decision making and provide emotional and practical support (Xiaolian et al. 2002), but who may also be a source of conflict and suffering (Lyons et al. 1995).

In a report on the evidence of systemic family therapy, Stratton (2005) indicated that systemic therapy started on a common ground, but has over the last 50 years grown in various directions, with the most significant specific interventions belonging to the work of Bateson and the Palo Alto team (Jackson 1968a, b), the family structural therapy by Minuchin (1974), the strategic family therapy developed by Haley (1976) and Madanes (1981), and the approaches of Selvini Palazzoli and the Milan team (1978, 1991). The most recent developments include solution-focused therapy (Molnar and de Shazer 1987; de Shazer and Dolan 2007), narrative therapy (White and Epston 1990) and collaborative approaches (Anderson 2012) inspired by the social constructionism paradigm.

Being a systemic therapist does not imply that clinical care is restricted to families, couples or groups; systemic therapists also treat individual patients, but they are sensitive to maintain an integrated systemic perspective in the analysis of the patient's problem and address systematically intergenerational and intrafamilial issues and resources. Family response to illness play an important role in the systemic therapy with the physically ill: for example family beliefs about a family member, such as "he has always been quickly irritated and prone to give up"—and family myths, such as "we function best by denying disagreements and avoiding difficulties".

Examples of scientifically evaluated systemic therapies in the medical and oncology setting are the Medical Family Therapy (Doherty et al. 1994) and the Family-Focused-Grief Therapy (FFGT), a preventive intervention for high-risk families (Kissane et al. 2006). FFGT is based on the assumption that the family is the primary provider of care for the terminally ill, that the type of functioning of the family is essential (Kissane et al. 1996a, b) and that to optimize family functioning and to share grief is beneficial for the patient and the family. FFGT is a time-limited intervention (four to eight sessions of 90 min each), over a 9–18 month period, based on a manual with specific guidelines and clinical illustrations; its efficacy has been demonstrated in a randomized controlled trial (Kissane et al. 2006).

One of the more recent systemic approaches, mostly qualitatively researched, is narrative therapy, developed by White and Epston (1990). Narrative therapy is based on the social constructionism paradigm that implies that our language is not only descriptive but also performative and, as such, is a tool that builds our conception of reality. The stories told by others or by ourself about our identity therefore shape our perception of ourself and the world. What we call reality is thus a co-construction between different individuals, and the relational consensus about a narrative leads to its perception as acceptable or not. Thus, not only the mind creates impressions based on observations, but confirmations of these impressions are sought with members of the society, the family or other systems, and this interpersonal exchange finally colors the way we perceive life. In narrative therapy the patient could, for example, be invited to question the relationship he maintains with his disease through a process called externalizing conversations: the goal is to draw a comprehensive map of the effects and "intentions" of the disease on the patient and his relations, to enlarge his view, to invite him to take position, to enlarge his potential choices, and thus empower him.

Narration is part of any psychotherapy, not only narrative approaches, and it is therefore surprising to define and label a specific form of psychotherapy as "narrative" psychotherapy. The point here is that the therapist focuses more on problematic narratives or stories than on problematic behaviours or inherent individual characteristics of the patient. Narrative therapy has the potential to also address narratives which circulate as dominant discourses among health care professionals and within society. As examples may serve the narratives among palliative care professionals concerning "good death" and "good palliative care patient" (Stiefel et al. 2016, in press) or the "good" and "bad" cancer (patients) (Stiefel and Bourquin 2015). Dominant discourses within society and medicine can negatively impact the individual patient (Bell 2012) and narrative therapy could contribute to link individual and social discourses, to question these discourses and to liberate patients from such injunctions; in other words: the potential of narrative therapy lies in an expansion of the patient's range of possibilities in the way he perceives his disease and his identity.

Finally, systemic psychotherapy plays a role in childhood cancer, childhood cancer survivors and their families. For example, Kazak (1989) found that multi-family group interventions reduced posttraumatic stress and anxiety in childhood cancer survivors and their families.

2.6 Cognitive Behavioural Psychotherapy

Cognitive-behavioural therapy (CBT) is a general term for several forms of therapies with similar characteristics, such as cognitive therapy, behaviour therapy, rational emotive therapy, schema focused therapy, dialectical behaviour therapy, mindfulness, motivational therapy or cognitive-behavioural stress management. These interventions intend to reduce psychological distress and enhance adaptive coping by modifying maladaptive thoughts and behaviours, by raising awareness of emotional states and their connection with thoughts and behaviours, and by providing new skills (Eyles et al. 2015; Hollon and Beck 2004).

CBT assumes that thoughts, behaviours and emotions are at the origin of persistence of human well-being but also of psychological distress and disorders. For example, individual responses to illness are influenced by cognitive factors such as symptom perception (Lacroix et al. 1991), variability in emotional reactions and self-care behaviours can be partly explained by disease-specific illness representations (Petrie et al. 1996; Prohaska et al. 1987), and the same situation encountered when feeling sad or happy will be followed by very different thoughts and behaviours (Segal et al. 2002). As it becomes more and more current in western healthcare to promote active self-management (Tattersall 2002), CBT, which focuses on an analysis of the function of the symptoms, skills acquisition and autonomy, has also been proposed for patients with physical and psychological comorbidity.

CBT offers several types of interventions for the somatic setting and for patients with chronic medical problems, such as the "Mind over Mood" framework of Greenberger and Padesky (1995, 2016) or Acceptance and Commitment Therapy (ACT), an approach developed by Steven Hayes and colleagues (Hayes et al. 1999). Both interventions are part of the "third wave" of CBT (the first wave concentrated on the behavioural approaches, the second on the cognitive approaches, while the third is more focused on emotion, meta-cognition and integration). For example, ACT is based on the idea that (i) instead of controlling our thoughts and feelings, one can choose to observe and accept them as they are and (ii) instead of putting energy in avoiding problems, one can direct it into actions which pursue personal values. For example, a patient with cancer might consider that his situation is desperate and he avoids engaging in life: in ACT he would be invited to identify his emotions and thoughts inducing his disengagement, and to reflect on whether they help him or not to realize personal values. By investigating his values he might find reasons and motivation to relate to life again, for example by connecting to other people, sharing his thoughts and emotions, or by discovering new aspects of life. Or he might conclude that he wishes to distance himself from life and then might do so on a more solid and coherent basis, for example by understanding that this now favours tranquility, contemplation or self-reflection.

CBT can be used as an individual or group treatment and therapists feel free to follow a specific model or integrate different techniques (e.g. relaxation, exposure, meaning seeking), adapted to the needs of the patient.

CBT strives to be evidence based, which results in an important body of scientific research. In patients with cancer, CBT has been demonstrated to improve anxiety and depressive symptoms, self-esteem, immune functions, quality of life, optimism, self-efficacy, compliance, coping, psychological flexibility, and satisfaction and to decrease cancer-related fatigue, cortisol levels, pain and distress (Andersen et al. 2007; Chambers et al. 2014; Daniels and Kissane 2008; Greer et al. 1992; Hopko et al. 2005; Hubert-Williams and Storey, 2016; Lee et al. 2006; Manne et al. 2007; Mefford et al. 2007; Moorey et al. 1998; Osborn et al. 2006; Penedo et al. 2007; Spencer and Wheeler 2016; Tatrow 2006; Witek-Janusek et al. 2008; Wojtyna et al. 2007).

2.7 Specific Psychotherapies Proposed for the Oncology (Palliative Care) Setting

Over the last decades, several specific psychotherapies for the cancer/palliative care setting have been developed. These therapies are based on single concepts or directed towards very specific goals, e.g. meaning-centered therapy (Breitbart et al. 2012, 2015), spiritual interventions (Casellas-Grau et al. 2014) or approaches using new technologies (Leykin et al. 2012). Attempts to introduce specific interventions in the oncology setting, including those proposing substances such as LSD (Gasser et al. 2015), can be understood in light of the existential threat of cancer and the limited life expectancy. While these two issues certainly play a major role in the psychotherapeutic treatment of (advanced) cancer patients, it has to be reminded that highly specific interventions leave little room for the patient to negotiate a therapy adapted to his needs and that the singularity of the patient—since such interventions are manualized and standardized—might be evacuated.

The emergence of new therapeutic approaches enables us to continue the development and conceptualization of psychotherapy. However, a critical stance must be advocated concerning the pertinence and efficacy of these "new label" psychotherapies. Indeed, psychotherapy research has repeatedly demonstrated that unspecific elements of the therapeutic process (e.g., therapeutic alliance) are most important and these elements are not always given room in the "new label" psychotherapies. Nevertheless, between "re-inventing the wheel", marketing strategies to promote new psychotherapy for the cancer setting, and advocating that we do not need to look further because there is enough proof for the benefits of the already existing there is room for scientific curiosity and creativity. Indeed reading, studying and thinking about our evolving societies will help health professionals keep the pace in a changing world.

2.8 Psychotherapy Integration

Integrative approaches are more and more practiced, with one-half to two-thirds of clinicians working with a variety of concepts derived from distinct theoretical frameworks (Lambert et al. 2004). A survey, conducted among 1143 therapists from various therapeutic orientations, found that self-declared monotherapists of all orientations actually use interventions from other theoretical approaches (Trijsburg et al. 2004).

Nowadays neither monism (psychotherapeutic modalities have unique qualities differentiating them) or specificity (one intervention has one intended result), nor eclecticism (interventions are effective irrespective of the particular theory from which they derive) or universality (common factors among psychotherapeutic treatments) can adequately reflect clinical reality in its totality; instead it is considered that specific interventions reinforce common factors and common factors reinforce the effects of specific interventions (Strupp and Hadley 1979).

Several integrative psychotherapeutic approaches have been developed (e.g., Common Factor Model of Arkowitz 1992; Interpersonal Therapy by Klerman et al. 1984; Cognitive analytic therapy by Ryle and Kerr 2002; Systematic Eclectic psychotherapy by Beutler and Consoli 1992; Multimodal therapy by Lazarus 1989, 2005; Kissane's cognitive-existential group therapy 1997). This work could benefit psycho-oncology, for which encouraging results have been found endorsing the common factors theory in cancer care and the effectiveness of technical eclecticism and theoretical integration (Liossi and White 2001; McLean et al. 2013; Schnur and Montgomery 2010). Moreover, integration of different psychotherapeutic approaches seems especially important in oncology, since patients' needs are various and evolving over the course of disease (Krenz et al. 2014).

3 Outcome of Psycho-oncological Interventions

Even though the above mentioned psychotherapeutic approaches have shown positive outcome for (cancer) patients (e.g., improving anxiety and depressive symptoms, immune functions, quality of life, and satisfaction and decreasing cancer-related fatigue, cortisol levels, and pain), outcomes of psycho-oncological interventions are not always easy to determine. Some patients value a decrease of distressing symptoms, such as feelings of depressed mood, while others emphasize personal growth, finding meaning in a situation perceived as chaotic or improving interpersonal relationships and communication. Up to now, most studies evaluated outcome by means of psychometric assessments, which do not always reflect the therapeutic process and might not be relevant to all patients and psychotherapeutic approaches (Krenz et al. 2014; Lurati et al. 2012). Several authors have therefore underlined that symptoms as sole outcome lack validity and have advocated to enlarge the view by other measures, such as body image (Fingeret et al. 2014), motivations of patients to seek treatment (Salander 2010) or well-being (Steinert et al. 2016).

The measured impact of psychotherapeutic interventions in cancer care is often modest. This seems partly due to the fact that many interventions have not been targeted at the most distressed patients (Goerling et al. 2011; Linden and Girgis 2012; Ludwig et al. 2014). However, other issues need attention: for example markers for response have to be identified and studied (Hubert-Williams and Storey 2016, Knapp et al. 2015), physicians' characteristics, such as their own level of stress and self-regulation of emotions, should be taken into account (De Vries et al. 2014, 2017), patients' characteristics, such as alexithymia, self-compassion, self-critical judgement and psychopathology in relationship to outcome in patients with cancer should be investigated (De Vries et al. 2012; Pinto-Gouveia et al. 2014). Integrated, collaborative care approaches seem in this respect to be a promising concept (Sharpe et al. 2014).

In addition, outcomes for partners and family members have also been neglected, as well as their mutual influences with patients' outcome. New outcome for significant others, who are often caregivers, have therefore to be identified and studied.

Finally psycho-oncological interventions seem to influence treatment adherence, but its relevance for survival is controversial (Barrera and Spiegel 2014; Chow et al. 2004; Smedslund and Ringdal 2004; Spiegel et al. 1989). However, a systematic Cochrane review examining the effectiveness of psychosocial interventions in breast cancer patients on long-term survival outcome showed insufficient evidence for such an effect (Mustafa et al. 2013). Possible pathways for prolonging survival, taking into account symptom alleviation, adherence to treatment, self-care or enhanced immune system, might deserve attention, since it has been reported that mood disturbance is associated with poorer response to chemotherapy (Walker et al. 1999), and that feelings of helplessness or hopelessness are associated with poorer survival (Watson et al. 1999).

References

Andersen BL, Farrar WB, Golden-Kreutz D et al (2007) Distress reduction from a psychological intervention contributes to improved health for cancer patients. Brain Behav Immun 21 (7):953–961

Anderson H, Gehart D (2012) Collaborative therapy: relationships and converstations that make a difference. Routledge, New York

Ando M, Tsuda A, Morita T (2007) Life review interview on the spiritual well-being of terminally ill cancer patients. Support Care Cancer 15:225–231

Arkowitz H (1992) A common factors therapy for depression. In: Norcorss JC, Goldfried MR (eds) Handbook of psychotherapy integration. Basic Books, New York, pp 402–432

Barrera I, Spiegel D (2014) Review of psychotherapeutic interventions on depression in cancer patients and their impact on disease progression. Int Review of Psychiat 26:31–43

Bell K (2012) Remaking the self: trauma, teachable moments, and the biopolitics of cancer survivorship. Cult Med Psychiat 36:584–600

Beutler LE, Consoli AJ (1992) Integration through fundamental similarities and useful differences among schools. In: Norcross JC, Goldfried MR (eds) Handbook of psychotherapy integration. Basic Books, New York, pp 202–231

Breitbart W, Poppito S, Rosenfeld B et al (2012) Pilot randomized controlled trial of individual meaning-centered psychotherapy for patients with advanced cancer. J Clin Oncol 30: 1304–1309

Breitbart W, Rosenfeld B, Pessin H et al (2015) Meaning-centered group psychotherapy: an effective intervention for improving psychological well-being in patients with advanced cancer. J Clin Oncol 33:749–754

Bressoud A, Real del Sarte O, Stiefel F et al (2007) Impact of family structure on long-term survivors of osteosarcoma. Sup Care Cancer 15:525–531

Casellas-Grau A, Font A, Vives J (2014) Positive psychology interventions in breast cancer. A systematic review. Psycho-Oncology 23:9–19

Chambers SK, Girgis A, Occhipinti S et al (2014) A randomized trial comparing two low-intensity psychological interventions for distressed patients with cancer and their caregivers. Oncol Nursing Forum 41:256–266

Chow E, Tsao MN, Harth T (2004) Does psychosocial intervention improve survival in cancer? A meta-analysis. Palliat Med 18:25–31

Daniels J, Kissane DW (2008) Psychosocial interventions for cancer patients. Cur Opin Oncol 20:367–371

De Shazer S, Dolan Y (2007) More than miracles: the state of the art of solution-focused brief therapy. Routledge, New York

De Vries AMM, Stiefel F (2014) Psycho-oncological interventions and psychotherapy in the oncology setting. Recent Results Cancer Res 197:121–135

De Vries AMM, Forni R, Voellinger R et al (2012) Alexithymia in cancer patients: review of the literature. Psychother Psychosom 81:79–86

De Vries AMM, de Roten Y, Meystre C et al (2014) Clinician characteristics, communication, and patient outcome in oncology: a systematic review. Psycho-Oncology 23:375–381

De Vries AMM, Gholamrezaee MM, Verdonck-de Leeuw IM et al (2017) Patient satisfaction and alliance as a function of the physician's self-regulation, the physician's stress, and the content of consultation in cancer care. Psycho-Oncology, accepted for publication. doi:10.1002/pon. 4233

Devine EC, Westlake SK (1995) The effects of psychoeducational care provided to adults with cancer: meta-analysis of 116 studies. Oncol Nurs Forum 22:1369–1381

Doherty WJ, McDaniel SH, Hepworth J (1994) Medical family therapy: an emerging arena for family therapy. J Fam Ther 16:31–46

Eyles C, Leydon GM, Hoffman CJ et al (2015) Mindfulness for the self-management of fatigue, anxiety, and depression in women with metastatic breast cancer: a mixed methods feasibility study. Integrat Cancer Ther 14:42–56

Faulkner A, Maguire P (1994) Talking to cancer patients and their relatives. Oxford University Press, New York

Fingeret MC, Teo I, Epner DE (2014) Managing body image difficulties of adult cancer patients: lessons from available research. Cancer 120:633–641

Franck JD, Frank JB (1991) Persuasion and healing: a comparative study of psychotherapy. John Hopkins Universtiy Press, Baltimore

Frank J (1988) [1979] What is psychotherapy?. In: Bloch S (ed) An Introduction to the psychotherapies. Oxford University Press, Oxford

Gasser P, Kirchner K, Passie T (2015) LSD-assisted psychotherapy for anxiety associated with a life-threatening disease: a qualitative study of acute and sustained subjective effects. J Psychopharmacol 29:57–68

Goerling U, Foerg A, Sander S et al (2011) The impact of short-term psycho-oncological interventions on the psychological outcome of cancer patients of a surgical-oncology department—a randomized controlled study. Eur J Cancer 47:2009–2014

Greenberger D, Padesky CA (1995) Mind over mood: a cognitive therapy treatment manual for clients. Guilford press, New York

Greenberger D, Padesky CA (2016) Mind over mood: change how you feel by changing the way you think. Guilford Publications, New York

Greer S, Moorey S, Baruch JD et al (1992) Adjuvant psychological therapy for patients with cancer: a prospective randomised trial. BMJ 304:675–680

Guex P, Stiefel F, Rousselle I (2000) Psychotherapy for the patient with cancer. Psychother Rev 2:269–273

Haley J (1976) Problem-solving therapy: new strategies for effective family therapy. Josey Bass, San Francisco

Hayes SC, Strosahl KD, Wilson KG (1999) Acceptance and commitment therapy: an experiential approach to behavior change. The Guilford Press, NewYork

Hellbom M, Brandberg Y, Glimelius B et al (1998) Individual psychological support for cancer patients: utilisation and patient satisfaction. Patient Edu Couns 34:247–256

Hollon SD, Beck AT (2004) Cognitive and cognitive behavioral therapies. In: Lambert MJ (ed) Bergin and Garfied's handbook of psychotherapy and behavior change, 5th edn. Wiley, New York

Hopko DR, Bell JL, Armento MEA et al (2005) Behavior therapy for depressed cancer patients in primary care. Psychother Theory Res Pract Train 42:236–243

Hulbert-Williams NJ, Storey L (2016) psychological flexibility correlates with patient-reported outcomes independent of clinical or sociodemographic characteristics. Supp Care Cancer 24:2513–2521

Jackson DD (1968a) Human communication, T.1: communication, family and marriage. Science and behavior books, Palo Alto

Jackson DD (1968b) Human communciation,T.2: communcation, family and marriage. Science and behavior books, Palo Alto

Kaplan HI, Sadock BJ (1998) Kaplan and Sadock's synopsis of psychiatry: behavioral sciense/clinical psychitary, 8th edn. Williams and Wilkins, Baltimore

Kazak AE (1989) Families of chronically ill children: a systems and social-ecological model of adaptation and challenge. J Consul Clin Psychol 57:25–30

Kerrihard T, Breitbart W, Dent R et al (1999) Anxiety in patients with cancer and human inmmunodeficiency virus. Semin Clin Neuropsychiat 4:114–132

Kissane DW, Bloch S, Dowe DL et al (1996a) The Melbourne Family Grief Study, I: perceptions of family functioning in bereavement. Am J Psychiat 153:650–658

Kissane DW, Bloch S, Dowe DL et al (1996b) The Melbourne Family Grief Study, II: psychosocial morbidity and grief in bereaved families. Am J Psychiat 153:659–666

Kissane DW, Bloch S, Miach P et al (1997) Cognitive-existential group therapy for patients with primary breast cancer—techniques and themes. Psycho-Oncology 6:25–33

Kissane DW, Grabsch B, Love A et al (2004a) Psychiatric disorder in women with early stage and advanced breast cancer: a comparative analysis. Aust N Z J Psychiat 38:320–326

Kissane DW, Wein S, Love A et al (2004b) The demoralization scale. A report of its development and preliminary validation. J Palliat Care 20:269–276

Kissane DW, McKenzie M, Bloch S et al (2006) Family Focused Grief Therapy: a randomized, controlled trial in palliative care and bereavement. Am J Psychiat 163:1208–1218

Klerman G, Weissman M, Rousevill B et al (1984) Interpersonal psychotherapy of depression. Basic Books, New York

Knapp P, Kieling C, Beck AT (2015) What do psychotherapist do? A systematic review and meta-regression of surveys. Psychother Psychosom 84:377–378

Krenz S, Sodel C, Stagno A et al (2014) Psychodynamic interventions in cancer care II: a qualitative analysis of the therapists' reports. Psycho-Oncology 23:75–80

Lacroix JM, Martin B, Avendano M et al (1991) Symptom schemata in chronic respiratory patients. Health Psychol 10:268–273

Lacy TJ, Higgins MJ (2005) Integrated medical-psychiatric care of a dying patient: a case of dynamically informed 'practical psychotherapy'. J Am Acad Psychoanal Dynamic Psychiat 33:619–636

Lambert MJ, Ogles BM (2004) The efficacy and effectiveness of psychotherapy. In: Lambert MJ (ed) Bergin and Garfield's handbook of psychotherapy and behavior change, 5th edn. Wiley, New York

Lambert MJ, Bergin AE, Garfield SL (2004) Introduction and historical overview. In: Lambert MJ (ed) Bergin and Garfield's handbook of psychotherapy and behavior change, 5th edn. New York, Wiley, pp 3–15

Lazarus AA (1989) The practice of multimodal therapy. Systematic, comprehensive, and effective psychotherapy. Johns Hopkins University Press, Baltimore

Lazarus AA (2005) Multimodal therapy. In: Norcross JC, Goldfried MR (eds) Handbook of psychotherapy integration, 2nd edn. New York, Oxford, pp 105–120

Lee V, Cohen SR, Edgar L et al (2006) Meaning—making intervention during breast or colorectal cancer treatment improves self-esteem, optimism, and self-efficacy. Soc Sci Med 62:3133–3145

Lewin K (2005) The theoretical basis of dynamic psychiatry. In: Gabbard GO (ed) Psychodynamic psychiatry in clinical practice: the DSM-IV edition. American Psychiatric Press, Washington

Leykin Y, Thekdi SM, Shumay DM et al (2012) Internet interventions for improving psychological well-being in psycho-oncology: review and recommendations. Psycho-Oncology 21:1016–1025

Linden W, Girgis A (2012) Psychological treatment outcomes for cancer patients: what do meta-analyses tell us about distress reduction? Psycho-Oncology 21:343–350

Liossi C, White P (2001) Efficacy of clinical hypnosis in the enhancement of quality of life of terminally ill cancer patients. Contemporary Hypnosis 18:145–160

Ludwig S, Krenz S, Zdrojewski C et al (2014) Psychodynamic interventions in cancer care I: psychometric results of a randomized controlled trial. Psycho-Oncology 23:65–74

Lurati C, Riva M, Resega R et al (2012) A mono-institutional prospective study on the effectiveness of a specialist psychotherapeutic intervention (POI) started at the diagnosis of cancer. Supp Care Cancer 20:475–481

Ludwig S, Verdu B, Stiefel F (2011) Konzeptuelle Überlegungen zur psychodynamisch orientierten Konsiliar- und Liaison-Psychiatrie. Die Psychodynamische Psychotherapie 10:69–77

Lyons RF, Sullivan MJL, Ritvo PG (1995) Relationships in chronic illness and disability. Sage publications, Thousand oaks

Madanes C (1981) Strategic family therapy. Josey Bass, San Francisco

Manne SL, Rubin S, Edelson M et al (2007) Coping and communication-enhancing intervention versus supportive counseling for women diagnosed with gynecologic cancers. J Consult Clin Psychol 75:615–628

Massie MJ (2004) Prevalence of depression in patients with cancer. J Natl Cancer Inst Monogr 32:57–71. doi:10.1093/jncimonographs/lgh014

McLean LM, Walton T, Rodin G et al (2013) A couple-based intervention for patients and caregivers facing end-stage cancer: outcomes of a randomized controlled trial. Psycho-Oncology 22:28–38

McLoon J, Menzies S, Meiser B et al (2013) Psycho-educational interventions for melanoma survivors: a systematic review. Psycho-Oncology 22:1444–1456

Mefford K, Nichols JF, Pakiz B et al (2007) A cognitive behavioral therapy intervention to promote weight loss improves body composition and blood lipid profiles among overweight breast cancer survivors. Breast Cancer Res Treat 104:145–152

Meyer TJ, Mark MM (1995) Effects of psychosocial interventions with adult cancer patients: a meta-analysis of randomized experiments. Health Psychol 14:101–108

Minuchin S (1974) Families and family therapy. Harvard University, Cambridge

Minuchin P (1988) Relationships within the family: a systems perspective on development. In: Hinde RA, Stevenson-Hinde J (eds) Relationships within families: mutual influences. Wiley, New York

Mitchell AJ, Chan M, Bhatti H et al (2011) Prevalence of depression, anxiety, and adjustment disorder in oncological, heamatological, and palliative-care settings: a meta-analysis of 94 interview-based studies. Lancet Oncol 12:160–174

Molnar A, de Shazer S (1987) Solution-focused therapy: toward the identification of therapeutic tasks. J Marital Fam Ther 13:349–358

Moorey S, Greer S, Bliss J et al (1998) A comparison of adjuvant psychological therapy and supportive counselling in patients with cancer. Psycho-oncology 7:218–228

Mustafa M, Carson-Stevens A, Gillespie D et al (2013) Psychological interventions for women with metastatic breast cancer. Cochrane Database Syst Rev Issue 6: Art. No. CD004253. doi:10.1002/14651858.CD004253.pub4

Osborn RL, Demoncada AC, Feurerstein M (2006) Psychosocial interventions for depression, anxiety, and quality of life in cancer survivors: meta-analyses. Int J Psychiat Med 36:13–34

Penedo FJ, Traeger L, Dahn J et al (2007) Cognitive behavioral stress management intervention improves quality of life in Spanish monolingual Hispanic men treated for localized prostate cancer: results of a randomized controlled trial. Int J Behav Med 12:164–172

Petrie KJ, Weinman J, Sharpe N et al (1996) Roles of patients' view of their illness in predicting return to work and functioning after myocardial infarction: longitudinal study. BMJ 312:1191–1194

Pinto-Gouveia J, Duarte C, Matos M et al (2014) The protective role of self-compassion in relation to psychopathology symptoms and quality of life in chronic and in cancer patients. Clinic Psychol Psychother 21:311–323

Pirl WF (2004) Evidence report on the occurrence, assessement, and treatment of depression in cancer patients. J Natl Cancer Inst Monogr 32:32–39. doi:10.1093/jncimonographs/lgh026

Prohaska TR, Keller ML, Leventhal EA et al (1987) Impact of symptoms and aging attribution on emotions and coping. Health Psychol 6:495–514

Razavi D, Stiefel F (1994) Common psychiatric disorders in cancer patients. I. Adjustment disorders and depressive disorders. J Supp Care cancer 2:223–232

Redding KK (2005) When death becomes the end of an analytic treatment. Clin Work Soc J 33:69–79

Rodin G, Gillies LA (2000) Individual psychotherapy for the patient with advanced disease. In: Ghochinov HM, Breitbart WGO (eds) Handbook of psychiatry in palliative medicine. Oxford University Press, New York

Ryle A, Kerr I (2002) Introducing cognitive analytic therapy: principles and practice. Wiley, Chichester

Salander P (2010) Motives that cancer patients in oncological care have for consulting a psychologist—an empirical study. Psycho-Oncology 19:248–254

Sameroff AJ (1983) Developmental systems: context and evolution. In: Mussen PH, Kessen W (ed) Handbook of child psychology: history, theory, and methods, 4th edn. Wiley, New York

Schnur JB, Montgomery GH (2010) A systematic review of therapeutic alliance, group cohesion, empathy, and goal consensus/collaboration in psychotherapeutic interventions in cancer: Uncommon factors? Clin Psychol Rev 30:238–247

Segal Z, Teasdale J, Williams M (2002) Mindfulness-based cognitive therapy for depression. Guilford Press, New York

Selvini Palazzoli M (1978) Self starvation: from the individual to family therapy. Aronson, New York

Selvini Palazzoli M (1991) Team consultation: an indispensable tool for the process of knowledge. J Fam Ther 13:31–53

Sharpe M, Walker J, Holm Hansen C et al (2014) Integrated collaborative care for comorbid major depression in patients with cancer (SMaRT Oncology-2): a multicentre randomized controlled effectiveness trial. Lancet 384:1099–1108

Sheard T, Maguire P (1999) The effect of psychological interventions on anxiety and depression in cancer patients: results of two meta-analyses. Br J Cancer 80:1770–1780

Smedslunc G, Ringdal GI (2004) Meta-analysis of the effects of psychosocial interventions on survival time in cancer patients. J Psychosom Res 57:123–131

Spencer JC, Wheeler SB (2016) A systematic review of motivational interviewing interventions in cancer patients and survivors. Pat Educ Couns 99:1099–1105

Spiegel D, Bloom JR, Kraemer HC et al (1989) Effect of psychosocial treatment on survival of patients with metastatic breast cancer. Lancet 2:888–891

Steinert C, Kruse J, Leichsenring F (2016) Long-term outcome and non-response in psychotherapy: are we short-sighted? Psychother Psychosom 85:235–237

Stiefel F, Bernard M (2008) Psychotherapeutic interventions in palliative care. In: Lloyd-Williams M (ed) Psychosocial issues in palliative care. Oxford University Press, New York

Stiefel F, Bourquin C (2015) Good cancers-bad cancers good patients-bad patients? J Thoracic Oncol 10(3):407–408

Stiefel F, Nakamura K, Terui T et al (2016). Collusions between patients and clinicians in end-of-life care: why clarity matters. J Pain Symptom Manag (accepted)

Stratton P (2005) Report on the evidence base of systemic family therapy. Association for family therapy and systemic practice. Available at: http//www.aft.org.uk

Strupp HH, Hadley SW (1979) Specific vs. Nonspecific factors in psychotherapy. Arch Gen Psychiat 36:1125–1136

Tatrow K, Montgomery GH (2006) Cognitive behavioral therapy for distress and pain in breast cancer patients: a meta-analysis. J Behav Med 29:17–27

Tattersall RL (2002) The expert patient: a new approach to chronic disease management for the twenty-first century. Clin Med 2:227–229

Tepper MC, Dodes LM, Wool CA et al (2006) A psychotherapy dominated by separation, termination, and death. Harv Rev Psychiat 14:257–267

Trijsburg RW, Lietaer G, Colijn S et al (2004) Construct validity of the comprehensive psychotherapeutic interventions rating scale. Psychother Res 14:346–366

Viederman M (1983) The psychodynamic life narrative: a psychotherapeutic intervention useful in crisis situations. Psychiat 46:236–246

Viederman M (2000) The supportive relationship, the psychodynamic life narrative, and the dying patient. In: Chochinov HM, Breitbart WGO (eds) Handbook of psychiatry in palliative medicine. Oxford University Press, New York

Viederman M, Perry SW (1980) Use of a psychodynamic life narrative in the treatment of depression in the physically ill. Gen hosp Psychiat 2:177–185

Walker LG, Walker MB, Ogston K et al (1999) Psychological, clinical and pathological effects of relaxation training and guided imagery during primary chemotherapy. Br J Cancer 80:262–268

Wampold BE (2001) The great psychotherapy debate: models, methods and findings. Lawrence Erlbaum Associates, Mahwah NJ

Watson M, Haviland JS, Greer S et al (1999) Influence of psychological response on survival in breast cancer: a population-based cohort study. Lancet 354:1331–1336

White M, Epston D (1990) Narrative means to therapeutic ends. WW Norton, New York

Witek-Janusek L, Albuquerque K, Chroniak KR et al (2008) Effect of mindfulness based stress reduction on immune function, quality of life and coping in women newly diagnosed with early stage breast cancer. Brain Behav Immun 22:969–981

Wojtyna E, Zycinska J, Stawiarska P (2007) The influence of cognitive-behaviour therapy on quality of life and self-esteem in women suffering from breast cancer. Rep Pract Oncol Radiother 12:109–117

Xiaolian J, Chaiwan S, Panuthai S et al (2002) Family support and self-care behaviour of Chinese chronic obstructive pulmonary disease patients. Nursing Health Sci 4:41–49

Zabora J, Brintzenhogeszoc K, Love A et al (2001) The prevalence of psychosocial distress by cancer site. Psycho-oncology 10:19–28

Quality of Life in Oncology

Anna Stickel and Ute Goerling

> Sittin' on the front porch
> ice cream in my hand
> meltin' in the sun
> all that chocolate on my tongue
> and that's
> good enough reason to live
> good enough reason to live…
> And if I die young, at least I got some chocolate on my
> tongue… (The Wood Brothers 2006)

Abstract

Continuous improvements in the diagnosis and treatment of cancer lead to improved cure rates and longer survival. However, in many patients, the disease becomes chronic. In this context, the patients' quality of life (QOL) becomes a crucial issue. After an introduction about QOL, results from different areas of cancer treatment are presented considering their impact on QOL. Finally, implications are discussed for researchers, clinicians, and patients.

Keywords

Psycho-oncology · Quality of life · Cancer treatment

A. Stickel · U. Goerling (✉)
Charité - Universitätsmedizin Berlin, corporate member of Freie Universität Berlin,
Humboldt-Universität zu Berlin, and Berlin Institute of Health,
Charité Comprehensiver Cancer Center, Charitéplatz 1, 10115 Berlin, Germany
e-mail: Ute.goerling@charite.de

A. Stickel
e-mail: Anna.stickel@charite.de

© Springer International Publishing AG 2018
U. Goerling and A. Mehnert (eds.), *Psycho-Oncology*, Recent Results
in Cancer Research 210, https://doi.org/10.1007/978-3-319-64310-6_10

1   Introduction

Quality of life (QOL)—everyone knows what it is, but it probably means something different to each individual. For some, being able to travel to foreign countries is important for their appraisal of good QOL, for others, it is having time for their hobbies or enjoying little things like the pleasure of chocolate melting on one's tongue.

In the face of a chronic disease, QOL is an issue of special value. Cancer and its treatment are debilitating and thus have an impact on QOL, depending on the individual's perception of the situation. Cancer care has become more successful, yet also more complicated. Therefore, understanding what cancer survival means to patients is an important intention in current research (see also Chapter "Cancer Survivorship in adults"). Not only the efficacy of treatments but also their toxicity and associated problems for patients are receiving increasing attention.

Many parameters elucidating the effects of cancer are not quantifiable with laboratory tests or imaging procedures. Therefore, variables such as social functioning, sense of well-being, fatigue, or global QOL are ascertained by self-reports. These self-reports add to the picture of biomedical outcomes and are important for gaining a better understanding of the consequences of cancer and its treatments (Osoba 2011).

Thus, apart from objective criteria like survival time, time to recurrence, side effects, etc., the interest in patients' experiences has grown and their subjective perceptions of living with cancer are valued more.

2   What Exactly Is Quality of Life?

2.1   Terms and Definitions

Different terms and definitions revolve around the rather elusive multidimensional construct: Patient function, health status, life satisfaction, quality of life, health related quality of life, or patient-reported outcomes. Yet there is no universal definition (Leplège and Hunt 1997).

QOL is always highly individual. It depends on the present lifestyle, past experiences, future hopes, dreams, and ambitions. QOL should include all aspects of life and experiences in life and take account of disease and treatment. An individual has a good QOL, when experiences are in accordance to hopes. The opposite is true when the experiences the individual makes do not match the hopes that he/she cherishes. QOL is time-dependent and gives information about the difference between hopes or expectations of the individual and his/her experiences at a given moment (Calmann 1984).

Already Aristotle (384–322 BC) refers to the fundamental problem of QOL-research: "and often the same person changes his mind: when he becomes ill, it is health, and as long as he is healthy it is money." Patients may change their personal scale about what is important in the course of their disease and the question is how?

In 1993, the World Health Organization published following definition:

"Quality of life is defined as an individual's perception of their position in life in the context of the culture and value systems in which they live and in relation to their goals, expectations, standards and concerns. It is a broad ranging concept affected in a complex way by the person's physical health, psychological state, level of independence, social relationships, and their relationship to salient features of their environment." (WHOQOLGroup 1993, p. 153).

To distinguish QOL of the general population from the QOL of patients the term "health related quality of life (HRQOL)" was introduced. A more inclusive term, however, is "patient reported outcomes" (PRO) which comprises any feedback given directly by the patient, e.g., satisfaction with care (Osoba 2011).

2.2 Measures in Quality of Life

A proper estimation of QOL is challenging. Already 100 years ago, there were efforts to include aspects of QOL in the use and evaluation of medical treatment. "Health is a state of complete physical, mental and social well-being and not merely the absence of disease or infirmity" (WHO 1946).

Early evaluation instruments of QOL focused on physical aspects of disease (Fayers and Bottomley 2002). In 1948, the American oncologist David A. Karnofsky developed an index that allows the doctor to give an estimation of the patient's physical condition on a scale (Karnofsky index, Karnofsky and Burchenal 1949). Another observer-rated assessment of QOL in oncology was developed by Spitzer. The doctor can value the activity, daily life, health, social support, and future perspective of the patient and create a total score. However, this time economic method has a significant drawback: it is open to different interpretations (Spitzer et al. 1981). Later the patients' expectations, perceptions as well as values received increasing attention and emotional and social aspects were added in assessments (Schumacher et al. 1991).

Today, self-reports are considered more appropriate than observer ratings of QOL. The questionnaires need to be short but nevertheless sensitive. They should allow cross-disease comparisons but also assess the specific nature of a certain disease. Finally, they must be reliable and valid.

Since 1964 certain projects in the United States assessing the needs and QOL of healthy individuals aim at resolving long-term deficits. The National Cancer Institute confirms that all clinical trials should include QOL as an outcome measure since 1991.

In the endeavor to improve QOL-research, several institutions created groups to give advice on the design, implementation, and analysis of QOL studies. For example, the Quality of Life Group (QLG) of the European Organisation for Research and Treatment of Cancer (EORTC) was established in 1980 (Fayers and

Bottomley 2002). One of the group's main achievements is the development and continual improvement of the Quality of Life Questionnaire. Its 30-item core measure (QLQ-C 30) includes a global health status/QOL scale, functional scales, symptom scales, and several single questions on frequently reported symptoms and financial concerns (see Table 1). In order to identify clinically relevant symptom burden or impairment, thresholds have recently been estimated for the key domains: physical functioning, emotional functioning, fatigue and pain using anchor items assessing burden, limitation and need for help (Giesinger et al. 2016b). Further, a single summary score has been suggested in order to reduce the risk of type I errors due to multiple testing (Giesinger et al. 2016a). Especially for palliative care, the QLG developed the 15-item EORTC QLQ-C15-PAL (Groenvold et al. 2006).

The QLQ-C 30 should be supplemented by modules specific to a tumor site, treatment modality, or additional QOL dimensions. The modules which have already been validated are presented in Table 2. The QLQ-C30 and QLQ modules are applicable cross-culturally as they are available in many different languages and are the most extensively used questionnaires in clinical trials in Europe (Fayers and Bottomley 2002).

In North America, the predominantly used tool is the Functional Assessment of Cancer Therapy Scale. Its general version (FACT-G, Version 3) has 27 items from which the subscales physical, social, emotional, and functional well-being can be derived (Cella et al. 2002, 1993) and which can be summed to a total score. Additionally, a broad range of tumor-, treatment-, or symptom-specific modules can be used (Luckett et al. 2011).

Table 1 The EORTC core questionnaire

		Number of items
QLQ-C30	Global health status	2
	Functional scales	
	Physical functioning	5
	Role functioning	2
	Emotional functioning	4
	Social functioning	2
	Cognitive functioning	2
	Symptom scales	
	Fatigue	3
	Nausea and vomiting	2
	Pain	2
	Dyspnoea	1
	Insomnia	1
	Appetite loss	1
	Constipation	1
	Diarrhea	1
	Financial impact	1

Table 2 The EORTC modules

Modules (validated)	Name[a]
Bone metastases	QLQ-BM 22
Brain cancer	QLQ-BN 20
Breast cancer	QLQ-BR 23
Cervical cancer	QLQ-CX 24
Colorectal cancer	QLQ-CR 29
Colorectal Liver metastases	QLQ-LMC 21
Elderly Cancer patients	QLQ-ELD 14
Endometrial	QLQ-EN 24
Gastric cancer	QLQ-STO 22
Head and neck	QLQ-H&N 35
Hepatocellular carcinoma	QLQ-HCC 18
Information	QLQ-INFO 25
Lung	QLQ-LC 13
Multiple myeloma	QLQ-MY 20
Neuroendocrine carcinoid	QLQ-GINET 21
Oesophageal cancer	QLQ-OES 18
Oesophago-gastric cancer	QLQ-OG 25
Oral health	QLQ-OH 15
Ovarian	QLQ-OV 28
Prostate	QLQ-PR 25

[a]The number after the abbreviation indicates the number of items

These two most widely used tools (EORTC QLQ-C30 and FACT-G) differ in scale structure, social domains, and tone. Their psychometric properties are comparable and thus cannot be used as a criterion in selecting one of these questionnaires (Luckett and King 2010). However, a direct comparison of similar scales from both questionnaires showed differences in their responsiveness, statistical efficiency, and power (King et al. 2014).

Furthermore, item banks and computerized adaptive testing (CAT) have been developed to gain a more comprehensive coverage of QOL issues (Cella et al. 2007). The Patient-Reported Outcomes Measurement Information System (PROMIS) was funded by the National Institutes of Health (NIH) and aims to enable an efficient, flexible, and precise measurement of PROs (http://www.nihpromis.org/). A computerized adaptive testing (CAT) version of the EORTC QLQ-C30 is also currently being developed (http://groups.eortc.be/qol/eortc-cat).

3   Quality of Life During Oncological Treatment

Treatments differ in their impact on QOL. In the case of various treatment options with curative objective, relapse free survival was previously considered as the only target criterion. Again, QOL must be seen as an important parameter and should be discussed with the patient. Efforts in early diagnosis, state of the art diagnostics, and multimodal therapy concepts prolong survival time, but what is the price the patient has to pay? Which of the therapies offering an improved life expectancy is superior considering their impact on QOL? Is a treatment which is less effective but also less detrimental to QOL more preferable than an aggressive therapy? The same thoughts apply to palliative treatment options. How much QOL does a person need to endure survival eight weeks longer?

Thus, the selection of tools for assessing QOL should also be determined by the treatment choice. For example, one questionnaire was developed specifically for patients after high-dose chemotherapy or palliative care (Sprangers et al. 1998) or a module was created to detect cancer-related fatigue, which can occur as a side effect but also as a long-term consequence of the antitumor therapy (Weis et al. 2013).

Below we will briefly discuss QOL-research in selected areas of oncologic therapy. This—by no means exhaustive—overview aims to demonstrate the complexity, diversity, and problems of QOL issues.

3.1   Surgery

The influence of surgical approaches on QOL has been examined in the context of different tumor entities. Interventions changing the body image are of particular interest. A number of studies, for example, examine the impact the creation of an anus praeter has on QOL (Grumann et al. 2001; Mrak et al. 2011). For almost 100 years, the abdominoperineal extirpation represented the standard therapy in surgery of rectal cancer (Pachler and Wille-Jorgensen 2012). In the context of the development and improvement of surgical techniques, and depending on the location of the tumor, an anterior sphincter-preserving resection then became the preferred treatment. This decision was not least due to the assumption that QOL is significantly better for patients whose sphincter function is preserved. In a systematic review on this topic, Pachler and Wille-Jorgensen (2012) evaluated 35 studies, matching their inclusion criteria, involving 5127 patients. None of the selected studies were randomized, 20 were retrospective and 15 prospective. Disease-specific instruments (e.g., EORTC-C30 and QLQ-C38, FACTC) were used in 23 studies. Seven studies used general questionnaires and five combined general with disease-specific questionnaires. Contrary to general expectations, a total of 14 studies showed that patients after abdominoperineal extirpation do not have poorer QOL compared to patients after an anterior resection. A small influence due to a stoma could be found in three trials. In 12 studies, patients who experienced an abdominoperineal extirpation showed a significantly poorer QOL on one or more subscales. However, in five studies, a significantly better QOL was found in some subscales after anterior resection. One study describes an improved QOL in patients after abdominoperineal extirpation. A recent systematic review focused on ostomy-related problems and their impact on QOL of colorectal cancer ostomates. Sexual problems, a depressed mood, gas, constipation, dissatisfaction with appearance, change in clothing, travel difficulties, feeling exhausted, and worried about noises were issues associated with impaired QOL (Vonk-Klaassen et al. 2016).

Comparisons of open versus laparoscopic surgery and robot-assisted surgery are further topics in literature (Bertani et al. 2011). King et al. (2006) compared the laparoscopic resection with the open resection of colorectal cancer in a randomized trial and came to the conclusion that patients have a shorter residence time in the hospital after laparoscopic resection. However, the groups did not differ concerning QOL.

A review on the outcome of oncoplastic breast-conserving surgery evaluated 88 studies (Haloua et al. 2013). Only one trial used QOL as an outcome measure (Veiga et al. 2010). This study compared the results of oncoplastic breast-conserving surgery with breast-conserving surgery, and concluded that oncoplastic surgery has a positive impact on QOL of women with breast cancer.

Little to no attention seems to be given to studies on the impact of palliative surgery on QOL. In a review, De Mestier et al. pointed out that QOL has not been evaluated in studies examining the impact of tumor resection in patients with colorectal cancer and unresectable synchronous liver metastases (de Mestier et al. 2014).

3.2 Chemotherapy

Studies on QOL during chemotherapy with curative objective address nausea, vomiting, and fatigue, among other aspects. The negative impact of chemotherapy-induced nausea and vomiting despite antiemetic therapy could be shown in a multicenter study in various tumor entities (Fernández-Ortega et al. 2012). Chemotherapy in women with breast cancer was found to have a negative impact on cognition and fatigue (de Ruiter et al. 2011). The latter showed a poorer QOL compared to the patients with no indication for adjuvant chemotherapy. A further study comparing younger versus older adults with acute myeloid leukemia receiving an intensive chemotherapy showed a diminished QOL and physical function. However, the patients' age had no influence on QOL (Mohamedali et al. 2012). A recent trial including patients with different tumors undergoing cancer chemotherapy showed that especially difficulties managing everyday tasks have a negative impact on QOL (Wagland et al. 2016).

Several studies can be found in the literature on the effect of therapy on QOL in systemic cancers in childhood, enabling an extended follow-up period (Kanellopoulos et al. 2013).

Drug trials often explore QOL in various treatment arms. Thus given the same overall survival rate in different arms, treatment decisions can be made according to the results of QOL assessments. The question of using chemotherapy in palliative situations is especially challenging. Studies have demonstrated the willingness of patients to accept side effects while gaining relief from disease associated symptoms (Archer et al. 1999).

3.3 Radiotherapy

Radiotherapy is a further essential element in cancer treatment in curative, as well as palliative care, however, once again not without consequences for the patients' QOL. Fatigue is one of the most common side effects and late sequelae of radiotherapy. Research indicates that up to 80% of the patients suffer from fatigue during and after radiotherapy (Jereczek-Fossa et al. 2002).

Due to the fact, that radiotherapy often is organ-preserving, the maintenance of a good QOL is expected. However, prospective studies on this subject are still rare. A review on the use of intensity-modulated radiotherapy in patients with head and neck cancer was able to detect only 10 studies in which QOL data was collected, out of 65 studies matching the search criteria (Scott-Brown et al. 2010). Only one study was randomized. According to its results, the expected positive impact of intensity-modulated radiotherapy versus conventional radiotherapy could not be detected. The authors assume that there is no relationship between loss of function and global QOL.

A further study with over 500 patients with head and neck cancer demonstrated that a quarter of patients treated with radiotherapy had more than 10% weight loss, which was associated with a diminished QOL (Langius et al. 2013).

In a secondary analysis comparing different radiation doses (74 Gy vs. 60 Gy), patients (n = 360) with unresectable stage III non-small cell lung cancer receiving concurrent chemotherapy showed significantly worse QOL in the high-dose arm at 3 months. Interestingly, the provider-reported toxicities were similar in both treatment arms (Movsas et al. 2016).

4   Relevance of Quality of Life

4.1   Relevance for Researchers

> … oncology has generated some of the most productive research in medicine for the development and utilisation of QoL measures. (Fallowfield 2009, p. 2)

Although QOL issues have gained increasing attention in recent years, QOL outcomes are still often not presented. A recent study analyzed protocols of 173 cancer trials and corresponding publications (Schandelmaier et al. 2015). About half of the protocols included specified QOL outcomes, and for only 20% of the trails data on QOL was reported in associated publications. The most frequent reasons for this the lack of reporting were non-specification of QOL outcomes in the protocol, non-publication of the whole study, and non-publication of the results considering QOL.

However, the methodology in HRQOL research has improved and the compliance with its measurement has grown (Bottomley et al. 2005; Efficace et al. 2003). Several reviews about QOL studies examine their reporting standard, presentation, and interpretation for QOL (Bottomley et al. 2005; Brundage et al. 2011; Cocks et al. 2008). Different researchers have proposed guidelines for developing and evaluating study protocols (Cocks et al. 2011; Efficace et al. 2003) and are working on international standards for the analysis of QOL outcomes (Bottomley et al. 2016). Also statistical challenges have been addressed (Bonnetain et al. 2016).

The presentation of results in QOL-research has increasingly become a matter of debate as the meaningfulness of statistical significance has been questioned in the clinical context. Statistical significance cannot be equated with clinical significance, especially if the later was not defined a priori and used to determine the sample size for a trail (Cocks et al. 2008). Different guidelines have been published on how to rate the importance of change (Cocks et al. 2012; King 1996, 2001; Osoba et al. 1998). It has been proposed that a change of 10 points on a scale from 0 to 100 (Osoba et al. 2005) or the 0.5 standard deviation (Norman et al. 2003) is clinically meaningful. However, the clinical interpretation of QOL differences is lacking as clinical significance is mostly not addressed in papers (Cocks et al. 2008). A recent review described signs of improvement over time in the publication of data on clinical significance (Rees et al. 2015).

A further problem is that QOL results are often published in separate papers. However, self-reports should complement standard biological endpoints (like tumor regression, time to progression, survival) and be described in a single publication (Osoba 2011).

Conflicting findings in comparative analyses of research results make unequivocal treatment decisions difficult for clinicians. Divergent results may occur through the use of different questionnaires. Hence, a generic questionnaire may not be sensitive to differences, for example, in certain surgical procedures. Many studies lack the pre-therapeutic assessment of QOL. Furthermore, the influence of important factors such as social status, and gender differences remain unconsidered. In order to give careful consideration to these aspects, prospective, methodologically well planned, and comprehensive studies are needed.

But how can we interpret results of QOL-research? Why does a patient with a colostomy rate his QOL as good as or better as a patient, whose natural anus could be preserved? Why does a woman after mastectomy evaluate her QOL as comparably good as a woman after breast-conserving surgery? These issues are known as the paradox of QOL-research in literature (Herschbach 2002).

As described above various dimensions are assessed in QOL-research. However, the patient's preference is often ignored, i.e., which dimensions are given more weight by which patient. Their ratings can vary considerably (Osoba 1994). Furthermore, the weighting of the dimensions may change over time. Ultimately, the patient's expectations to the outcome of cancer therapy play a significant role, which arise from the comparison of the actual state and the desired state.

4.2 Implications for Clinicians

It has been criticized that study results are not receiving enough attention from clinicians and the routine assessment of QOL has not been implemented into clinical practice. There are fears that this might be too expensive or time-consuming. However, research has shown that the regular use of QOL measurements increases the practitioner's awareness, facilitates the conversation about QOL issues, and thus has been shown to be of value for doctor–patient communication (Detmar et al. 2002; Velikova et al. 2004, 2010). Communication between doctor and patient is an essential aspect in the treatment of oncological patients. The majority of patients want support from their doctor. Thus, talking about QOL helps the doctor give the right kind of support. Patients receiving adequate information and who are content with the practitioner interaction show a better QOL (Velikova et al. 2004).

In addition, evidence for a positive relationship between QOL data and duration of survival in cancer patients has been reported in different reviews (Gotay et al. 2008; Montazeri 2009; Quinten et al. 2009, 2011). A recent review of PROs in radiation oncology presented evidence for the prognostic value of QOL instruments for outcome (e.g., local control and survival) (Siddiqui et al. 2014). In patients with non-small cell lung cancer, certain domains on QOL, measured at diagnosis (Fiteni et al. 2016) and after the initial treatment (Lemonnier et al. 2014), have been shown to be related to survival.

Different parameters such as pain, physical functioning and appetite loss can provide prognostic information beyond clinical measures. This was described across different disease sites and therefore taking into account QOL parameters can improve survival prediction of cancer patients (Quinten et al. 2009). Fiteni et al. discussed that data on QOL possibly may also be useful in determining subgroups of patients who will benefit from doublet chemotherapy (Fiteni et al. 2016).

Thus, clinicians may benefit from the possible predictive value of QOL assessments in the treatment of cancer patients, as they may be used as early warning systems. Although patient and clinician ratings of clinical symptoms have been shown to differ, both are described as valuable in the estimation of overall survival (Quinten et al. 2011). Future research should examine whether and to what extent improvements in QOL have the potential to increase survival.

In palliative situations, healthcare providers have the opportunity to effectively improve the QOL of their patients, especially in early stages of palliative care. Early support through specialized palliative interventions has been shown to lead to a greater improvement in QOL compared to usual care in patients newly diagnosed with non-small-lung cancer. Patients in the intervention group reported less depression and additionally showed a longer median survival (Temel et al. 2010).

A further issue of discussion is the facilitation of using QOL information for clinical doctors. Bezjak et al. (2001) recommend increasing the knowledge of oncologists on QOL literature by presenting findings in a comprehensible manner and emphasizing their clinical relevance. Furthermore, doctors should address QOL issues and explore the patients' perceptions of QOL. Finally, the application and interpretation of QOL questionnaires should be facilitated, e.g., by using modern technology displaying clear and simple graphics with current and previous as well as normative QOL data.

4.3 Significance for People Affected by Cancer

In a European population based survey (n = 9344), random households were asked what they would prioritize in the face of a serious illness like cancer: improving their QOL, prolonging survival or both. Across different countries 57–81% chose improving QOL, 2–6% preferred extending life and 15–40% described both as being equally important (Higginson et al. 2013). Thus, QOL issues seem to be of great value to the population.

Patients need to be informed about their disease, possible treatments, and the outcome of medical care. Information on the impact of a disease or treatment on their QOL is essential to patients especially while participating in decision-making about the cancer care they undergo (Bottomley et al. 2005; Cella et al. 2002; de Haes and Stiggelbout 1996). Both the psychosocial impairments (see Chapter "Psychosocial Impact of Cancer") and the worry and fear of recurrence or progression of the disease (see Chapter "Fear of Progression in Cancer Patients and Survivors") have a negative impact on QOL.

But also moving beyond active treatment, QOL remains an important topic for cancer survivors. Research has reported different results on the QOL of cancer survivors. Although cancer survivors have generally not been described as more vulnerable to the effects of day-to-day hassles, Costanzo et al. proposed a higher sensitivity to interpersonal tensions (Costanzo et al. 2012).

Cancer survivors may also be preoccupied with fears of recurrence, existential and spiritual problems, and experience difficulties in making new decisions considering their future life (Hewitt et al. 2005). Further challenges may be the adjustment to long-term and late effects like infertility and fatigue or changes in their social network, for example, the loss of friendship due to the lack of support during treatment (Cella 1988). Each of these issues can have a major influence on QOL in the individual. A recent study in patients suffering from thyroid cancer pointed out that fatigue-related issues are highly relevant across different cultures (Singer et al. 2016).

In a study with cervical cancer survivors (n = 173) 5, 10 and 15 years after diagnosis Le Borgne et al. (2013) showed a similarly good global QOL in cancer survivors compared to healthy controls. However, survivors 15 years after diagnosis reported more psychological burdens and—in case of prior radiotherapy—also more physical sequelae like sexual dysfunctions. Low income and comorbidities were further factors impairing QOL. A comparison of patients in a cancer rehabilitation program (n = 1879) with healthy controls (n = 2081) showed an impaired QOL in cancer patients. The differences between cancer patients and control were most striking in younger patients (Peters et al. 2016). Knowing different risk factors helps patients and healthcare professionals arrange appropriate interventions.

On the other hand, it has been reported that cancer survivors often benefit from the cancer experience. A new appreciation of life, deeper spirituality, personal improvement, improved relationships, help orientation, and increased attention to their own health have been described as advantages of cancer survivorship in literature (Documet et al. 2012). Positive psychological change in the face of challenging life events, so-called posttraumatic growth, has been shown to develop relatively quickly after the diagnosis of breast cancer (Danhauer et al. 2013). An exploratory study with 39 breast cancer survivors 4.5–5 years after diagnosis showed that 2/3 described their lives as good or even better than before the diagnosis (Salander et al. 2011). Thus, cancer survival also seems to bring many opportunities to improve QOL (Hewitt et al. 2005). The development of a healthy lifestyle can give survivors a sense of control and more self-awareness as well as setting new priorities can help increase life satisfaction.

5 Challenges in Quality of Life-Measurements

A review of 794 randomized trials showed that in 25.4% (200/794) HRQOL was a primary outcome (Brundage et al. 2011). 14% of the trials published their findings on QOL in a further publication. In general, the question remains, which and how many papers on QOL where actually accepted for publication (publication bias). Planning and conducting clinical trials is associated with strict ethical requirements. How is the QOL of seriously ill people? Are patients with extremely impaired QOL even able to provide a realistic assessment of their situation? How do researchers deal with missing data? Missing data lead to less power, i.e., the fewer study participants, the lower the probability to detect differences.

Another possibility of bias in longitudinal assessments is the so-called response shift effect. In the context of QOL measurement and cancer patients, response shift implies changes in patients' internal standards, values, and understanding or perception of QOL while adapting to their disease and its treatment (Dabakuyo et al. 2013). Part of the psychological adaption in the process of disease, for example, may be a change in the patient's concept of "worst pain imaginable." Furthermore, patients may set new priorities and develop a new concept of QOL (Luckett and King 2010). Thus, the correct interpretation of results in QOL measurement may require the assessment and adjustment for response shift effects.

More specific measurements assessing particular symptoms may be more responsive to change than a global measure of QOL. Further disadvantages of a global measure are its greater vulnerability to response shift effects and its inability to show changes in single dimensions of QOL. Nevertheless, if the relative burden of one disease is to be compared with others, the assessment of overall QOL may be more appropriate and also more convenient (Luckett and King 2010).

Furthermore, other sources of error in studies cannot be excluded: social desirability is a phenomenon which occurs repeatedly. There is a possibility that patients answer in ways not to offend their doctor. On the other hand, patients may perceive QOL assessments as time-consuming and sometimes as an additional burden.

In literature, one repeatedly encounters studies in which the QOL of cancer patients after treatment is compared with the QOL of healthy subjects due to missing control groups. It appears questionable if such comparisons are appropriate.

6 Quality of Life of Health Care Providers

The impact cancer has especially on the family of patients is described in Chapter "Family Caregivers to Adults with Cancer: The Consequences of Caring *Psychosocial burden of family caregivers to adults with cancer.* But what would oncology be without the professional health care providers? "Cancer is often seen as precipitating an existential crisis; a crisis of spirit and an opportunity for meaning. This is true not only for the patient with cancer and his or her family and loved ones, but also, interestingly enough, for oncologists and cancer care providers." (Breitbart 2006).

We have performed extensive literature searches on QOL. Alone, the keyword search in PubMed "quality of life and cancer" reveals over 61,200 entries. Healthcare providers appear only in the context of QOL-research, when it comes to observer-rated assessments of QOL of patients.

In a very impressive paper, Laurie Lyckholm (2001) reports on handling stress, burnout, and grief in the practice of oncology. Causes of stress are seen in insufficient personal or vacation time, a sense of failure, unrealistic expectations, anger, frustration, as well as feelings of inadequacy or self-preservations, reimbursement and other issues related to managed care and third-party payers, and last but not least grieving. Burnout can manifest itself in substance abuse, marital conflict, overeating and substantial weight gain, higher frequency of mistakes in clinical care, inappropriate emotional outbursts, interaction problems, depression and anxiety disorders, and even suicide. Lack of or inadequate training of communication and management skills are also considered causes of burnout (Ramirez et al. 1996). In a survey of 7288 physicians in the United States, 45.8% reported at least one of the following symptoms of burnout: loss of enthusiasm for work, feelings of cynicism (depersonalization), and low sense of personal accomplishment (Shanafelt et al. 2012). A recent review reports alarmingly higher rates (> 50%) of burnout among surgeons (Dimou et al. 2016). High prevalence of burnout has also been shown for oncologists (Cass et al. 2016; Deng et al. 2016).

Thus few but meaningful results on QOL of healthcare providers make further research in this area necessary, in order to provide effective interventions and strategies for these individuals. Ultimately, this would, in turn, be advantageous for the patients.

7 Summary

Cancer itself has a negative impact on the QOL of patients. However, individual conditions, values and resources influence this impact. Generally and in various definitions HRQOL is considered as a multifactorial concept. In the assessment of QOL, observer-rated assessments were increasingly replaced by self-reports of patients. Meanwhile, validated assessment tools for different research questions and treatment settings exist in different languages. Many improvements have been made in QOL-research. However, there are still many trials with study designs of low quality (not randomized or prospective, etc.) and where QOL is missing as an outcome measure. Furthermore, the variety of research results is often inconsistent, making it difficult to draw clear conclusions.

Nevertheless, information on possible changes in QOL is not only relevant for researchers, as described above, but also has implications for clinicians and for people affected by cancer. Ideally, it forms a basis for shared decision-making.

Last but not least more attention must be paid to the QOL of healthcare providers, which in turn would be beneficial to the patients and their families.

"...and that's good enough reason to live..." (The Wood Brothers 2006)

References

Archer VR, Billingham LJ, Cullen MH (1999) Palliative chemotherapy: no longer a contradiction in terms. Oncologist 4(6):470–477

Bertani E, Chiappa A, Biffi R et al (2011) Assessing appropriateness for elective colorectal cancer surgery: clinical, oncological, and quality-of-life short-term outcomes employing different treatment approaches. Int J Colorectal Dis 26(10):1317–1327

Bezjak A, Ng P, Skeel R et al (2001) Oncologists' use of quality of life information: results of a survey of eastern cooperative oncology group physicians. Qual Life Res 10(1):1–14

Bonnetain F, Fiteni F, Efficace F et al (2016) Statistical challenges in the analysis of health-related quality of life in cancer clinical trials. J Clin Oncol 34(16):1953–1956

Bottomley A, Flechtner H, Efficace F et al (2005) Health related quality of life outcomes in cancer clinical trials. Eur J Cancer 41(12):1697–1709

Bottomley A, Pe M, Sloan J et al (2016) Analysing data from patient-reported outcome and quality of life endpoints for cancer clinical trials: a start in setting international standards. The Lancet Oncol 17(11):e510–e514

Breitbart W (2006) Communication as a bridge to hope and healing in cancer care. In: Stiefel F (ed) Recent results in cancer research: communication in cancer care. Springer, Berlin

Brothers (2006) Chocolate on my tongue. In: Ways not to loose. http://wwwsongmeanings.net/songs/view/3530822107858616716/

Brundage M, Bass B, Davidson J et al (2011) Patterns of reporting health-related quality of life outcomes in randomized clinical trials: implications for clinicians and quality of life researchers. Qual Life Res 20 (5):653–664

Calmann KC (1984) Quality of life in cancer patients–an hypothesis. J Med Ethics 10(3):124–127

Cass I, Duska LR, Blank SV et al (2016) Stress and burnout among gynecologic oncologists: a society of gynecologic oncology evidence-based review and recommendations. Gynecol Oncol 143(2):421–427

Cella D, Gershon R, Lai J-S et al (2007) The future of outcomes measurement: item banking, tailored short-forms, and computerized adaptive assessment. Qual Life Res 16(1):133–141

Cella D, Hahn E, Dineen K (2002) Meaningful change in cancer-specific quality of life scores: differences between improvement and worsening. Qual Life Res 11(3):207–221

Cella DF (1988) Quality of life during and after cancer treatment. Compr Ther 14(5):69–75

Cella DF, Tulsky DS, Gray G et al (1993) The functional assessment of cancer therapy scale: development and validation of the general measure. J Clin Oncol 11(3):570–579

Cocks K, King MT, Velikova G et al (2012) Evidence-based guidelines for interpreting change scores for the European Organisation for the research and treatment of cancer quality of life questionnaire core 30. Eur J Cancer 48(11):1713–1721

Cocks K, King MT, Velikova G et al (2008) Quality, interpretation and presentation of European organisation for research and treatment of cancer quality of life questionnaire core 30 data in randomised controlled trials. Eur J Cancer 44(13):1793–1798

Cocks K, King MT, Velikova G et al (2011) Evidence-based guidelines for determination of sample size and interpretation of the European organisation for the research and treatment of cancer quality of life questionnaire core 30. J Clin Oncol 29(1):89–96

Costanzo ES, Stawski RS, Ryff CD et al (2012) Cancer survivors' responses to daily stressors: implications for quality of life. Health Psychol 31(3):360–370

Dabakuyo TS, Guillemin F, Conroy T et al (2013) Response shift effects on measuring post-operative quality of life among breast cancer patients: a multicenter cohort study. Qual Life Res 22(1):1–11

Danhauer SC, Case LD, Tedeschi R et al (2013) Predictors of posttraumatic growth in women with breast cancer. Psycho-oncology 22(12): 10.1002/pon.3298

de Haes JCJM, Stiggelbout AM (1996) Assessment of values, utilities and preferences in cancer patients. Cancer Treatment Rev 22, Supplement A (0):13–26

de Mestier L, Manceau G, Neuzillet C et al (2014) Primary tumor resection in colorectal cancer with unresectable synchronous metastases: a review. World J Gastrointest Oncol 6(6):156–169

de Ruiter MB, Reneman L, Boogerd W et al (2011) Cerebral hyporesponsiveness and cognitive impairment 10 years after chemotherapy for breast cancer. Human Brain Mapp 32(8):1206–1219

Deng Y-t, Liu J, Zhang J et al (2016) A multicenter study on the validation of the burnout battery: a new visual analog scale to screen job burnout in oncology professionals. Psycho-Oncol:n/a–n/a

Detmar S, Muller M, Schornagel J et al (2002) Health-related quality-of-life assessments and patient-physician communication: a randomized controlled trial. JAMA 288(23):3027–3034

Dimou FM, Eckelbarger D, Riall TS (2016) Surgeon Burnout: A Systematic Review. J Am Coll Urgeons 222(6):1230–1239

Documet P, Trauth J, Key M et al (2012) Breast cancer survivors' perception of survivorship. Oncol Nurs Forum 39(3):309–315

Efficace F, Bottomley A, Osoba D et al (2003) Beyond the development of Health-Related Quality-of-Life (HRQOL) measures: a checklist for evaluating HRQOL outcomes in cancer clinical trials—does HRQOL evaluation in prostate cancer research inform clinical decision making? J Clin Oncol 21(18):3502–3511

Fallowfield L (2009) What is…? series. In: Hayward Medical Communications, a division of Hayward Group Ltd., pp 1–8

Fayers P, Bottomley A (2002) Quality of life research within the EORTC—the EORTC QLQ-C30. Eur J Cancer 38, Supplement 4(0):125–133

Fernández-Ortega P, Caloto MT, Chirveches E et al (2012) Chemotherapy-induced nausea and vomiting in clinical practice: impact on patients' quality of life. Supp Care Cancer 20 (12):3141–3148

Fiteni F, Vernerey D, Bonnetain F et al (2016) Prognostic value of health-related quality of life for overall survival in elderly non-small-cell lung cancer patients. Eur J Cancer 52:120–128

Giesinger JM, Kieffer JM, Fayers PM et al (2016a) Replication and validation of higher order models demonstrated that a summary score for the EORTC QLQ-C30 is robust. J Clin Epidemiol 69:79–88

Giesinger JM, Kuijpers W, Young T et al (2016b) Thresholds for clinical importance for four key domains of the EORTC QLQ-C30: physical functioning, emotional functioning, fatigue and pain. Health Qual Life Outcomes 14:87

Gotay CC, Kawamoto CT, Bottomley A et al (2008) The prognostic significance of patient-reported outcomes in cancer clinical trials. J Clin Oncol 26(8):1355–1363

Groenvold M, Petersen MA, Aaronson NK et al (2006) The development of the EORTC QLQ-C15-PAL: a shortened questionnaire for cancer patients in palliative care. Eur J Cancer 42(1):55–64

Grumann M, Noack EM, Hoffmann I et al (2001) Comparison of quality of life in patients undergoing abdominoperineal extirpation or anterior resection for rectal cancer. Ann Surg 233 (2):149–156

Haloua MH, Krekel N, Winters HAH et al (2013) A systematic review of oncoplastic breast-conserving surgery: current weaknesses and future prospects. Ann Surg 257(4):609–6020

Herschbach P (2002) Das "Zufriedenheitsparadox" in der Lebensqualitätsforschung. Psychother Psych Med 52(03/04):141–150

Hewitt M, Greenfield S, Stovall E (2005) From cancer patient to cancer survivor: lost in transition. The National Academies Press, USA

Higginson IJ, Gomes B, Calanzani N et al (2013) Priorities for treatment, care and information if faced with serious illness: a comparative population-based survey in seven European countries. Palliative Medicine

Jereczek-Fossa BA, Marsiglia HR, Orecchia R (2002) Radiotherapy-related fatigue. Crit Rev Oncol/Hematol 41(3):317–325

Kanellopoulos A, Hamre HM, Dahl AA et al (2013) Factors associated with poor quality of life in survivors of childhood acute lymphoblastic leukemia and lymphoma. Pediatr Blood Cancer 60 (5):849–855

Karnofsky DA, Burchenal JH (1949) The clinical evaluation of chemotherapeutic agents in cancer. In: MacLeod CM (ed) Evaluation of chemotherapeutic agents. Columbia University Press, New York, p 196

King MT (1996) The interpretation of scores from the EORTC quality of life questionnaire QLQ-C30. Qual Life Res 5(6):555–567

King MT (2001) Cohen confirmed? Empirical effect sizes for the QLQ-C30. Qual Life Res 10 (3):278

King MT, Bell ML, Costa D et al (2014) The quality of life questionnaire core 30 (QLQ-C30) and Functional Assessment of Cancer-General (FACT-G) differ in responsiveness, relative efficiency, and therefore required sample size. J Clin Epidemiol 67(1):100–107

King PM, Blazeby JM, Ewings P et al (2006) Randomized clinical trial comparing laparoscopic and open surgery for colorectal cancer within an enhanced recovery programme. Br J Surg 93 (3):300–308

Langius JAE, van Dijk AM, Doornaert P et al (2013) More than 10% weight loss in head and neck cancer patients during radiotherapy is independently associated with deterioration in quality of life. Nutr Cancer 65(1):76–83

Le Borgne G, Mercier M, Woronoff A-S et al (2013) Quality of life in long-term cervical cancer survivors: a population-based study. Gynecol Oncol 129(1):222–228

Lemonnier I, Guillemin F, Arveux P et al (2014) Quality of life after the initial treatments of non-small cell lung cancer: a persistent predictor for patients' survival. Health and Qual Life Outcomes 12:73

Leplège A, Hunt S (1997) The problem of quality of life in medicine. JAMA 278(1):47–50

Luckett T, King MT (2010) Choosing patient-reported outcome measures for cancer clinical research—practical principles and an algorithm to assist non-specialist researchers. Eur J Cancer 46(18):3149–3157

Luckett T, King MT, Butow PN et al (2011) Choosing between the EORTC QLQ-C30 and FACT-G for measuring health-related quality of life in cancer clinical research: issues, evidence and recommendations. Ann Oncol 22(10):2179–2190

Lyckholm L (2001) Dealing with stress, burnout, and grief in the practice of oncology. Lancet Oncol 2(12):750–755

Mohamedali H, Breunis H, Timilshina N et al (2012) Older age is associated with similar quality of life and physical function compared to younger age during intensive chemotherapy for acute myeloid leukemia. Leukemia Res 36(10):1241–1248

Montazeri A (2009) Quality of life data as prognostic indicators of survival in cancer patients: an overview of the literature from 1982 to 2008. Health and Qual Life Outcomes 7(1):102

Movsas B, Hu C, Sloan J et al (2016) Quality of life analysis of a radiation dose–escalation study of patients with non–small-cell lung cancer: a secondary analysis of the radiation therapy oncology group 0617 randomized clinical trial. JAMA Oncol 2(3):359–367

Mrak K, Jagoditsch M, Eberl T et al (2011) Long-term quality of life in pouch patients compared with stoma patients following rectal cancer surgery. Colorectal Dis 13(12):403–410

Norman GR, Sloan JA, Wyrwich KW (2003) Interpretation of changes in health-related quality of life: the remarkable universality of half a standard deviation. Med Care 41(5):582–592

Osoba D (1994) Lessons learned from measuring health-related quality of life in oncology. J Clin Oncol 12(3):608–616

Osoba D (2011) Health-related quality of life and cancer clinical trials. Therapeutic Adv Med Oncol 3(2):57–71

Osoba D, Bezjak A, Brundage M et al (2005) Analysis and interpretation of health-related quality-of-life data from clinical trials: basic approach of The National Cancer Institute of Canada Clinical Trials Group. Eur J Cancer 41(2):280–287

Osoba D, Rodrigues G, Myles J et al (1998) Interpreting the significance of changes in health-related quality-of-life scores. J Clin Oncol 16(1):139–144

Pachler J, Wille-Jorgensen P (2012) Quality of life after rectal resection for cancer, with or without permanent colostomy. Cochrane Database of Systematic Reviews (12). doi:10.1002/14651858. CD004323.pub4

Peters E, Mendoza Schulz L, Reuss-Borst M (2016) Quality of life after cancer—How the extent of impairment is influenced by patient characteristics. BMC Cancer 16:787

Quinten C, Coens C, Mauer M et al (2009) Baseline quality of life as a prognostic indicator of survival: a meta-analysis of individual patient data from EORTC clinical trials. The Lancet Oncol 10(9):865–871

Quinten C, Maringwa J, Gotay CC et al (2011) Patient self-reports of symptoms and clinician ratings as predictors of overall cancer survival. J Natl Cancer Inst 103(24):1851–1858

Ramirez AJ, Graham J, Richards MA et al (1996) Mental health of hospital consultants: the effects of stress and satisfaction at work. Lancet 347:724–728

Rees JR, Whale K, Fish D et al (2015) Patient-reported outcomes in randomised controlled trials of colorectal cancer: an analysis determining the availability of robust data to inform clinical decision-making. J Cancer Res Clin Oncol 141(12):2181–2192

Salander P, Lilliehorn S, Hamberg K et al (2011) The impact of breast cancer on living an everyday life 4.5–5 years post-diagnosis—a qualitative prospective study of 39 women. Acta Oncol 50(3):399–407

Schandelmaier S, Conen K, von Elm E et al (2015) Planning and reporting of quality-of-life outcomes in cancer trials. Ann Oncol 26(9):1966–1973

Schumacher M, Olschewski M, Schulgen G (1991) Assessment of quality of life in clinical trials. Statistics in Med 10(12):1915–1930

Scott-Brown M, Miah A, Harrington K et al (2010) Evidence-based review: quality of life following head and neck intensity-modulated radiotherapy. Radiother Oncol 97(2):249–257

Shanafelt TD, Boone S, Tan L et al (2012) Burnout and satisfaction with work-life balance among us physicians relative to the general us population. Arch Intern Med 172(18):1377–1385

Siddiqui F, Liu AK, Watkins-Bruner D et al (2014) Patient-reported outcomes and survivorship in radiation oncology: overcoming the cons. J Clin Oncol 32(26):2920–2927

Singer S, Husson O, Tomaszewska IM et al (2016) Quality-of-life priorities in patients with thyroid cancer: a multinational european organisation for research and treatment of cancer phase i study. Thyroid 26(11):1605–1613

Spitzer WO, Dobson AJ, Hall J et al (1981) Measuring the quality of life of cancer patients: a concise QL-Index for use by physicians. J Chronic Dis 34(12):585–597

Sprangers MAG, Cull A, Groenvold M et al (1998) The European organization for research and treatment of cancer approach to developing questionnaire modules: an update and overview. Qual Life Res 7(4):291–300

Temel JS, Greer JA, Muzikansky A et al (2010) Early palliative care for patients with metastatic non-small-lung-cancer. N Engl J Med 363:733–742

Veiga DF, Veiga-Filho J, Ribeiro LM et al (2010) Quality-of-Life and self-esteem outcomes after oncoplastic breast-conserving surgery 125(3):811–817

Velikova G, Booth L, Smith AB et al (2004) Measuring quality of life in routine oncology practice improves communication and patient well-being: a randomized controlled trial. J Clin Oncol 22 (4):714–724

Velikova G, Keding A, Harley C et al (2010) Patients report improvements in continuity of care when quality of life assessments are used routinely in oncology practice: Secondary outcomes of a randomised controlled trial. Eur J Cancer 46(13):2381–2388

Vonk-Klaassen SM, de Vocht HM, den Ouden MEM et al (2016) Ostomy-related problems and their impact on quality of life of colorectal cancer ostomates: a systematic review. Qual Life Res 25:125–133

Wagland R, Richardson A, Ewings S et al (2016) Prevalence of cancer chemotherapy-related problems, their relation to health-related quality of life and associated supportive care: a cross-sectional survey. Supp Care Cancer 24(12):4901–4911

Weis J, Arraras JI, Conroy T et al (2013) Development of an EORTC quality of life phase III module measuring cancer-related fatigue (EORTC QLQ-FA13). Psycho-Oncol 22(5):1002–1007

WHO (1946) In: Preamble to the Constitution of the World Health Organization as adopted by the International Health Conference, New York, 19–22 June 1946; signed on 22 July 1946 by the representatives of 61 States (Official Records of the World Health Organization, no 2, p 100) and entered into force on 7 April 1948

WHOQOL Group (1993) Study protocol for the World Health Organization project to develop a Quality of Life assessment instrument (WHOQOL). In: Research QoL, pp 153–159

Psychosocial Impact of Personalized Therapies in Oncology

Georgia Schilling and Frank Schulz-Kindermann

Abstract

Personalized medicine is a keyword in modern oncology summarizing biomarker-driven targeted therapies. Those novel agents enhance our therapeutic portfolio and offer new options for our patients. But the term is often misleading and implicates a tailored therapy to the individual person, but it rather means a treatment stratified on genetic characteristics of the tumor. Molecular therapies raise expectations of curability or long-term treatments making former life-threatening diseases to more chronic ones but this is true only for some patients. So we have to carefully communicate with our patients about the options and limitations of those modern therapies not to trigger disappointments.

Keywords

Molecular stratified medicine · Chances · Limitations · Improved patient care

G. Schilling (✉)
Department of Oncology with Section Hematology, Asklepios Klinik Altona,
Asklepios Cancer Center Hamburg, Paul-Ehrlich-Str. 1, 22763 Hamburg, Germany
e-mail: g.schilling@asklepios.com

F. Schulz-Kindermann
Institute of Medical Psychology, University Hospital Hamburg-Eppendorf,
Martinistr. 52, W26, 20246 Hamburg, Germany
e-mail: schulzk@uke.de

© Springer International Publishing AG 2018
U. Goerling and A. Mehnert (eds.), *Psycho-Oncology*, Recent Results
in Cancer Research 210, https://doi.org/10.1007/978-3-319-64310-6_11

181

1 "Personalized Medicine" in Oncology

The terms individualized, tailored, personalized, and targeted describe modern therapies in oncology. It may be more appropriate to use the expression stratified medicine as the treatment is based on stratification by genetic characteristics of the tumor. They are detected by new molecular methods and tests and are used for therapeutic decision-making or rather predicting treatment response. The path is clearly mapped out: away from a shotgun method toward specific treatment on the basis of genetic characteristics.

That is to treat different tumors sharing the same pathogenetic relevant molecular alteration, a so-called "driver mutation," with one single drug. As an example, pilocytic astrocytoma, hairy cell leukemia and malignant melanoma: all three entities may bear the B-RAF mutation $^V600^E$, against the B-RAF inhibitor Vemurafenib is targeted with therapeutic success.

Tumors which seemed to be homogenous based on morphological and histological findings are divided into clinically distinct, mostly very small subgroups today. For instance, colon carcinoma, which was to be treated in the same way in all patients only depending on the tumor stage, does not exist any longer: with regard to 100 patients suffering from a colon carcinoma, you now have to deal with several sub-entities, all treated in different ways (De Roock et al. 2010). Latest findings indicate, that a right-sided colon carcinoma responds to specific therapies unlike a tumor on the left side of the colon. The reasons therefore are molecular changes which have not been revealed yet.

The latest concept characterized by the American expert in biomedicine Leroy Hood is, P4 medicine (Hood and Friend 2011) meaning preventive, personalized, participative, and precise. It takes into account cancer prevention and early diagnosis programs as well as the participation of the patient in the therapeutic shared decision-making, besides genetic characteristics of the disease and increasingly specific diagnostics.

The aim of personalized medicine is an improvement of systemic treatment due to preferably exact molecular characterization of the individual tumor and the use of highly specific drugs.

2 History of Personalized Medicine

Certain genetic alterations are responsible for malignant processes like immortalization, neo-angiogenesis, disturbed apoptosis, continuous activated proliferative signaling pathways, genetic instability, or the ability for invasion and metastasis formation. There are so-called activating (driver) mutations in protooncogenes or rather inactivation of tumor suppressor genes leading to malignant cell transformation. The better understanding of these molecular processes enables us to target tumor treatment nowadays:

Chronic Myeloid Leukemia (CML) is a prime example or rather a model disease for the development of personalized medicine. Rudolf Virchow has described the disease as "white blood" for the first time in 1845. In 1960 Peter Nowell and David

Hungerford discovered the so-called "Philadelphia"-chromosome to be the first recurrent chromosomal aberration in a malignant disease (Nowell and Hungerford 1960). Few years later, in 1972, Janet Rowley was able to show that this tiny chromosome arises out of a translocation between chromosomes 9 and 22 (Rowley 1973).

The mentioned translocation results in a fusion gene, an altered protein with increased tyrosine kinase activity is being transcribed from. This change finally ends up in an increased proliferative activity of haematopoietic stem cells and a tremendous proliferation of myeloid cells.

The development of drugs against this modified tyrosine kinase (tyrosine kinase inhibitors = TKIs) was enabled by tracing back the pathogenesis of CML to this unique molecular mechanism.

Since the beginning of the 2000s, Imatinib is available on the market, a first generation TKI competitively inhibiting the activity of the new emerging kinase. The IRIS trial (O'Brien et al. 2003), investigating Imatinib as sole medication for CML, revealed an 8-year survival rate of >85% and thus revolutionized the treatment of the disease—20 years earlier, the 8-year survival rate was at below 15%. By now we use second and third generation TKIs capable to improve CML treatment even when Imatinib is not effective anymore. TKIs are the gold standard by now. Allogeneic stem cell transplantation today is reserved for only a few young patients who are non-responders to TKI therapy.

This might have been the birth of modern molecular oncology: the identification of a driver mutation and the targeted inhibition of the resulting structurally and functionally altered protein.

3 Chances Offered by Personalized Medicine

Through decoding the human genome and the availability of high throughput molecular analyses, the so-called "omics"-technologies, biomarkers could be identified. They are of prognostic value: this means that a patient at high risk of relapse can be identified as well as a patient who benefits from a more intense or multimodal treatment. Biomarkers may also be predictive: they are capable to foresee the response of individual patients to certain systemic therapies. In addition there are pharmacodynamic biomarkers, giving us information on possible side effects due to slower or accelerated degradation processes in individual patients during certain treatments. Adopting this knowledge, we will be able to avoid ineffective, unnecessary, or even harmful therapies and actually treat patients really in an individualized manner.

There are numerous entities insufficiently treated by conventional chemotherapies so far. One example is malignant melanoma, a disease which can be treated targeted today and thereby prolonging survival rates significantly. Moreover, prognostic tests allow us to tailor treatments for distinct cases and avoid over- and undertreatment. They can predict the individual risk of relapse on the basis of gene expression analyses: e.g., Oncotype DX®, Endopredict®, or Mammaprint® is used in early breast cancer for determining the adjuvant therapy in borderline cases.

4   Limitations of Personalized Medicine

CML, is a prime example of individualized treatment. It is a success story for targeted therapy but still an exception among malignant diseases so far. Although the decoding of molecular signal transduction pathways and possible therapeutic targets led to a better understanding of the pathogenesis of different tumor entities, tailored treatment has not nearly been as successful as in CML:

In Her2/neu positive breast cancer (15–20% of breast cancers), distinguished by a more unfavorable prognosis and a faster growth, the monoclonal antibody Trastuzumab has been used for many years. By this, the overall survival rate of the patients in the adjuvant setting could be improved significantly, but still approximately half of the patients with a Her2/neu positive tumor does not benefit from this treatment. It is still unknown why not every patient gains a survival advantage by the use of Trastuzumab despite the presence of the molecular target. A biomarker identifying these women is still missing.

After an initial good response to targeted treatment however, e.g., endocrine therapy in hormone-receptor positive breast cancer or TKI therapy in non-small-cell lung cancer (NSCLC), the disease proceeds. This demonstrates the complexity of interlinked and multiple feedback signaling pathways being significantly higher in solid tumors than in CML. The reasons for the development of resistance mechanisms are the genetic instability of the tumor or the variable response mechanisms of tumor cells in order to bypass the deactivation of target structures. Several mutations in genes, leading to activation of signaling pathways more downstream or of alternative signaling pathways, are known. This hampers sustainable success of one single targeted treatment. Due to the genetic heterogeneity of the tumor itself and the presence of several distinct cell clones, only parts of the tumor could be destroyed by targeted therapies. Other subclones derive a survival advantage which results in recurrence or disease progression after a while. Genetic characteristics found in the primary tumor do not necessarily have to be present in its metastases.

Due to recent molecular high throughput analyses we receive lots of information, which we have to use properly for individualized therapy.

A malignant tumor bears 30–60 mutations on an average (Vogelstein et al. 2013): "driver" mutations, being responsible for the malignant transformation and providing a growth advantage must be differentiated from neutral *bystander-* or *passenger*-mutations. The latter are not causative for the pathogenesis of the tumor and thus are not suitable as therapeutic "targets."

Just as today we are able to predict which patients have a higher risk for developing an Oxaliplatin-induced polyneuropathy or an Anthracycline-induced cardiomyopathy by the detection of tiny genetic changes [Single Nucleotide Polymorphisms (SNPs)]. Nevertheless, despite this knowledge, we cannot refuse a life-saving drug to the patient if an alternative treatment is (still) missing.

Last but not least the costs for a wider application of high throughput screenings as well as for resulting therapies will certainly be huge and will raise a number of socioeconomic issues we will have to face on in our health care system.

5 Molecular Therapies and Quality of Life

Often being conducted over years until disease progression, these therapies are supposed to impair patients' quality of life as little as possible. This was hoped for targeted therapies, but unfortunately it has not come true in many cases. The same signaling pathways or metabolic processes, against targeted drugs are directed, also take place in normal cells. Serious side effects can occur just as tremendous as those known by chemotherapy. For example, skin toxicity of EGFR-targeted therapies may be at least as impairing as the side effects of chemotherapy leading to social withdrawal and isolation (Charles et al. 2013).

Currently there is still little data on quality of life during targeted therapies, particularly in comparison to chemotherapy. In molecular defined groups, like EGFR-mutated lung cancer, a targeted therapy may have less side effects than a platinum-based chemotherapy regimen (Druker et al. 2006). Patient reported outcomes (PROs) of patients with relapsed head and neck tumors demonstrate evidence of improved functionality and quality of life, taking the immunotherapeutic drug Nivolumab compared to a standard second line treatment with a single cytostatic drug. Additional it showed a significant overall survival advantage (Ferris et al. 2016).

Considering Imatinib, there are only small differences in quality of life compared to an age-appropriate control population, especially for patients older than 60 years, even when treated for many years. On the contrary, younger patients, aged 18–39 years, state a reduced ability to work and a change of their social role as one major burden among other things. Main side effect was fatigue, independent of age and gender; it was stated by up to 82% (O'Brien et al. 2003). Fortunately, some side effects decreased over the years despite long term intake of Imatinib (Druker et al. 2006). Further long term data considering the quality of life among targeted therapy are missing, especially for solid tumors.

By investigating patient preferences, we can better evaluate the question, how stressful a treatment is assessed by the individual patient. For good counseling and care of our patients in practice we need further research on these topics. Doing so, we will rather be able to realize true individualized therapy—independent of media and pharmaceutical marketing—without raising false expectations.

6 What Does "Personalized" or "Individualized" in Oncological Treatment Really Mean?

The terms "individualized" or "personalized" might imply that these therapies are tailored in a very special way to an individual patient. But compared to surgical interventions, where tumor localization, size, and possible metastasis, etc., in every patient are assessed precise and subtle, modern therapies are hardly "more" individualized. Since they merely focus on certain molecular features which can be assigned to certain clusters associated with a high likelihood for a tumor response to a specific treatment for example.

Charles Bardes commented on this development as follows: "As a rhetorical slogan, it takes a position in contrast to which everything else is both doctor-centered and suspect on ethical, economic, organizational, and metaphoric grounds." (Bardes 2012).

But even therapies in oncology which seem to fit like a key into a lock, do not relieve us from a thorough processing and perception of all associated (bio)psychosocial burdens. The advantage of using a more innovative, effective, safe, and poor in side effects treatment not necessarily implies the discharge from all negative impact from a patients' perspective.

In this sense combining oncological treatment range and comprising personal wellbeing—health—is not something static but a dynamic interactive process. The personal integrity of the patient thereby serves as a corrective. That is how we see modern medicine since the paradigm shift of Georg Engel to a biopsychosocial understanding of disease and treatment. Engel's proposal for a biopsychosocial model would take into account the patient, the social context in which he lives, and the complementary system devised by society to deal with the disruptive effects of illness (Engel 1977).

We further recognize, that a malignant disease, especially one that cannot be cured, challenges the person as a whole. The threat due to suffering not only affects the physical but quite the existential dimension. This clarification is of utmost importance because less clearly definable aspects, e.g., spiritual and existential needs or the "personal identity" are included. When faced with cancer, most patients experience a fundamental threat to their life and livelihood. All that makes up a human being is totally questioned: the self-determined, dignified life in principle, which follows a certain chronology and coherence.

The term "person" designates uniqueness, dignity, and freedom of every individual, as well as the relation to a counterpart and to the community (Kriz 2014). The real confrontation with a more or less close end of life may bring up final and hidden resources and a—sometimes desperate—will to survive. Those patients often have already been through a number of crucial treatments but will finally have to recognize that all those attempts would not be able to cure them.

In this situation, the offer of "personalized" therapies seems to be very tempting: they promise a treatment which really addresses "me," the person standing with one's back to the wall in this desperate situation. Expectations considering a last minute rescue are raised. The euphoria coming with "personalized therapies," might be explained in part by this psychological constellation.

7 "Individualization" of Psychosocial Aspects?

One aspect, being raised by discussing modern therapies in oncology, is the further individualization or rather stratification of patients' characteristics. As well as any chemotherapy or radiation therapy does not make sense for any kind of cancer, one psychosocial intervention does not fit for all possible psychosocial concerns. We know that a substantial proportion of cancer patients suffer from psychosocial distress, we are aware of distinct psycho-oncological patterns of distress and it is well known that more than one third of all patients with cancer may develop mental disorders of pathological significance during the course of the disease (Faller et al. 2013; Mehnert et al. 2014).

But at the same time, we are aware that a broad majority of all cancer patients doesn't show any equivalent burden or disorder. In our opinion a significant error in definition is made while discussing "individualization": an exact consideration or a screening for certain characteristics is a fundamental precondition for an appropriate treatment, whether oncological or psychosocial. This provides the basis for the decision who needs treatment at all and for whom treatment is not appropriate—either it is not necessary or it likely would not be effective.

Having made this fundamental decision, further multilevel investigations and considerations have to be taken into account before initiating an optimum therapy.

From psychotherapy research it is well known, that we have to deal with general and specific factors determining the success of a psychotherapeutic intervention: general features like characteristics of the person, certain variables of the therapist, those of the therapeutic relationship and the specific therapeutic method. Even when manualizing meticulously, the impact of the specific factors rarely exceeds the unspecific ones (Asay and Lambert 2008).

But these "unspecific" factors affect mainly those concerning "the individual" and "the person." This involves personal conditions, terms of the therapist–patient relationship or the social setting, the access to the therapeutic offers, etc. Many of those "unspecific impact factors" have been defined in "person centered psychotherapy" by Rogers (Rogers 1961).

In the field of advanced disease we also increasingly perceive aspects focusing the "person." When confronted with finiteness, dying and death, authors like Cassel, Saunders, or Kissane emphasizes the threat to the "whole person" or existential distress (Kissane 2000). But this describes, what patients (just like relatives) expect from "personalized therapy": fully addressing aspects nor measurable in quality of life data neither in categories of psychiatric disorders but meeting the needs of the patient's person.

In contrary, there do exist specific indications for certain interventions for a long time in the field of psycho-oncology derived rather from medical treatment or disease setting than from psychosocial characteristics of the patient. This includes, e.g., side effects or consequences of the treatment like mucositis associated pain or fatigue (Kühne et al. 2016). Systemic interventions address, e.g., the family and focus on the burden of minor children of the patients (Herschbach and Dinkel

2014), other programs focus on fear of recurrence (Romer 2014) or existential distress faced with a palliative treatment situation (Scheffold et al. 2016).

Thus, psycho-oncology seems to be well equipped for the challenges of modern oncological therapies: on the one hand, emphasizing the meaning of the "whole person," always comprises a whole of individual features. On the other hand, checking carefully diverse indications and conditions of psycho-oncological impact and initiating appropriate interventions. And finally taking into account all general impact factors of all psychosocial professions showing far stronger effects than highly engineered and manualized methods. Thereby, psycho-oncological support is of vital importance to confrontation with the so-called "personalized therapies."

8 Challenges and Conclusions for the Future

We should focus on further development of the principles of personalized therapy in the preceding years. The evaluation of benefits of new drugs in the setting of classical clinical trials must certainly be questioned; patient related outcomes should be a core element of the evaluation.

Molecular therapies may gain considerable achievements in certain indications, but also raise expectations of curability rather due to the hope of escaping the restrictions of conventional treatment in oncology. The expectation to be perceived as a whole "person" may hardly be met by drugs as they reduce the uniqueness of an individual to more refined specifics of genetic constitutions. This is to be expected the less when such kinds of therapy are initiated in very palliative settings or during disease progression.

Thus, we recommend embedding these modern therapies into a very careful process of communication with a genuine relationship between the patient and the therapist in which the patient may become visible as a real person. By this, we would come closer to the patient's expectation: that "personalized therapy" really stands for person centered empathetic treatment.

References

Asay TP, Lambert MJ (2008) The empirical case for the common factors in therapy: quantitative findings. In: Hubble MA, Duncan BL, Miller SD (eds) The heart and soul of change: what works in therapy. American Psychological Association, Washington, pp 23–55

Bardes CL (2012) Defining patient-centered medicine. N Engl J Med 366:782–783

Charles C, Sultan S, Bungener C, Mateus C, Lanoy E, Dauchy S, Verschoore M, Robert C (2013) Impact of cutaneous toxicities associated with targeted therapies on quality of life. Results of a longitudinal exploratory study. Bull Cancer 100:213–222

De Roock W, Claes B, Bernasconi D, De Schutter J, Biesmans B, Fountzilas G, Kalogeras KT, Kotoula V, Papamichael D, Laurent-Puig P, Penault-Llorca F, Rougier P, Vincenzi B, Santini D, Tonini G, Cappuzzo F, Frattini M, Molinari F, Saletti P, De Dosso S, Martini M, Bardelli A, Siena S, Sartore-Bianchi A, Tabernero J, Macarulla T, Di Fiore F, Gangloff AO, Ciardiello F, Pfeiffer P, Qvortrup C, Hansen TP, Van Cutsem E, Piessevaux H, Lambrechts D, Delorenzi M, Tejpar S (2010) Effects of KRAS, BRAF, NRAS, and PIK3CA mutations on the efficacy of cetuximab plus chemotherapy in chemotherapy-refractory metastatic colorectal cancer: a retrospective consortium analysis. Lancet Oncol 11(8):753–762

Druker BJ, Guilho F, O'Brien SG, Gathmann I, Kantarjian H, Gattermann N, Deininger MW, Silver RT, Goldman JM, Stone RM, Cervantes F, Hochhaus A, Powell BL, Gabrilove JL, Rousselot P, Reiffers J, Cornelissen JJ, Hughes T, Agis H, Fischer T, Verhoef G, Shepherd J, Saglio G, Gratwohl A, Nielsen JL, Radich JP, Simonsson B, Taylor K, Baccarani M, So C, Letvak L, Larson RA (2006) IRIS Investigators. Five-year follow-up of patients receiving imatinib for chronic myeloid leukemia. N Engl J Med 355(23):2408–2417

Engel GL (1977) The need for a new medical model: a challenge for biomedicine. Science 196:129–136

Faller H, Schuler H, Richard M, Heckl U, Weis J, Küffner R (2013) Effects of psycho-oncologic interventions on emotional distress and quality of life in adult patients with cancer: systematic review and meta-analysis. J Clin Oncol 31(6):782–793

Ferris RL, Blumenschein G Jr, Fayette J, Guigay J, Colevas AD, Licitra L, Harrington K, Kasper S, Vokes EE, Even C, Worden F, Saba NF, Iglesias Docampo LC, Haddad R, Rordorf T, Kiyota N, Tahara M, Monga M, Lynch M, Geese WJ, Kopit J, Shaw JW, Gillison ML (2016) Nivolumab for recurrent squamous-cell carcinoma of the head and neck. N Engl J Med 375(19):1856–1867

Herschbach P, Dinkel A (2014) Fear of progression. Recent Results Cancer Res 197:11–29

Hood L, Friend SH (2011) Predictive, personalized, preventive, participatory (P4) cancer medicine. Nat Rev Clin Oncol 8(3):184–187

Kissane DW (2000) Psychospiritual and existential distress. The challenge for palliative care. Aust Fam Physician 11(29):1022–1025

Kriz J (2014) Grundkonzepte der Psychotherapie. Beltz, Weinheim

Kühne F, Meinders C, Mohr H, Kieseritzky K, Rosenberger C, Härter M, Schulz-Kindermann F, Klinger R, Nestoriuc AY (2016) Psychological treatments for pain in cancer patients: a systematic review on the current state of research. Schmerz 30(6):496–509

Mehnert A, Brähler E, Faller H, Härter M, Keller M, Schulz H, Wegscheider K, Weis J, Boehncke A, Hund B, Reuter K, Richard M, Sehner S, Sommerfeldt S, Szalai C, Wittchen H-U, Koch U (2014) Four-week prevalence of mental disorders in patients with cancer across major tumor entities. J Clin Oncol 32(31):3540–3546

Nowell PC, Hungerford DA (1960) Chromosome studies on normal and leukemic human leukocytes. J Natl Cancer Inst 25:85–109

O'Brien SG, Guilhot F, Larson RA, Gathmann I, Baccarani M, Cervantes F, Cornelissen JJ, Fischer T, Hochhaus A, Hughes T, Lechner K, Nielsen JL, Rousselot P, Reiffers J, Saglio G, Shepherd J, Simonsson B, Gratwohl A, Goldman JM, Kantarjian H, Taylor K, Verhoef G, Bolton AE, Capdeville R, Druker BJ (2003) IRIS investigators. imatinib compared with interferon and low-dose cytarabine for newly diagnosed chronic-phase chronic myeloid leukemia. N Engl J Med 348(11):994–1004

Rogers C (1961) On becoming a person. Houghton Mifflin, Boston

Romer G (2014) Children of somatically ill parents: psychological stressors, ways of coping and perspectives of mental health prevention. Prax Kinderpsychol Kinderpsychiatr 56(10):870–890

Rowley JD (1973) Letter: a new consistent chromosomal abnormality in chronic myelogenous leukaemia identified by quinacrine fluorescence and Giemsa staining. Nature 243 (5405):290–293

Scheffold K, Phillipp R, Engelmann D, Schulz-Kindermann F, Rosenberger C, Oechsle K, Härter M, Wegscheider K, Lordick F, Lo C, Hales S, Rodin G, Mehnert A (2016) Efficacy of a brief manualized intervention Managing Cancer and Living Meaningfully (CALM) adapted to German cancer care settings: study protocol for a randomized controlled trial. Br J Cancer 2015, 15:592

Vogelstein B, Papadopoulos N, Velculescu VE, Zhou S, Diaz LA Jr, Kinzler KW (2013) Cancer genome landscapes. Science 339(6127):1546–1558

COMSKIL Communication Training in Oncology—Adaptation to German Cancer Care Settings

Tim J. Hartung, David Kissane and Anja Mehnert

Abstract

Medical communication is a skill which can be learned and taught and which can substantially improve treatment outcomes, especially if patients' communication preferences are taken into account. Here, we give an overview of communication training research and outline the COMSKIL program as a state-of-the-art communication skills training in oncology. COMSKIL has a solid theoretical foundation and teaches core elements of medical communication in up to ten fully operationalized modules. These address typical situations ranging from breaking bad news to responding to difficult emotions, shared decision-making, and communicating via interpreters.

Keywords

Neoplasms · Communication · Medical psychology · Physician-patient relations · Continuing medical education

1 Background

Identifying patients' communication needs and preferences represent a complex and challenging task for doctors and other members of the multidisciplinary team; it requires high cognitive and communication skills. Accurate perception of patients' needs is crucial for effective doctor–patient communication. Such needs include not only

T.J. Hartung · A. Mehnert (✉)
Department of Medical Psychology and Medical Sociology, University Medical Center Leipzig, Philipp-Rosenthal-Strasse 55, 04103 Leipzig, Germany
e-mail: anja.mehnert@medizin.uni-leipzig.de

D. Kissane
Department of Psychiatry, Monash University, Melbourne, Australia

© Springer International Publishing AG 2018
U. Goerling and A. Mehnert (eds.), *Psycho-Oncology*, Recent Results in Cancer Research 210, https://doi.org/10.1007/978-3-319-64310-6_12

preferences and expectations regarding medical issues but also general interpersonal needs (Hack et al. 2005). A trusting relationship can influence important outcome parameters of medical treatment as well as psychosocial distress, the ability to cope with the illness and treatment adherence (Fallowfield and Jenkins 1999; Watson et al. 2005). Therefore, interventions which improve medical communication also bear the potential of improving cancer treatment outcomes (Butow et al. 1999).

Evidence from medical psychology research suggests that doctor–patient communication is a skill which can be learned and taught effectively by well-structured communication training programs (Barth and Lannen 2011). Nonetheless, there are very few programs which include patients' communication preferences as a central element. One of these programs is COMSKIL, which was developed at Memorial Sloan-Kettering Cancer Center (MSKCC) in New York (Brown and Bylund 2008; Bylund et al. 2010; Kissane et al. 2012). Here we will give an overview of communication training research and outline the COMSKIL program as a state-of-the-art communication skills training. It provides a core curriculum for oncology training programs (Kissane et al. 2017) and creates a glossary of communication skills, which empower the clinician to constructively reflect on their communication and improve whenever needed.

2 State of the Research

Numerous psycho-oncological studies have found that a substantial proportion of cancer patients show psychosocial distress in need of treatment, which is not recognized or treated adequately in clinical practice (Mallinger et al. 2005; Mehnert et al. 2014; Mitchell et al. 2011). In light of these findings, optimal doctor–patient communication represents the corner stone of patient information, provision, support and compassionate care, thus improving treatment adherence and thereby successful treatment (Fallowfield and Jenkins 1999; Maguire 2002; Rehse and Pukrop 2003; Thorne et al. 2008). Particularly, difficult conversations include breaking the bad news about the diagnosis, informing patients about invasive treatment, cancer recurrence or the transfer to palliative treatment. Doctors experience such consultations as highly distressing (Brown and Bylund 2010; Fallowfield and Jenkins 2004; Parker et al. 2010).

There are many reasons for enhancing clinicians' communication skills. It is not only patients who criticize doctors' communication behavior, but also physicians who have emphasized a need for improvement (Back et al. 2005; Brown et al. 2007; Butow et al. 2004; Mallinger et al. 2005; Parker et al. 2010). In reaction, a variety of expert recommendations have been drafted (Baile et al. 2000; Epstein and Street Jr. 2007; Holland and Alici 2010; Lee and Wu 2002; Okamura et al. 1998), which were the basis for a wide range of communication trainings from individual lectures to programs for continued medical education which last several days (Barth and Lannen 2011; Butler et al. 2005; Cegala and Lenzmeier Broz 2002; Rao et al. 2007; Uitterhoeve et al. 2010). A general difficulty of such interventions is that a clear conceptualization of communication skills

Table 1 Overview of communication training programs

Region	Program	Topics	Target audience	Teaching structure	Duration	Outcome parameters
New York (USA)	COMSKIL (implemented at MSKKC since 2005)	Conceptual introduction, communicating bad news, discussing the prognosis, dealing with anger, conversation with patients and significant others, communication via translator, shared decision making, obtaining informed consent for clinical studies	Doctors, nurses	Short lectures, role play with actors, video analyses, feedback, small groups (6 participants)	2 days	Self-report regarding skills and satisfaction, video analyses
Texas (USA)	Oncotalk (developed in 2002)	Communicating with palliative care patients	Doctors during residency	Short lectures, role play with actors, feedback, small groups (5 participants)	3.5 days	Self-report regarding skills and satisfaction, audio analyses
Switzerland	Communication training program (introduced as obligatory by the Swiss Society for Medical Oncology in 2001)	4 elements of communication: structure, exchange of information, emotion, relationship aspects	Doctors during oncological residency, nurses	Case discussions, role play with actors, audio recordings (pre/post), small groups (10 participants)	2 days, 4-6 single supervisions, half-day workshop	Self-report regarding skills and satisfaction, audio analyses by blinded raters
Australia	Several programs, traditionally a small workshop model for one specific topic	E.g., basic communication skills, breaking bad news, improving communication in an interdisciplinary team	All oncological health care professionals	Short lectures, role play with actors, small groups (4-6 participants)	3–4 h	Self-report regarding skills and satisfaction
Great Britain	Postgraduate course for palliative care specialists at Cardiff University	Internet-based portfolio e-learning system and communication trainings with different content	All oncological health care professionals	E.g., short lectures, role play with actors, video analyses, supervision, visitations with colleagues	2 years	N/A

(continued)

Table 1 (continued)

Region	Program	Topics	Target audience	Teaching structure	Duration	Outcome parameters
Brussels (Belgium)	Training programs of varying scope	Basics of communication, dealing with patients' anxiety and distress, identifying distressed patients, discussing the prognosis, dealing with death and dying	Nurses, social workers, work therapists	Lectures, role play with actors, audio recordings (including real patients), small groups (12 participants)	12 h 1 day 2.5 days 105 h	Self-report regarding skills and satisfaction, audio analyses, patient satisfaction and quality of life
	Basic communication and consolidation work shop	Aims, purpose and specifics of communication, dealing with patient distress, conversations where significant others are present	Doctors	Lectures, actor patients, video recordings (incl. real doctor–patient consultations), role play, small groups (6 participants)	40 h 3 h	Self-report regarding skills and satisfaction, distress, video analyses, patient satisfaction and quality of life
Germany	Kompass (compact course plus consolidation work shop)	Breaking bad news, shared decision making, transition from curative to palliative care, support in dealing with the disease, conversations about death, dying, ethical problems	Doctors	Lectures, patient actors, video recordings, role play, small groups (10 participants)	2.5 days 1 day	Self-report regarding skills and satisfaction, distress, video analyses
	COM-ON-p or COM-ON-rct	Transition from curative to palliative care or information about randomized controlled trials (RCT)	Doctors	Lectures, role play with patient actors, video recordings, small groups (8-9 participants)	1.5 days	Self-report regarding skills and satisfaction, video analyses

has been lacking. Therefore, outcome variables for operationalization and efficacy studies have not been defined well (Cegala and Lenzmeier Broz 2002). These methodological limitations are also evident in the majority of studies evaluating training programs (Barth and Lannen 2011; Fellowes et al. 2004; Gysels et al. 2004, 2005). These reviews conclude that the best results are achieved by those programs that comprise a combination of different learner-centered methods and a mixture of theoretical and practical elements. Table 1 shows an overview of international initiatives to improve medical communication skills.

Complex training programs have been able to improve communication skills, although these changes have been mostly assessed by subjective self-report (Barth and Lannen 2011; Bylund et al. 2010; Delvaux et al. 2005; Fallowfield et al. 2002, 2003; Jenkins and Fallowfield 2002; Lenzi et al. 2011; Merckaert et al. 2005; Razavi et al. 2003). With regard to patient-related outcome parameters, studies have found an increase in patient satisfaction and trained doctors have shown greater awareness of patients' psychosocial issues (Delvaux et al. 2005; Merckaert et al. 2005; Uitterhoeve et al. 2010; Visser and Wysmans 2010). Evidence for improved mental health reduced patient distress or enhanced coping skills has been scarce (Barth and Lannen 2011; Uitterhoeve et al. 2010). Furthermore, although training programs aim to consider individual patient needs, the immense variety and diversity of such issues have made the development of a comprehensive curriculum challenging (Dale et al. 2004; Echlin and Rees 2002; Girgis et al. 1999; Mallinger et al. 2006). In their review of the literature, Kiesler and Auerbach found that

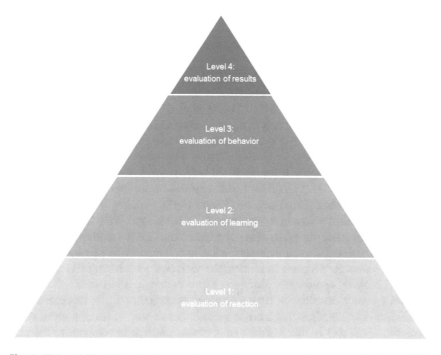

Fig. 1 Kirkpatrick's Triangle showing levels of assessment for communication training programs; adapted from Hutchinson (1999)

successful communication between doctor and patient depends little on accordance with recommendations and guidelines; it is rather the result of congruence between the patient's needs and the doctor's response (Kiesler and Auerbach 2006). This emphasizes the need for training programs which teach how to identify changing communication needs throughout the trajectory of care.

Common outcome criteria in this field are: patient satisfaction with doctors' communication, patient competence and knowledge of their illness, and doctors' empathy as perceived by the patient, consideration of patients' communication preferences during the consultation, doctor satisfaction with the training, improvements in communication skills, doctors' feeling of being overwhelmed, and change of communication behavior (Barth and Lannen 2011).

One of the most widely used assessment models for training programs Kirkpatrick's Triangle, (Kirkpatrick 1967; Konopasek et al. 2010). It consists of four levels of evaluation (Fig. 1) to assess the impact of a training program. The first level focuses on immediate reactions to the training, offering an opportunity for trainees to voice their opinions, self-efficacy, and level of satisfaction with the training. The second level assesses new knowledge and skills in a standardized way. The third level measures changes in actual behavior in the clinical setting when communicating with real rather than simulated patients. At the fourth and highest level, the overall impact in terms of benefits to patients and other members of the care system is assessed. The COMSKIL Coding System is one way to assess and code the use of communication skills and strategies taught during the program(Bylund et al. 2008).

3   COMSKIL: Theoretical Foundations and Structure

The COMSKIL communication training was developed at Memorial Sloan-Kettering Cancer Center (MSKCC), New York, USA in 2005 (Banerjee et al. 2015; Brown and Bylund 2008; Bylund et al. 2010; Kissane et al. 2012). It is a multidisciplinary curriculum, which applies not only to doctors but also to nurses and other members of the health care team. It aims to overcome many of the methodological limitations of other programs and studies by teaching the core elements of doctor–patient communication in a thoroughly operationalized way and with a solid theoretical foundation (Brown et al. 2009). COMSKIL was developed from three theoretical models: goals, plans, and action (GPA) theories (Berger 1997), sociolinguistic theory (Miller 2007) and Leventhal's common sense model (Donovan and Ward 2001). Based on the premise that goals and plans guide communication, GPA theorists have ordered components of interpersonal communication in a hierarchy from goals, the most abstract component, via plans to actions, the most concrete element (Berger 1997). This goal-centered approach is combined with a communication style, which sociolinguistic theory describes as person-centered communication. In this model, the practitioner acknowledges that there is more than one way to reach a given communication goal and is able to adapt their communication in response to the perspectives, feelings, and intentions of others (Miller 2007). A third aspect stems from the view that illness is understood through common sense. Patients may develop a comprehensive concept of an illness by incorporating information provided by the physician and thereby questioning and deepening their common sense concept. Patients' representations of illness and treatment are thus continually modified, cross-checked and updated in a process that becomes self-regulating (McAndrew et al. 2008). It is the clinician's responsibility to understand and review the patient's explanatory model and guide the patient's understanding toward the clinician's medical model. By incorporating these theoretical constructs, COMSKIL aimed to increase the practitioner's flexibility and to expand the range of their communication skills such that they can consciously apply a skill as the situation requires it.

COMSKIL has five core components which will be explained in turn: goals, strategies, skills, process tasks, and cognitive appraisal (Fig. 2). A communication goal is a desired state that the individual is trying to attain. The other core elements serve to achieve such communication goals. Thus, to reach a shared treatment decision, the communication goal is "to help the patient make a fully informed treatment choice, based on a detailed understanding of their illness, the benefit and burden of each treatment option, and its impact on their lifestyle and values, so that their choice optimally suits the patient."

Communication strategies are more concrete than goals and are defined as plans which direct behavior toward the realization of a goal. Using several strategies in the sequence may serve to realize different aspects of a goal, e.g., an emotional and an information-related aspect. The order of execution of these strategies can be varied to meet individual needs and achieve patient-centered communication. Table 2 illustrates these strategies in specific modules of the curriculum.

Communication skills are the most concrete elements and are defined as discrete units of speech which can further the clinical dialog. Skills are concrete, teachable, and observable. They contain elements such as checking a patient's understanding of the information conveyed, validating a patients' feelings or explaining and

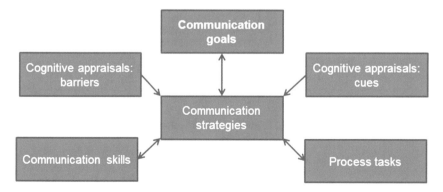

Fig. 2 Core components of COMSKIL modules. Communication goals are achieved through a series of sequenced strategies, which in turn are accomplished via skills and process tasks. Cues from the patient produce cognitive appraisals in the clinician, whereas barriers block open communication and can arise in either party; adapted from Kissane et al. (2012)

Table 2 COMSKIL modules and main strategies

Module	Strategies
Breaking bad news	1. Establish consultation framework 2. Tailor the consultation to the patient's needs 3. Provide information in a way that it will be understood and recalled 4. Respond empathically to emotion 5. Check readiness to discuss management options 6. Close the consultation
Discuss prognosis and risk	1. Ascertain the patient's need for prognostic information 2. Negotiate the type and format of prognostic information 3. Provide information in a manner that is sensitive to the patient's needs and promotes hopefulness 4. Respond empathically to emotion 5. Respond to patient information cues
Shared decision making	1. Establish the consultation framework 2. Establish the physician–patient team 3. Develop an accurate, shared understanding of the patient's situation 4. Present established treatment options 5. Discuss the patient's values and lifestyle factors that may impact on the standard treatment decision 6. Present a clear statement of the recommended treatment option and invite patient choice 7. Close the consultation
Responding to difficult emotions	1. Allow the patient to recount concerns or grievances 2. Work toward a shared understanding of the patient's emotional experience 3. Empathically respond to the emotion/experience 4. Explore attitudes and expectations leading to the difficult emotion 5. Facilitate coping and connect to social support
Communicating with patients using avoidance or denial	1. Exclude misunderstanding and determine if avoidance is adaptive or maladaptive 2. Provide information tailored to the patient 3. Explore emotional reactions with empathy 4. Challenge inconsistencies explore factors enhancing adherence to recommended treatments 5. Respect patient's stance and follow-up to monitor carefully
Communicating about survivorship	1. Introduce survivorship care plan for patient and their general practitioner 2. Review diagnostic features and summarize treatments delivered 3. Identify any long term effects and strategies to manage these (e.g., sexual, reproductive) 4. List on a survivorship care plan any late effects and strategies to recognize early (e.g., secondary cancers) 5. Review any cancer screening and health promotion strategies to reduce risk for late effects 6. Ensure genetic counseling and family advice covered 7. Consider insurance, employment and financial implications

(continued)

Table 2 (continued)

Module	Strategies
	8. Check for any unmet needs or unanswered questions
	9. Describe follow-up plan for future appointments and with whom
Communicating about recurrence of cancer	1. Review understanding of tests, extent of spread and need for treatment
	2. Respond empathically to emotion
	3. Ascertain interest in discussion of prognosis and tailor response
	4. Acknowledge uncertainty
	5. Discuss treatment options, future clinical trials and preferences for management
	6. Summarize action plan and check understanding
Conducting a family meeting	7. Planning and prior set up to arrange the family meeting
	8. Welcome and orient the family to the goals of the meeting
	9. Check each family member's understanding of the illness and its prognosis
	10. Check for consensus about the current goals of care
	11. Identify family concerns about their management of key symptoms or care needs
	12. Clarify the family's view of what the future holds
	13. Clarify how family members are coping and feeling emotionally
	14. Identify family strengths and affirm their level of commitment and mutual support for each other
	15. Close the family meeting by final review of agreed goals of care and future plans
Discussing palliative care and the process of dying	1. Recognize patient's cue or emergent clinical reality
	2. Establish understanding of disease progression, treatment efficacy and prognosis
	3. Discuss patient's values and lifestyle factors that may impact on goals of care; negotiate appropriate if need be new goals of care
	4. Respond empathically to emotion
	5. Negotiate the shift to discuss the process of dying
	6. Promote understanding of change–illness transitions–and role of courage in accepting one's dying
	7. Address caregiver's concerns
	8. Effect referral to palliative care service whenever appropriate
	9. Close consultation
Communicating with patients via interpreters	1. Introduce the content and expectations of the consultation with the interpreter
	2. Elicit interpreter's knowledge about the patient
	3. Establish the doctor–patient–interpreter team
	4. Explore culturally held health beliefs
	5. Promote effective interpretation throughout the consultation
	6. Review the consultation with the interpreter

Each strategy is implemented through concrete process tasks and individual skills summarizing information. Skills can be applied to all areas of health care. There are six broad clusters of these skills, agenda setting, questioning skills, information giving, checking understanding, reaching shared decisions, and empathic responses (Brown and Bylund 2008).

In addition, there are contextual aspects which bear relevance to the initiation and maintenance of doctor–patient consultations. These are called process tasks. Process tasks can be verbal or nonverbal behaviors or dialogs, which create an atmosphere that is beneficial for effective communication. Process tasks can be very simple, e.g., creating a quiet and undisturbed setting for breaking bad news, but they can also be complex, e.g., avoid premature reassurance.

By observing and internally processing patients' verbal and nonverbal behavior, clinicians can form hypotheses about patients' unstated needs and intentions. This process of cognitive appraisal determines which communication strategies, skills, and process tasks the practitioner may choose to achieve the communication goal at hand. Although doctors use cognitive appraisal continuously throughout the communication process, COMSKIL focuses on two particular aspects: patient cues and patient barriers.

Patient cues are indirect behaviors which, if recognized, prompt the clinician to address a certain issue. In this way, a patient may state that they know little about a particular treatment (informational cue) or mention that they cry frequently (emotional cue) without directly asking for information or emotional support.

Patient barriers are concealed perceptions which prevent the patient from communicating openly about an issue and may thus thwart an effective decision-making process. For instance, a patient may have an exaggerated or particularly threatening impression of a treatment's side effects and, as a consequence, avoid discussing this treatment with their doctor.

The COMSKIL communication program consists of ten modules (Table 2) (Bialer et al. 2011; Brown et al. 2010a, b; Di Lubrano Ciccone et al. 2010; Gueguen et al. 2009; Kissane et al. 2017; Levin et al. 2010b). The program is usually taught in small groups during a 2-day workshop, where each group can be optimally facilitated by two instructors, one from the discipline of the trainees and the other from a psychosocial discipline. The emphasis lies with practicing communication skills through role play with simulated patients. For every module, there is a booklet, which forms the basis of the workshop and helps participants prepare. In the first module, the general framework of COMSKIL is laid out and general communication skills necessary for successful communication are explained. The other modules focus on specific but common clinical encounters, which have different goals and therefore require different skills by the doctor. Besides concrete examples to illustrate specific situations, there will be a variety of clinical scenarios available, which serve as the basis for the role playing exercises. A particular advantage is the use of specially trained actors as simulated patients to ensure that the role play is as realistic as possible, while preserving a protected space in which doctors can experiment with different techniques without risk of harm to a real patient. In this small group work, to create a protected, validating setting, which enables an intensive learning experience, there should be no more than six participants. This also makes it possible for clinicians to reflect upon their personal experiences in the role playing exercises. However, when the module focuses on running family meetings, and four simulated patients may form the family for this experiential exercise, a fish bowl setting is utilized, in which the members of the small breakout groups are combined to form a larger observing group. Trainees are then rotated to take turns facilitating the family meeting.

4 Facilitator Training

Educators who provide CST to oncology trainees need to build their own skill base in the effective delivery of this experiential training (Bylund et al. 2008). Using a train-the-trainer model, instructors engage facilitators to define learning goals for each trainee and to build their literacy in the skills, strategies, and tasks that equip them to become optimal communicators. Facilitators establish guidelines for the safety and confidentiality of CST. They brief as necessary the simulated patients to role-play accurately and bring forth nuanced segments of desired intensity that will suit the learner's personal goals (Heinrich 2017). They use a stop–start technique that runs short segments of role-play, video recording for playback and learner review to promote reflection. They facilitate small group appraisal to identify strengths and opportunities for improved communication in the encounter (Manna et al. 2017). Most importantly, they guide the learner to rerun the segment, compare the outcomes, and thus experience a growing sense of mastery of the communication goal. Learners often have an "a-ha" moment as they gain new insight through the use of strategies, skills and process tasks that help them to more competently pursue the communication challenge at hand (Levin et al. 2010a).

Empirical work has established how facilitators can be trained and standardized to generate reproducible facilitation skills and sustain competence in creating a worthwhile learning experience for their trainees (Bylund et al. 2009). Facilitators from the trainee's discipline bring local expertise in the science of that discipline, while psychosocial facilitators bring wisdom and guidance in empathic communication to build an appropriate blend of skills to the advantage of each learner. Facilitators take responsibility for the safety of role-play and guide the small group feedback to be nurturing and constructive for the benefit of each learner.

5 Conclusion

Communication training is vital in oncology and palliative care to develop effective skills in clinicians serving our patients. The existential threat of cancer, related uncertainty, and the complexity of available treatments make this especially pertinent to this field. Experiential training of sufficient dose is critical to this skill development. The COMSKIL model provides a structured CST process wherein trainees learn a language and a reflective method to equip them with an approach that will continue to serve them as their career unfolds. The curriculum has expanded to cover all phases of a patient's journey with cancer. The empirical evidence to support such CST grows ever stronger and more robust. A nursing curriculum has now emerged (Kissane et al. 2017). A number of applied modules have been developed to deal with unexpected adverse surgical outcomes, enrolment in clinical trials, treatment adherence, communicating genetic risk, discussing unproven therapies, communicating with ethnically diverse populations, and so on. The importance of the facilitator's skill and art for the learner is now clear (Lim 2017). CST is established as a crucial and clinically meaningful dimension of advanced training in quality cancer care.

References

Back AL, Arnold RM, Baile WF, Tulsky JA, Fryer-Edwards K (2005) Approaching difficult communication tasks in oncology. CA: A Cancer J Clin 55:164–177. doi:10.3322/canjclin.55.3.164

Baile WF, Buckman R, Lenzi R, Glober G, Beale EA, Kudelka AP (2000) SPIKES-A six-step protocol for delivering bad news: application to the patient with cancer. The Oncol 5(4):302–311

Banerjee SC, Matasar MJ, Bylund CL, Horwitz S, McLarney K, Levin T et al (2015) Survivorship care planning after participation in communication skills training intervention for a consultation about lymphoma survivorship. Trans Behav Med 5:393–400. doi:10.1007/s13142-015-0326-z

Barth J, Lannen P (2011) Efficacy of communication skills training courses in oncology: a systematic review and meta-analysis. Ann Oncol 22:1030–1040. doi:10.1093/annonc/mdq441

Berger CR (1997) Planning strategic interaction: [attaining goals through communicative action] (LEA's communication series). L. Erlbaum Associates, Mahwah, N.J

Bialer PA, Kissane D, Brown R, Levin T, Bylund C (2011) Responding to patient anger: development and evaluation of an oncology communication skills training module. Palliat Supp Care 9:359–365. doi:10.1017/S147895151100037X

Brown RF, Bylund CL (2008) Communication skills training: describing a new conceptual model. Acad Med 83:37–44. doi:10.1097/ACM.0b013e31815c631e

Brown R, Bylund CL (2010) Theoretical models of communication skills training. In: Kissane DW (ed) Handbook of communication in oncology and palliative care. Oxford University Press, Oxford

Brown RF, Butow PN, Boyle F, Tattersall MHN (2007) Seeking informed consent to cancer clinical trials; evaluating the efficacy of doctor communication skills training. Psycho-Oncol 16:507–516. doi:10.1002/pon.1095

Brown RF, Bylund CL, Kline N, La Cruz A, de Solan J, Kelvin J et al (2009) Identifying and responding to depression in adult cancer patients: evaluating the efficacy of a pilot communication skills training program for oncology nurses. Cancer Nurs 32:E1–7. doi:10.1097/NCC.0b013e31819b5a76

Brown R, Bylund CL, Eddington J, Gueguen JA, Kissane DW (2010a) Discussing prognosis in an oncology setting: initial evaluation of a communication skills training module. Psycho-Oncol 19:408–414. doi:10.1002/pon.1580

Brown RF, Bylund CL, Kissane DW (2010b) Principles of communication skills training in cancer care. In: Holland J, Breitbart W, Jacobsen P, Lederberg M, Loscalzo M, McCorkle R (eds) Psycho-Oncology, 2nd edn. Oxford University Press, New York, pp 597–604

Butler L, Degner L, Baile W, Landry M (2005) Developing communication competency in the context of cancer: a critical interpretive analysis of provider training programs. Psycho-Oncol 14:861–72; discussion 873–4. doi:10.1002/pon.948

Butow P, Devine R, Boyer M, Pendlebury S, Jackson M, Tattersall MHN (2004) Cancer consultation preparation package: changing patients but not physicians is not enough. J Clin Oncol 22:4401–4409. doi:10.1200/JCO.2004.66.155

Butow PN, Coates AS, Dunn SM (1999) Psychosocial predictors of survival in metastatic melanoma. J Clin Oncol 17:2256–2263. doi:10.1200/JCO.1999.17.7.2256

Bylund CL, Brown RF, Di Ciccone BL, Levin TT, Gueguen JA, Hill C et al (2008) Training faculty to facilitate communication skills training: development and evaluation of a workshop. Patient Educ Couns 70:430–436. doi:10.1016/j.pec.2007.11.024

Bylund CL, Brown RF, Di Lubrano Ciccone B, Diamond C, Eddington J, Kissane DW (2009) Assessing facilitator competence in a comprehensive communication skills training programme. Med Edu 43:342–349. doi:10.1111/j.1365-2923.2009.03302.x

Bylund CL, Brown R, Gueguen JA, Diamond C, Bianculli J, Kissane DW (2010) The implementation and assessment of a comprehensive communication skills training curriculum for oncologists. Psycho-Oncol 19:583–593. doi:10.1002/pon.1585

Cegala DJ, Lenzmeier Broz S (2002) Physician communication skills training: a review of theoretical backgrounds, objectives and skills. Med Edu 36, 1004–1016 (2002). doi:10.1046/j.1365-2923.2002.01331.x

Dale J, Jatsch W, Hughes N, Pearce A, Meystre C (2004) Information needs and prostate cancer: the development of a systematic means of identification. BJU Int 94:63–69. doi:10.1111/j.1464-410X.2004.04902.x

Delvaux N, Merckaert I, Marchal S, Libert Y, Conradt S, Boniver J et al (2005) Physicians' communication with a cancer patient and a relative: a randomized study assessing the efficacy of consolidation workshops. Cancer 103:2397–2411. doi:10.1002/cncr.21093

Di Lubrano Ciccone B, Brown RF, Gueguen JA, Bylund CL, Kissane DW (2010) Interviewing patients using interpreters in an oncology setting: initial evaluation of a communication skills module. Ann Oncol Official J Eur Soc Med Oncol 21:27–32. doi:10.1093/annonc/mdp289

Donovan HS, Ward S (2001) A representational approach to patient education. J Nurs Scholarsh 33:211–216. doi:10.1111/j.1547-5069.2001.00211.x

Echlin KN, Rees CE (2002) Information needs and information-seeking behaviors of men with prostate cancer and their partners: a review of the literature. Cancer Nurs 25(1):35–41

Epstein RM, Street Jr RL (2007) Patient-centered communication in cancer care: promoting healing and reducing suffering (NIH Publication No. 07-6225). National Cancer Institute, Bethesda

Fallowfield L, Jenkins V (1999) Effective communication skills are the key to good cancer care. Eur J Cancer 35:1592–1597. doi:10.1016/S0959-8049(99)00212-9

Fallowfield L, Jenkins V, Farewell V, Solis-Trapala I (2003) Enduring impact of communication skills training: results of a 12-month follow-up. Br J Cancer 89:1445–1449. doi:10.1038/sj.bjc.6601309

Fallowfield L, Jenkins V (2004) Communicating sad, bad, and difficult news in medicine. The Lancet 363:312–319. doi:10.1016/S0140-6736(03)15392-5

Fallowfield LJ, Jenkins VA, Beveridge HA (2002) Truth may hurt but deceit hurts more: communication in palliative care. Palliat Med 16:297–303. doi:10.1191/0269216302pm575oa

Fellowes D, Wilkinson S, Moore P (2004) Communication skills training for health care professionals working with cancer patients, their families and/or carers. The Cochrane Database Syst Rev CD003751. doi:10.1002/14651858.CD003751.pub2

Girgis A, Sanson-Fisher RW, Schofield MJ (1999) Is there consensus between breast cancer patients and providers on guidelines for breaking bad news? Behav Med 25:69–77. doi:10.1080/08964289909595739

Gueguen JA, Bylund CL, Brown RF, Levin TT, Kissane DW (2009) Conducting family meetings in palliative care: themes, techniques, and preliminary evaluation of a communication skills module. Palliat Support Care 7:171–179. doi:10.1017/S1478951509000224

Gysels M, Richardson A, Higginson IJ (2004) Communication training for health professionals who care for patients with cancer: a systematic review of effectiveness. Support Care Cancer 12:692–700. doi:10.1007/s00520-004-0666-6

Gysels M, Richardson A, Higginson IJ (2005) Communication training for health professionals who care for patients with cancer: a systematic review of training methods. Support Care Cancer 13:356–366. doi:10.1007/s00520-004-0732-0

Hack TF, Degner LF, Parker PA (2005) The communication goals and needs of cancer patients: a review. Psycho-Oncol 14:831–45; discussion 846–7. doi:10.1002/pon.949

Heinrich P (2017) The role of the actor in medical education. In: Kissane DW, Bultz BD, Butow PN, Bylund CL, Noble S, Wilkinson S (eds) Oxford textbook of communication in oncology and palliative care (Oxford medicine online). Oxford University Press, Oxford

Holland JC, Alici Y (2010) Management of distress in cancer patients. J Support Oncol 8(1):4–12

Hutchinson L (1999) Evaluating and researching the effectiveness of educational interventions. BMJ 318:1267–1269. doi:10.1136/bmj.318.7193.1267

Jenkins V, Fallowfield L (2002) Can communication skills training alter physicians' beliefs and behavior in clinics? J Clin Oncol 20:765–769. doi:10.1200/JCO.2002.20.3.765

Kiesler DJ, Auerbach SM (2006) Optimal matches of patient preferences for information, decision-making and interpersonal behavior: evidence, models and interventions. Patient Edu Couns 61:319–341 (2006). doi:10.1016/j.pec.2005.08.002

Kirkpatrick DL (1967) Evaluation of training. In: Craig RL, Bittel LR (eds) Training and development handbook. McGraw-Hill, New York

Kissane DW, Bylund CL, Banerjee SC, Bialer PA, Levin TT, Maloney EK et al (2012) Communication skills training for oncology professionals. J Clin Oncol 30:1242–1247. doi:10.1200/JCO.2011.39.6184

Kissane DW, Bultz BD, Butow PN, Bylund CL, Noble S, Wilkinson S (eds) (2017) Oxford textbook of communication in oncology and palliative care (Oxford medicine online). Oxford University Press, Oxford

Konopasek L, Rosenbaum M, Encandela J, Cole-Kelly K (2010) Evaluating communication skills training courses. In: Kissane DW (ed) Handbook of communication in oncology and palliative care. Oxford University Press, Oxford

Lee A, Wu HY (2002) Diagnosis disclosure in cancer patients–when the family says "no!". Singapore Med J 43(10):533–538

Lenzi R, Baile WF, Costantini A, Grassi L, Parker PA (2011) Communication training in oncology: results of intensive communication workshops for Italian oncologists. Eur J Cancer Care 20:196–203. doi:10.1111/j.1365-2354.2010.01189.x

Levin T, Horner J, Bylund C, Kissane D (2010a) Averting adverse events in communication skills training: a case series. Patient Edu Couns 81:126–130. doi:10.1016/j.pec.2009.12.009

Levin TT, Moreno B, Silvester W, Kissane DW (2010b) End-of-life communication in the intensive care unit. Gen Hosp Psychiatry 32:433–442. doi:10.1016/j.genhosppsych.2010.04.007

Lim R, Dunn S (2017) Journeys to the centre of empathy: The authentic core of communication skills. In: Kissane DW, Bultz BD, Butow PN, Bylund CL, Noble S, Wilkinson S (eds) Oxford textbook of communication in oncology and palliative care (Oxford medicine online). Oxford University Press, Oxford

Maguire P (2002) Key communication skills and how to acquire them. BMJ 325:697–700. doi:10.1136/bmj.325.7366.697

Mallinger JB, Griggs JJ, Shields CG (2005) Patient-centered care and breast cancer survivors' satisfaction with information. Patient Edu Couns 57:342–349. doi:10.1016/j.pec.2004.09.009

Mallinger JB, Shields CG, Griggs JJ, Roscoe JA, Morrow GR, Rosenbluth RJ et al (2006) Stability of decisional role preference over the course of cancer therapy. Psycho-Oncol 15:297–305. doi:10.1002/pon.954

Manna R, Bylund CL, Brown RF, Lubrano di Ciccone B, Konopasek L (2017) Facilitating communication role play sessions: Essential elements and training facilitators. In: Kissane DW, Bultz BD, Butow PN, Bylund CL, Noble S, Wilkinson S (eds) Oxford textbook of communication in oncology and palliative care (Oxford medicine online). Oxford University Press, Oxford

McAndrew LM, Musumeci-Szabo TJ, Mora P A, Vileikyte L, Burns E, Halm EA, et al (2008) Using the common sense model to design interventions for the prevention and management of chronic illness threats: from description to process. Br J Health Psychol 13:195–204. doi:10.1348/135910708X295604

Mehnert A, Brähler E, Faller H, Härter M, Keller M, Schulz H, et al (2014) Four-week prevalence of mental disorders in patients with cancer across major tumor entities. J Clin Oncol 32:3540–3546. doi:10.1200/JCO.2014.56.0086

Merckaert I, Libert Y, Delvaux N, Marchal S, Boniver J, Etienne A.-M et al (2005) Factors that influence physicians' detection of distress in patients with cancer: can a communication skills training program improve physicians' detection? Cancer 104:411–421. doi:10.1002/cncr.21172

Miller K (2007) Communication theories: Perspectives, processes, and contexts (2nd edn). Peking University Press; McGraw-Hill Education (Asia) Co, Beijing

Mitchell AJ, Chan M, Bhatti H, Halton M, Grassi L, Johansen C et al (2011) Prevalence of depression, anxiety, and adjustment disorder in oncological, haematological, and palliative-care settings: a meta-analysis of 94 interview-based studies. The Lancet Oncol 12:60–174. doi:10.1016/S1470-2045(11)70002-X

Okamura H, Uchitomi Y, Sasako M, Eguchi K, Kakizoe T (1998) Guidelines for telling the truth to cancer patients. Japanese National Cancer Center. Jpn J Clin Oncol 28(1):1–4

Parker PA, Ross AC, Polansky MN, Palmer JL, Rodriguez MA, Baile WF (2010) Communicating with cancer patients: what areas do physician assistants find most challenging? J Cancer Edu 25:524–529. doi:10.1007/s13187-010-0110-1

Rao JK, Anderson LA, Inui TS, Frankel RM (2007) Communication interventions make a difference in conversations between physicians and patients: a systematic review of the evidence. Med Care 45:340–349. doi:10.1097/01.mlr.0000254516.04961.d5

Razavi D, Merckaert I, Marchal S, Libert Y, Conradt S, Boniver J et al (2003) How to optimize physicians' communication skills in cancer care: results of a randomized study assessing the usefulness of posttraining consolidation workshops. J Clin Oncol 21:3141–3149. doi:10.1200/JCO.2003.08.031

Rehse B, Pukrop R (2003) Effects of psychosocial interventions on quality of life in adult cancer patients: Meta analysis of 37 published controlled outcome studies. Patient Edu Couns 50:179–186. doi:10.1016/S0738-3991(02)00149-0

Thorne SE, Hislop TG, Armstrong E-A, Oglov V (2008) Cancer care communication: the power to harm and the power to heal? Patient Edu Couns 71:34–40. doi:10.1016/j.pec.2007.11.010

Uitterhoeve RJ, Bensing JM, Grol RP, Demulder PHM, van Achterberg T (2010) The effect of communication skills training on patient outcomes in cancer care: a systematic review of the literature. Eur J Cancer Care 19:42–457. doi:10.1111/j.1365-2354.2009.01082.x

Visser A, Wysmans M (2010) Improving patient education by an in-service communication training for health care providers at a cancer ward: communication climate, patient satisfaction and the need of lasting implementation. Patient Edu Couns 78:402–408. doi:10.1016/j.pec.2010.01.011

Watson M, Homewood J, Haviland J, Bliss JM (2005) Influence of psychological response on breast cancer survival: 10-year follow-up of a population-based cohort. Eur J Cancer 41:1710–1714. doi:10.1016/j.ejca.2005.01.012

The Barrier to Informed Choice in Cancer Screening: Statistical Illiteracy in Physicians and Patients

Odette Wegwarth and Gerd Gigerenzer

Abstract

An efficient health care requires both informed doctors *and* patients. Our current healthcare system falls short on both counts. Most doctors and patients do not understand the available medical evidence. To illustrate the extent of the problem in the setting of cancer screening: In a representative sample of some 5000 women in nine European countries, 92% overestimated the reduction of breast cancer mortality by mammography by a factor of 10–200, or did not know. For a similar sample of about 5000 men with respect to PSA screening, this number was 89%. Of more than 300 US citizens who regularly attended one or more cancer screening test, more than 90% had never been informed about the biggest harms of screening—overdiagnosis and overtreatment—by their physicians. Among 160 German gynecologists, some 80% did not understand the positive predictive value of a positive mammogram, with estimates varying between 1 and 90%. In a national sample of 412 US primary care physicians, 47% mistakenly believed that if more cancers are detected by a screening test, this proves that the test saves lives, and 76% wrongly thought that if screen-detected cancers have better 5-year survival rates than cancers detected by symptoms, this would prove that the screening test saves lives. And of 20 German gynecologists, not a single one provided a woman with all information on the benefits and harms of cancer screening required in order to make an informed choice. Why is risk literacy so scarce in health care? One frequently discussed explanation assumes that people suffer from cognitive deficits that make them predictably irrational and basically hopeless at dealing with risks, so that they need to be "nudged" into healthy behavior. Yet research has

O. Wegwarth (✉) · G. Gigerenzer
Max Planck Institute for Human Development, Lentzeallee 94, 14195 Berlin, Germany
e-mail: wegwarth@mpib-berlin.mpg.de

© Springer International Publishing AG 2018
U. Goerling and A. Mehnert (eds.), *Psycho-Oncology*, Recent Results in Cancer Research 210, https://doi.org/10.1007/978-3-319-64310-6_13

demonstrated that the problem lies less in stable cognitive deficits than in *how* information is presented to physicians and patients. This includes biased reporting in medical journals, brochures, and the media that uses relative risks and other misleading statistics, motivated by conflicts of interest and defensive medicine that do not promote informed physicians and patients. What can be done? Every medical school should teach its students how to understand evidence in general and health statistics in particular. To cultivate informed patients, elementary and high schools should start teaching the mathematics of uncertainty—statistical thinking. Guidelines about complete and transparent reporting in journals, brochures, and the media need to be better enforced, and laws need to be changed in order to protect patients and doctors alike against the practice of defensive medicine instead of encouraging it. A critical mass of informed citizens will not resolve all healthcare problems, but it can constitute a major triggering factor for better care.

Keywords

Informed decision-making · Cancer screening · Medical risk illiteracy · Absolute risk · Relative risk · 5-year survival · Medical risk communication

1   Introduction

Patients appear to be the problem in modern high-tech health care: uninformed, anxious, noncompliant, and with unhealthy lifestyles. They demand drugs advertised by celebrities on TV, insist on unnecessary but expensive tests and treatments, and may eventually turn into plaintiffs. In light of skyrocketing health costs in Western countries, patients' lack of health literacy and the resulting costs and harms have received much attention. Consider a few cases. Almost 10 million U.S. women have had unnecessary Pap smears to screen for cervical cancer—unnecessary because each of them had had a complete hysterectomy and thus no longer had a cervix (Sirovich and Welch 2004). Unnecessary Pap tests may cause no harm but they waste millions that could be put to better use in health care. Every year, one million U.S. children have unnecessary computed tomography (CT) scans (Brenner and Hall 2007). An unnecessary CT scan is more than a waste of money; an estimated 29,000 cancers result from the approximately 70 million CT scans performed annually in the U.S. (Berrington de González et al. 2009). And when a random sample of 500 Americans was asked whether they would rather receive one thousand dollars in cash or a free full-body CT, three out of four wanted the CT (Schwartz et al. 2004). Why do people not protect their children or themselves from unnecessary doses of radiation? They probably would if they knew the risks involved. Uninformed patients are by no means restricted to the U.S. A representative study of over 10,000 citizens in nine European countries revealed that 89% of men and 92% of women, respectively, overestimated the benefit of PSA and mammography screening 10-fold, 100-fold and more, or did not know it (Gigerenzer et al. 2009). With more and better access to health information than ever, why are people so largely uninformed?

The answers proposed include that many patients are not intelligent enough or do not want to deal with numbers, even though most 12-year-olds in the U.S. already know baseball statistics, and their British peers can recite the relevant numbers of the Football Association (FA) Cup results. Scores of health psychologists and behavioral economists add to the list of suspected cognitive deficits by emphasizing patients' cognitive biases, weakness of will, and wishful thinking (Gigerenzer and Gray 2011). In this view, the problems facing health care are people who engage in self-harming behavior, focus on short-term gratification rather than long-term harms, suffer from the inability to predict their emotional states after a treatment, or simply do not want to think and prefer to trust their doctor (Wegwarth and Gigerenzer 2013). Consequently, the recommended remedies are some form of paternalism that "nudges" the inept patient in the right direction (Thaler and Sunstein 2008). Yet the most decisive reason for the lack of health literacy in patients is far more likely the widespread amount of misinformation, whose sources are risk illiterate physicians, intransparent patients' brochures, and the media.

2   How to Communicate the Benefit and Harms of Cancer Screening?

Imagine a 53-year-old woman who considers attending mammography screening for breast cancer. To make an informed decision about whether to attend, she needs to learn about the benefits and harms of that cancer screening. What is the current evidence? In 1996, results of four randomized trials on mammography screening including approximately 280,000 women (Nyström et al. 1996) showed that of 1000 women attending screening over 10 years, three women died of breast cancer, whereas of 1000 women not attending screening over 10 years, four women died of breast cancer. Further analysis showed similar effects: Here, breast cancer mortality was 4 out of 1000 women who attended mammography screening over a course of 10 years, compared to 5 out of 1000 who did not (Nyström et al. 2002). Thus, in both analyses the absolute reduction of breast cancer death due to mammography was 1 woman in 1000. Subsequent Cochrane reviews of these and further randomized trials enrolling approximately 500,000 women found the absolute risk reduction to be even smaller: Now it was estimated that mammography screening would save only 1 woman in 2000 (Gøtzsche and Nielsen 2006, 2011) from breast cancer death. In addition, authors quantified mammography's harms: overdiagnosis and overtreatment. Overdiagnosis refers to the detection of pseudodisease—screening-detected abnormalities that meet the pathologic definition of cancer but will never progress to cause symptoms or cancer death in the patient's lifetime. The consequence of overdiagnosis is overtreatment—surgery, chemotherapy, or radiation that provides the patient with no survival benefit but only side effects. For mammography it is estimated that for every 2000 women invited for screening throughout 10 years, 10 women who would not have been diagnosed with breast cancer if they had not been screened will be treated unnecessarily. Furthermore, more than 200 women out of these 2000 will experience important psychological distress, including anxiety and uncertainty for years because of false-positive findings.

Is the woman in question likely to learn about that evidence from her physician? To learn more about gynecologists' counseling on mammography, we conducted a study (Wegwarth and Gigerenzer 2011) in 2008, nearly 2 years after the first comprehensive Cochrane review about the benefits and harms of mammography was published (Gøtzsche and Nielsen 2006, 2011). One of us called gynecologists who were practicing in different cities across Germany and told them the following story: Our 55-year-old mother with no history of breast cancer in her family and without any symptoms had received an invitation to attend a mammography screening but doubted its effectiveness; we, in contrast, believed that it might be advisable to attend and would like to learn in more detail about its benefits and harms. Of the 20 gynecologists who were willing to talk to us, 17 strongly recommended mammography, emphasizing that it is a safe and scientifically well-grounded intervention. Only seven of these were able to provide numbers for the requested benefit of a reduced risk of breast cancer death, which ranged from 20 to 50%. Communication of the harms was even more discouraging: None of the gynecologists mentioned the risk of being overdiagnosed or overtreated as a consequence of mammography screening. Instead, the majority described the potential harms as "negligible" and "harmless." Only 3 out of the 20 gynecologists provided numbers for specific harms, out of which two numbers were wrong.

The results of these studies documented two issues: (1) People who consult their physicians on the benefits and harms of cancer screening are unlikely to receive correct numbers, if any, on the benefits and harms but instead verbal and subjective qualifiers, and (2) they are likely to be misled by *mismatched framing* (Gigerenzer et al. 2007). *Mismatched framing* refers to the act of reporting the benefits and harms of a medical intervention in difference "currencies": usually the benefits in relative risks (=large numbers) and the harms in absolute risks (=small numbers). The same risk reduction (for benefits) or risk increase (for harms) can be expressed as either a relative risk (RR), absolute risk (AR), or the number of people needed to be treated (screened) to prevent one death from cancer (NNT, which is 1/absolute risk reduction). For instance, taking the review on mammography screening (Gøtzsche and Nielsen 2006), where a breast cancer mortality reduction from 5 to 4 women in 2000 was observed, one can report these results as

RRR   If you have regular mammography screening, it will reduce your chances of dying from this cancer by around 20% over the next 10 years.

ARR   If you have regular mammography screening, it will reduce your chances of dying from this cancer from around 5 per 2000 to around 4 per 2000 over the next 10 years.

NNT   To save 1 woman from dying from breast cancer over the next 10 years, around 2000 woman have to have regular mammography screening.

Whereas absolute risks and NNT are typically small numbers, the corresponding relative risk tends to appear large. As a consequence, the format of relative risk leads not only laypersons but also doctors to overestimate the benefits of medical interventions. In our study about counseling on mammography screening, all numerical information we received from the gynecologists about the benefit were relative risk reductions, whereas the harms were quantified as absolute risk increase. For instance, the estimates we received for the benefit (reduction of breast cancer deaths) ranged from 20 to 50%. The 50% does not correspond to any findings of evidence-based studies on the effectiveness of mammography screening, but the 20% corresponds to results of earlier reviews (Nyström et al. 2002). To arrive at the 20%, all other information (e.g., how many women were in each of the studied groups = reference classes) is ignored and only the reduction from five breast cancer deaths (=100%) to four breast cancer deaths (=80% from 5) is considered. What this relative risk statement suggests to most readers is that of all people who are screened, 20% fewer die of breast cancer. Yet that is not what the 20% means. In fact, a relative risk of 20% can be compatible with a wide range of changes in the absolute risk reduction of death, such as a reduction from 50 to 40, from 1000 to 800, and from 0.0005 to 0.0004. Without specifying the underlying absolute risks, i.e., the absolute numbers of breast cancer deaths in the screening group and the non-screening group, as well as the sample size of each of the groups, the information is incomplete (Forrow et al. 1992). Effects presented in relative terms thus communicate very little about the true and absolute size of the effect of the medical mean.

3   Why Is the Misleading Relative Risk Information so Commonly Used?

As mentioned earlier, relative risk information typically yields large numbers and absolute risk information small numbers. This means that relative risk information appears much more impressive to physicians (Fahey et al. 1995; Naylor et al.1992), policy makers (Hux and Naylor 1995), and patients (Malenka et al. 1993; Schwartz et al. 1997). For instance, in a study in a Swiss hospital, 15 gynecologists were asked what the widely known 25% risk reduction through mammography actually means (Schüssler 2005). This number corresponds to the first review released in 1996 (Nyström et al. 1996) on the effects of mammography attendance, where the risk of dying from breast cancer was reduced from 4 to 3 (=25%) women in 1000. Asked how many fewer women die of breast cancer given the relative risk reduction of 25%, one physician thought that 25% meant 2.5 out of 1000, another 25 out of 1000; the total range of the answers was between 1 and 750 in 1000 women. At the beginning of a CME course in risk communication, another group of 150 gynecologists was also asked what the 25% risk figure meant (Gigerenzer et al. 2007). Using an interactive voting system, the physicians could choose between four alternatives

> Mammography screening reduces mortality from breast cancer by about 25%. Assume that 1000 women aged 40 and over participate in mammography screening. How many fewer women are likely to die of breast cancer?

1   [66%]

25   [16%]

100   [3%]

250   [15%]

The numbers in brackets show the percentage of gynecologists who gave the respective answer. Two-thirds understood that the best answer was 1 in 1000. Yet 16% believed that the figure meant 25 in 1000, and 15% responded that 250 fewer women in 1000 would die of breast cancer.

Where does this confusion come from? Next to the fact that more than 90% of all medical research is financed by the pharmaceutical industry—which has an obvious interest in making results look good—medical journals, even high-ranking ones, also play a role in spreading intransparent statistics. Studies on the coverage of medical findings in high-ranking medical journals revealed that nontransparent health statistics such as relative risk reduction are the rule rather than the exception. In their analysis of 359 articles that reported randomized trials in the years 1989, 1992, 1995, and 1998, published in *Annals of Internal Medicine, British Medical Journal (BMJ), Journal of the American Medical Association (JAMA), The Lancet*, and *The New England Journal of Medicine* Nuovo et al. (2002) found that only 25 articles reported absolute risk reduction and 14 of these 25 also included *the number needed to treat (NNT)*, which is simply the inverse of the absolute risk reduction. That is, only about 7% of the articles reported the results in a transparent way. The same journals, along with the *Journal of the National Cancer Institute*, were analyzed again in 2003/2004 (Schwartz et al. 2006). Sixty-eight percent of 222 articles failed to report the absolute risks for the first ratio measure (such as relative risks) in the abstract, and about half of these did not report the underlying absolute risks anywhere at all in the article. An analysis of *BMJ, JAMA*, and *The Lancet* from 2004 to 2006 found that in about half of the articles, absolute risks or other transparent frequency data were not reported (Sedrakyan and Shih 2007). The study further revealed that 1 out of 3 studies used mismatched framing when reporting their findings. In most cases, relative risks (=large numbers) were reported for benefits, and absolute risks (=small numbers) for harms. In 2010, we sought to find out whether the situation had since changed and investigated all free available research articles reporting drug interventions published in *BMJ* in 2009 (Gigerenzer et al. 2010). Of the 37 articles identified, 16 failed to report the underlying absolute numbers for the reported relative risk measures in the abstract. Among these, 14 reported the absolute risks elsewhere in the article, but 2 did not report them at all. Moreover, absolute risks or number needed to treat (NNT) were more often reported for harms (10/16 = 63%) than for benefits (14/27 = 52%). These analyses indicate that one reason why physicians, patients, and journalists talk about relative risk reductions is because most of the original studies regularly provide information in this form.

Leaflets—developed by the pharmaceutical industry to inform doctors and patients of medical products, tests, and treatments—are even worse. Comparing the summaries in 175 leaflets with the original studies (Kaiser et al. 2004), researchers from the German Institute for Quality and Efficiency in Health Care (IQWIG) found that in only 8% of the cases could the summaries be verified. In the remaining 92%, key results of the original study were systematically distorted or important details omitted. For instance, one pamphlet from Bayer stated that their potency drug Levitra (Vardenafil) works up to 5 h—without mentioning that this statistic was based on studies with numbed hares. Moreover, the cited sources were often either not provided or impossible to find. In general, leaflets exaggerated baseline risks and risk reduction, enlarged the period in which medication could safely be taken, or did not reveal severe side effects of medication pointed out in the original publications.

4   What Is the Lesson to Be Learned from This?

First, always be aware that not only treatments and drugs but also screening tests have benefits *and* harms. Second, when judging or communicating screening's benefits and harms, do not rely on percentages or ratio measures. Instead, find the absolute numbers of people involved in the intervention group (here, screening group) and control group (here, non-screening group) and the absolute numbers of the event (e.g., number of cancer deaths) in both groups. Third, to make the benefits and harms comparable to each other, adjust the numbers of events to the same and smallest possible denominator (e.g., 1000 people). The following fact box on mammography provides a good example of transparent risk communication of benefits and harms (Fig. 1).

5   Does a Positive Test Result of Cancer Screening Mean Having Cancer for Certain?

Doctors' understanding of a positive and a negative test result is essential for a patient who has taken a test. Not knowing and thereby miscommunicating the meaning of a positive result can lead to overdiagnosis, overtreatment, unnecessary fear, or sometimes even to suicide.

Mammography: Consider a woman who has just received a positive mammogram and who asks her doctor whether she has breast cancer for certain, and if not, what the chances are. One would assume that every gynecologist knows the answer.

Breast Cancer Early Detection
by Mammography

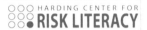

Mammography screening may reduce the number of women who die from breast cancer but this has no effect on overall cancer deaths. Among all women taking part in screening, some women will be overdiagnosed with non-progressive cancer and unnecessarily treated.

Numbers for women aged 50 years or older who did or did not participate in screening for about 10 years.

	1000 women without screening	1000 women with screening
Benefits		
How many women died from breast cancer?	5	4
How many women died from all types of cancer?	21	21
Harms		
How many women without cancer experienced false alarms or biopsies?	–	about 100
How many women with non-progressive cancer had unnecessary partial or complete breast removal?	–	5

Source: [1] Gøtzsche, PC, Jørgensen, KJ (2013). *Cochrane Database of Systematic Reviews* (6): CD001877.pub5
Numbers in the Fact Box are rounded. Where no data for women above 50 years of age are available, numbers refer to women above 40 years of age.
Date last updated: 13 March, 2014

Fig. 1 Fact box on effectiveness of mammography screening

But does the assumption hold true? At the beginning of one continuing education session, 160 gynecologists (Gigerenzer et al. 2007) were provided with the relevant health statistics needed for answering this question in the form of conditional probabilities, which is the form in which medical studies tend to report these health statistics

> Assume that you conduct breast cancer screening using mammography in a certain region. You know the following information about the women in this region:
>
> (1) The probability that a woman has breast cancer is 1% (prevalence).
> (2) If a woman has breast cancer, the probability that she tests positive is 90% (sensitivity).
> (3) If a woman does not have breast cancer, the probability that she nevertheless tests positive is 9% (false-positive rate).
>
> A woman tests positive. She wants to know from you whether this means that she has breast cancer for sure, or what the chances are. What is the best answer?
>
> (A) The probability that she has breast cancer is about 81%.
> (B) Out of 100 women with a positive mammogram, about 90 have breast cancer (90%).
> (C) Out of 100 women with a positive mammogram, about 10 have breast cancer (10%).
> (D) The probability that she has breast cancer is about 1%.

Gynecologists could either derive the answer from the health statistics provided or simply recall what they should have known anyhow. In either case, the best answer is (C). That is, only about 10 out of every 100 women who test positive in screening actually has breast cancer. The other 90 women are falsely alarmed, that is, have a false-positive test result because they do not have breast cancer. Only 21% of the gynecologists found the best answer; the majority (60%) disconcertingly chose the options of "90%" or "81%," thus grossly overestimating the probability of cancer. Another troubling result was the high variability in physicians' estimates, ranging between a 1% and 90% chance of cancer.

Fecal occult blood test (FOBT) screening: Hoffrage and Gigerenzer (1998) tested 48 physicians with an average professional experience of 14 years, including radiologists, internists, surgeons, urologists, and gynecologists. The sample had physicians from teaching hospitals slightly overrepresented and included heads of medical departments. They were given four problems, one of which concerned screening for colorectal cancer with the fecal occult blood test. Half of the physicians were given the relevant information in conditional probabilities (a sensitivity of 50%, a false-positive rate of 3%, and a prevalence of 0.3%). This group of physicians was then asked to estimate the probability of colorectal cancer given a positive test result. Their estimates ranged from a 1 to 99% chance of cancer after a positive test. Their modal answer was 50% (the sensitivity); four physicians deducted the false-positive rate from the sensitivity (arriving at 47%). When interviewed about how they arrived at their answers, several physicians claimed to be innumerate and hid this from patients by avoiding any mention of numbers.

Already back in 1978, a study (Casscells et al. 1978) documented that the majority of physicians struggled with making correct inferences from positive test results: Only 18% of the physicians and medical staff who participated could correctly infer the likelihood of having a disease given a positive test result (positive predictive value/PPV) from the given information. Somewhat later Eddy (1982) reported that 95 out of 100 physicians overestimated the probability of cancer after a positive screening mammogram by an order of magnitude. Similarly, Bramwell et al. (2006) found that only 1 out of 21 obstetricians was able to estimate the probability of an unborn child actually having Down Syndrome given a positive test, with those giving incorrect responses being fairly confident in their estimates. And in an Australian study, 13 of 50 physicians claimed they could describe the positive predictive value of a test, yet when directly interviewed, only 1 could do so (Young et al. 2002). Similar effects were reported for members of the U.S. National Academy of Neuropsychology (Labarge et al. 2003). Ghosh and Ghosh (2005) reviewed further studies that showed that few physicians were able to estimate the positive predictive value from the relevant health statistics.

6 Is There a Way Out of This Confusion?

A simple way of calculating the positive predictive value of a test is using *natural frequencies* (Gigerenzer and Hoffrage 1995). The principle of this approach rests on the assumption that our brains are shaped by evolution to the use of naturally gathered frequencies rather than probabilities, which were unknown before the late eighteenth century. Using that approach of natural frequencies entails "translating" all of the probabilistic information into frequencies. To illustrate, consider the example of the screening for colorectal cancer with the fecal occult blood test (FOBT) again with a sensitivity of 50%, a false-positive rate of 3%, and a prevalence of 0.3%.

- *Prevalence 0.3%*: Out of 10,000 people about 30 people actually have colorectal cancer. (*0.3% of 10,000*)
- *Sensitivity 50%*: Of these 30 people with colorectal cancer 15 will receive a true positive test result. (*50% of 30*) (*The other 15 will receive a false negative result*).
- *False-positive rate 3%*: Of the 9,970 people without colorectal cancer (10,000 minus 30 with colorectal cancer), 299 will receive a false-positive test result. (*3% of 9970*)

Altogether 314 people will receive a positive test result by the test, but for only 15 people is it correct. Thus, the likelihood of a person having colorectal cancer if their FOBT test is positive is about 5%. Given that physicians' estimates ranged from a 1 to 99% chance of colorectal cancer after a positive test with a modal answer of 50%, one can easily imagine how many patients will be unnecessarily frightened as a byproduct of their physicians' statistical illiteracy. Figure 2 illustrates the calculation within a natural frequency tree.

Conditional Probabilities   **Natural Frequencies**

one person   10,000 people

| 0.3% cancer | 99.7% no cancer | | 30 cancer | 9,970 no cancer |

| 50% positive | 50% negative | 3% positive | 97% negative | | 15 positive | 15 negative | 299 positive | 9,671 negative |

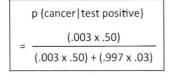

$$p\,(cancer\,|\,test\,positive)$$

$$=\frac{(.003 \times .50)}{(.003 \times .50) + (.997 \times .03)}$$

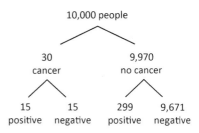

$$p\,(cancer\,|\,test\,positive)$$

$$=\frac{15}{15 + 299}$$

Fig. 2 The probability of colorectal cancer given a positive fecal blood test result. The *left* side illustrates the calculation with conditional probabilities, while the *right* side provides a more transparent calculation with natural frequencies

7   Does an Increase in 5-Year Survival Rates Mean that Lives Are Saved?

While running for president, Rudi Giuliani, former New York City mayor, said in a 2007 campaign advertisement:

> I had prostate cancer, 5, 6 years ago. My chance of surviving prostate cancer—and thank God, I was cured of it—in the United States? Eighty-two percent. My chance of surviving prostate cancer in England? Only 44 percent under socialized medicine (Dobbs 2007, October 30).

This difference in 5-year survival between the U.S. and the U.K. appears large. But is it really that different? It is not, although most people will not realize that they were misled by Giuliani. Giuliani presented higher 5-year survival rates as suggestive evidence for lower mortality due to screening, when in fact differences in survival rates are *uncorrelated* with differences in mortality rates (Welch et al. 2000). In reality, mortality from prostate cancer is about the same in the U.S. and the U.K., even though most American men take the PSA (Prostate-specific Antigen) test and most British men do not. There are two reasons why higher survival rates tell us nothing about lower mortality in the context of screening. First, screening results in early detection and thus inflates 5-year survival rates by simply setting the point of diagnosis earlier, without necessarily extending life (*lead time bias*). As a consequence, people may just live earlier (and longer) with the diagnosis than do people whose cancer is detected by symptoms but die no later than do people diagnosed by symptoms. As for the 5-year survival rate the clock starts ticking at the moment of the diagnosis, and thus people in the screening group are more likely to be still alive 5 years after the earlier diagnosis. Yet that does not mean that they have gained a single extra month of life compared to people without screening. Second, screening inflates survival rates by including people with non-progressive cancers that by definition do not lead to death (*overdiagnosis bias*; Gigerenzer et al. 2007). As a consequence the ratio between the number of people diagnosed with cancer (including the non-progressive types) and the number of diagnosed people still alive after 5 years automatically looks more favorable. Giuliani is not the only one to have misled the public with survival rates; other guilty parties include prestigious U.S. cancer centers such as MD Anderson (Gigerenzer et al. 2007) and high-profile charities such as The Susan G. Komen Association (Woloshin and Schwartz 2012).

8   What Do Physicians Know About the 5-Year Survival Statistic in the Context of Screening?

One might think that physicians would provide people with the right numbers precisely in order to avoid such misunderstandings and facilitate informed choice. Yet studies document that this is unlikely to happen. Few doctors themselves are aware that in screening, survival rates tell us nothing about mortality; nor do they know what lead time bias and overdiagnosis bias are (Wegwarth et al. 2011, 2012). More specifically, in a national sample of 412 US primary care physicians, 47% wrongly thought that if more cancers are detected by a screening test, this proves that the test saves lives, and 76% mistakenly believed that if screen-detected cancers have better 5-year survival rates than cancers detected by symptoms, this too proves that a test saves lives (Wegwarth et al. 2012). When provided with data on what appeared to be two screening tests, primary care physicians were more enthusiastic about the test supported by an increase in 5-year survival (increase of 31 percentage points) than about the test supported by reduced cancer mortality (reduction of 0.4 men in 1000): 69 versus 23%, respectively of the very same physicians said they would definitely recommend the test to their patients. In fact, all data came from medical evidence on the same cancer screening test—prostate cancer screening. These results demonstrate not only that physicians do not correctly understand cancer screening statistics but—even worse—that 46% of the physicians in our sample would have given their patients conflicting advice about a single cancer screening procedure, depending on what statistics they were confronted with.

If physicians do not understand medical statistics, clearly they cannot support informed decision-making in their patients. And if their physicians are of little help, do patients have a chance of making an informed choice after reading patient pamphlets or media reports? Not too likely. Reading through the pamphlet on prostate cancer published by *German Cancer Care* in 2009, for instance, a man will learn that according to experts, PSA tests are an important method for early detection, and that 10-year survival rates are higher than 80% (p. 15). He may also read a press release about the European randomized trial on prostate cancer screening, which states that PSA screening reduced mortality from prostate cancer by 20%. After having consulted different sources and seen various statistics, does the man now have all information to make an informed decision? No. But he may not even notice. To begin with, he may not find out that he has been misled by the 20% figure. What it refers to is a reduction from 3.7 to 3.0 in every 1000 men (age 50–69) who participate in screening, which is an absolute reduction of 0.7 in 1000, as reported in the original study (Schröder et al. 2009). Framing benefits in terms of *relative risks* (20%) is a common way to mislead the public without actually lying (see also pp. 5–9). Second, he may not know the subtle distinction between reduced cancer mortality and reduced prostate cancer mortality. The original study reported no difference in overall cancer mortality: In the screening group, 23.9 out of 1000 men died of cancer, compared to 23.8 in the non-screening group. The 0.7 out of 1000 who did not die of prostate cancer in the screening group died of another cancer. This information, however, is virtually never mentioned in health brochures, whose aim is often to increase attendance rates. Finally, chances are low that his urologist knows the scientific evidence and is able to explain to him the pros and cons of PSA screening. Only 2 out of a random sample of 20 Berlin urologists knew the benefits and harms of PSA screening (*Stiftung Warentest* 2/2004). Even if physicians know the evidence, they may practice defensive medicine in fear of litigation and recommend the test. For instance, although only half of 250 Swiss internists believed that the advantages of regular PSA screening outweigh its harms in men older than 50 years of age, 75% recommended regular PSA screening to their patients (Steurer et al. 2009).

What to learn from this? In the context of screening, changes in survival rates have no reliable relationship to changes in mortality, due to overdiagnosis and lead time bias. The only proof that a cancer screening test saves lives comes from mortality rates, because their calculation is not affected by the way in which diagnoses are made and thus are not biased by lead time and overdiagnosis.

9 Final Remarks

Statistical illiteracy is a big obstacle for informed decision-making. Studies document that a large number of physicians do not understand cancer screening statistics and that patient pamphlets and the media report misleading and incomplete statistics. As a consequence, a large number of patients are misinformed about cancer screenings' benefits and harms. What can be done to remedy this? Every medical school should teach its students how to understand evidence in general and health statistics in particular, and statistical literacy should be assessed in continuing medical education (CME). To cultivate informed patients, elementary and high schools should start teaching the mathematics of uncertainty—statistical thinking. Guidelines about complete and transparent reporting in journals, patient brochures, and the media need to be better enforced, and laws need to be changed in order to protect patients and doctors alike against the practice of defensive medicine instead of encouraging it. A critical mass of informed citizens will not resolve all healthcare problems, but it can constitute a major triggering factor for better care. Informed patients will ask questions that require doctors to become better informed about medical statistics, and in turn more easily see through biased reporting and attempts to create undue hopes and fears.

In the nineteenth century, people's health improved from a combination of clean water, better hygiene, and sufficient amounts of food. The twentieth century saw the professionalization of medicine and scientific breakthroughs, but it has left us with many uninformed physicians and patients. In the twenty-first century, we need a third revolution to promote clean information for better-informed doctors and patients (Wegwarth and Gigerenzer 2014).

References

Berrington de González A, Mahesh M, Kim KP, Bhargavan M, Lewis R, Mettler F, Land C (2009) Projected cancer risks from computed tomographic scans performed in the United States in 2007. JAMA Int Med 169(22):2071–2077

Bramwell R, West H, Salmon P (2006) Health professionals' and service users' interpretation of screening test results: experimental study. Br Med J 333:284–286

Brenner JT, Hall EJ (2007) Computed tomography—an increasing source of radiation exposure. N Engl J Med 357:2277–2284

Casscells W, Schoenberger A, Grayboys T (1978) Interpretation by physicians of clinical laboratory results. N Engl J Med 299:999–1000

Dobbs M (2007, October 30) Rudy wrong on cancer survival chances. Retrieved July 21, 2008 from http://blog.washingtonpost.com/

Eddy DM (1982) Probabilistic reasoning in clinical medicine: problems and opportunities. In: Kahneman D, Slovic P, Tversky A (eds) Judgment under uncertainty: heuristics and biases. Cambridge University Press, Cambridge, pp 249–267

Fahey T, Griffiths S, Peters TJ (1995) Evidence based purchasing: understanding results of clinical trials and systematic reviews. Br Med J 311(21 October):1056–1059

Forrow L, Taylor WC, Arnold RM (1992) Absolutely relative: how research results are summarized can affect treatment decisions. Am J Med 92:121–124

Ghosh AK, Ghosh K (2005) Translating evidence-based information into effective risk communication: current challenges and opportunities. J Lab Clin Med 145:171–180

Gigerenzer G, Gaissmaier W, Kurz-Milcke E, Schwartz LM, Woloshin S (2007) Helping doctors and patients make sense of health statistics. Psychol Sci Publ Interest 8:53–96

Gigerenzer G, Gray JAM (2011) Launching the century of the patient. In Gigerenzer G, Gray JAM (eds) Better doctors, better patients, better decisions: envisioning healthcare 2020. Strüngmann Forum Report. (vol 6, pp 1–19). MIT Press, Cambridge

Gigerenzer G, Hoffrage U (1995) How to improve Bayesian reasoning without instruction: frequency formats. Psychol Rev 102:684–704

Gigerenzer G, Mata J, Frank R (2009) Public knowledge of benefits of breast and prostate cancer screening in Europe. J Natl Cancer Inst 101(17):1216–1220

Gigerenzer G, Wegwarth O, Feufel M (2010) Misleading communication of risk: editors should enforce transaprent reporting in abstracts. Br Med J 341:791–792

Gøtzsche P, Nielsen M (2006) Screening for breast cancer with mammography. Cochrane Database of Syst Rev, 4(CD001877)

Gøtzsche P, Nielsen M (2011) Screening for breast cancer with mammography. Cochrane Database Syst Rev, 1(CD001877)

Hoffrage U, Gigerenzer G (1998) Using natural frequencies to improve diagnostic inferences. Acad Med 73:538–540

Hux J, Naylor C (1995) Communicating the benefits of chronic preventive therapy: does the format of efficacy data determine patient's acceptance of treatment? Med Decis Making 15:152–157

Kaiser T, Ewers H, Waltering A, Beckwermert D, Jennen C, Sawicki PT (2004) Sind die Aussagen medizinischer Werbeprospekte korrekt? Arznei-Telegramm 35:21–23

Labarge AS, McCaffrey RJ, Brown TA (2003) Neuropsychologists' ability to determine the predictive value of diagnostic tests. Clin Neuropsychol 18:165–175

Malenka DJ, Baron JA, Johansen S, Wahrenberger JW, Ross JM (1993) The framing effect of relative and absolute risk. J Gen Int Med 8:543–548

Naylor CD, Chen E, Strauss B (1992) Measured enthusiasm: does the method of reporting trial results alter perceptions of therapeutic effectiveness? Ann Int Med 117:916–921

Nuovo J, Melnikow J, Chang D (2002) Reporting number needed to treat and absolute risk reduction in randomized controlled trials. J Am Med Assoc 287:2813–2814

Nyström L, Andersson I, Bjurstam N, Frisell J, Nordenskjöld B, Rutqvist LE (2002) Long-term effects of mammography screening: updated overview of the Swedish randomised trials. The Lancet 359:909–919

Nyström L, Larsson LG, Wall S, Rutqvist LE, Andersson I, Bjurstam N, Tabár L (1996) An overview of the Swedish randomised mammography trials: total mortality pattern and the representativity of the study cohorts. J Med Screening 3:85–87

Schröder FH, Hugosson J, Roobol MJ, Tammela TL, Ciatto S, Nelen V, Auvinen A (2009) Screening and prostate-cancer mortality in a randomized European study. N Engl J Med 360 (13):1320–1328

Schüssler B (2005) Im Dialog: Ist Risiko überhaupt kommunizierbar, Herr Prof. Gigerenzer? Frauenheilkunde Aktuell 14:25–31

Schwartz L, Woloshin S, Dvorin EL, Welch H (2006) Ratio measures in leading medical journals: structured review of accessibility of underlying absolute risks. Br Med J 333:1248–1252

Schwartz LM, Woloshin S, Black WC, Welch HG (1997) The role of numeracy in understanding the benefit of screening mammography. Ann Int Med 127:966–972

Schwartz LM, Woloshin S, Fowler FJ, Welch HG (2004) Enthusiasm for cancer screening in the United States. J Am Med Assoc 291:71–78

Sedrakyan A, Shih C (2007) Improving depiction of benefits and harms: analyses of studies of well-known therapeutics and review of high-impact medical journals. Med Care 45:523–528

Sirovich B, Welch H (2004) Cervical cancer screening among women without a cervix. J Am Med Assoc 291:2990–2993

Steurer J, Held U, Schmidt M, Gigerenzer G, Tag B, Bachmann LM. (2009). Legal concerns trigger PSA testing. J Eval Clin Prac 15:390–392

Thaler RH, Sunstein CR (2008) Nudge: improving decisions about health, wealth, and happiness. Yale University Press, New Haven

Wegwarth O, Gaissmaier W, Gigerenzer G (2011) Deceiving numbers: survival rates and their impact on doctors' risk communication. Med Decis Making 31(3):386–394

Wegwarth O, Gigerenzer G (2011) "There is nothing to worry about": Gynecologists' counseling on mammography. Patient Educ Couns 84(2011):251–256

Wegwarth O, Gigerenzer G (2013) Trust-your-doctor: a simple heuristic in need of a proper social environment. In: Hertwig R, Hoffrage U, The ABC Research Group (eds) Simple heuristics in a social world. Oxford University Press, New York, pp. 67–102

Wegwarth O, Gigerenzer G (2014) Improving evidence-based practices through health literacy— in reply. JAMA Int Med 174(8):1413–1414

Wegwarth O, Schwartz LM, Woloshin S, Gaissmaier W, Gigerenzer G (2012) Do physicians understand cancer screening statistics? A national survey of primary care physicians in the U.S. Ann Int Med (156):340–349

Welch HG, Schwartz LM, Woloshin S (2000) Are increasing 5-year survival rates evidence of success against cancer? J Am Med Assoc 283(22):2975–2978

Woloshin S, Schwartz LM (2012) How a charity oversells mammography. BMJ 345:e5132

Young JM, Glasziou P, Ward JE (2002) General practitioners' self rating of skills in evidence based medicine: a validation study. BMJ 324:950–951

Future Research in Psycho-Oncology

Ute Goerling and Anja Mehnert

Abstract

Since the mid-1970s psycho-oncology and psycho-oncological research have been systematically developed in many industrialized countries and have produced nationally and internationally accepted guidelines. In this article developments and challenges are presented and discussed. From the perspective of various oncological treatment options, different needs for further psycho-oncological research are considered.

Keywords

Neoplasms · psycho-oncology · Medical psychology

1 Research in Psycho-Oncology: History and Recent Developments in Context

Since the mid-1970s psycho-oncology and psycho-oncological research have been systematically developed in many industrialized countries and since then, there are growing efforts to establish psycho-oncology in low- and middle-income countries

U. Goerling
Charité - Universitätsmedizin Berlin, Freie Universität Berlin,
Humboldt-Universität zu Berlin, Berlin Institue of Health, Charité Comprehensiver
Cancer Center, Berlin, Germany
e-mail: Ute.goerling@charite.de

A. Mehnert (✉)
Department of Medical Psychology and Medical Sociology,
University Medical Center Leipzig, University of Leipzig,
Philipp-Rosenthal-Strasse 55, 04103 Leipzig, Germany
e-mail: anja.mehnert@medizin.uni-leipzig.de

worldwide. Advances in the treatment of cancer that lead to a growing number of cancer survivors and changes in the healthcare system toward a greater emphasis on patients' needs for open communication on a level as partners as well as for emotional and psychosocial support have accelerated the development of psycho-oncology as a new discipline in oncology and psychosocial medicine (Koch et al. 2016).

In the previous years, psycho-oncological research has contributed to a wide spectrum of evidence-based knowledge on the psychosocial burden of cancer in patients and relatives as well as on effective interventions to reduce anxiety and depression and improve quality of life (Faller et al. 2013). Today, research objectives could be well based on the existing knowledge about physical symptom distress and its interaction with psychological well-being, coping and adaptation processes, social support, and quality of life. In addition, a wide range of validated screening and outcome measures is available. Thus, psycho-oncology has become an evidence-based subdiscipline within the psychosocial services in medical care and a model for the successful application of behavioral and social sciences in medicine (Holland and Weiss 2010; Watson et al. 2014).

From the international perspective, various developments contributed to the research in psycho-oncology including the Thanatology movement in the early decades of the last century, early (psychotherapy) research in palliative care, and quality of life as well as the growing establishment of psycho-oncological services within cancer care (Holland and Weis 2010). The formation of various national scientific psycho-oncology societies all over the world and the many activities initiated by the International Psycho-Oncology Society (IPOS) did not only promote psychosocial research in cancer but also the training of post-graduate, post-doc, and early career scientists in this field. Many psycho-oncology societies all over the world organize annual or bi-annual scientific meetings and increasingly experts present current psychosocial research findings at cancer conferences.

1.1 Specific Challenges Faced by Scientists in Psycho-Oncology

Research with physically severe ill patients confronts the researcher with a variety of challenges. First of all, research often requires an interdisciplinary approach taking into account the inpatient and outpatients settings patients are treated. Therefore, close collaborations with the healthcare team including physicians, nurses, psychologists and psychotherapists, social workers, and physiotherapists, for example, are often necessary to successfully recruit patients for a study. In addition to the institutional and patients safety requirements including research ethics, data protection, and privacy issues, time constraints between necessary clinical diagnostics and medical treatments can make it difficult to approach eligible patients. During primary treatments, a patient's ability to participate in the study can significantly fluctuate over daytime and depend, for example, on side effects such as nausea or fatigue. Thus, study participation is not only influenced by demographic factors such as younger age, higher education, and early disease stages, but also by physical and psychological well-being as well (Roick et al. 2017). These specific circumstances must be considered when interpreting research findings in terms of sample bias and limited generalization of findings.

Although a variety of validated outcome measures exist that can be used in psycho-oncological research, there is a lack of validated brief questionnaires that take limited physical and mental capacities of patients into account and are, at the same time, age and culture sensitive. Many and particularly clinical studies in psycho-oncology have small sample sizes and often include patients with specific tumor entities that are more easily accessible and motivated such as women with breast cancer. Small sample sizes allow only limited statistical methods and study findings are therefore limited as well in terms of interpretation and generalization. In longitudinal studies, problems of high drop-out rate due to medical reasons leading to sample bias and selection processes might also more often occur than in studies including physically healthy individuals.

The definition of appropriate comparison and control groups can be challenging in psycho-oncological research. To determine meaningful criteria for a comparison or a control group considering the specifics of the intervention group in terms of sociodemographic, cancer-related and medical characteristics is not an easy task. In addition, research designs such as wait-list control group designs can be considered unethical in patients with advanced disease, but different research designs specifically in randomized or cluster-randomized trials might be difficult to implement. Furthermore, in intervention and longitudinal studies in psycho-oncology, the investigator must be aware of limitations that include sudden changes in medical treatment regimes.

To summarize, it is important to acknowledge that psycho-oncological research strongly depends on institutional support, presupposing appropriate social and interactive competence of the researchers involved. Research competence does not only comprise methodological skills and detailed psychological and medical knowledge but also knowledge of the formal and informal structures and processes within the collaborating institutions (Koch et al. 2016). Well-developed communication skills can play a key role in conducting successful studies that enable the researcher to communicate effectively with the patient (and relatives) and with the multidisciplinary healthcare team involved.

1.2 Psycho-Oncology as a Mirror of Oncological Developments

Global disease burden has continued to shift away from communicable to non-communicable diseases and from premature death to years lived with disability (Murray et al. 2012). This is certainly the case for cancer. Recent developments including cancer vaccines, cancer immunotherapy, individualized cancer treatments, or advances in cancer surgery do influence not only oncology practice but also the mortality and morbidity of patients and caregivers. Research in psycho-oncology always needs to reflect new developments in oncology in order to provide and contribute to high-quality cancer care for patients and caregivers.

Scientific and practice innovations that are contributing to declining cancer mortality rates challenge the delivery of high-quality cancer care for every patient. New treatments and technology raise continuing concerns about costs. Can we actually pay all evidence-based treatments and technologies in the future where patients presumably life longer? Cancer patients survive longer with a variety of physical and psychosocial consequences for the individual and for our societies. Patient's aging will increase the demand for specific psychosocial care interventions and geriatric healthcare programs. We face an increase in cultural and social diversities that influence also our healthcare system. People are different, belong to different cultures, and have different personalities and their individual history, which leads to different perceptions of illness and needs for care. Furthermore, increasing urbanization and changes in urban and rural health care are increasingly challenging the demands for a humane and equitable healthcare system and healthcare services research.

Psycho-oncological research can significantly contribute to high-quality patient-centered cancer care and to overcome obstacles to successful outcomes including increasing healthcare costs, the discontinuity of care delivery as well as information overload that influences evidence- and value-based decision-making.

The current psycho-oncological research areas range from psychoneuroimmunology and the analysis of coping processes to more application-related clinical questions such as the communication of oncologists with patients or the development and evaluation of psycho-oncological intervention programs. Research areas in psycho-oncology can be, for example, categorized according to different criteria, i.e., according to the target groups, e.g., patients (children, adolescents, and adults), partners, and family caregivers as well as healthcare professionals; according to (behavioral and social) risk factors for cancer and the issues of cancer prevention; according to different treatments and survivorship phases (e.g., survivorship, palliative care, bereavement) and tumor entities (e.g., breast cancer); according to treatment side effects (e.g., pain, fatigue) and the consequences of the treatment for the individual and the society (e.g., work participation); and according to psychological and psychosocial sequels of the disease (e.g., emotional distress, coping efforts) and moderating and mediating factors as well as according to intervention and health services research in psycho-oncology. The heterogeneity of the research field and the necessary methodological pluralism make it, however, difficult to precisely define the psycho-oncological research from a content or methodological point of view.

2 Psycho-Oncology Research Needs

In this time we know that psychotherapy is effective and the outcomes achieved in randomized clinical trials are comparable with outcomes achieved in practice (Wampold and Imel 2015). The access is often hindered, particularly for patients with cancer accompanied by anxiety of stigmatizing. Nevertheless, until today in

Table 1 Reviews regarding psycho-oncology research

Nr.	Authors	Outcomes	Studies included	Time periods Search period	Number of studies included
1	Li M et al. Canada (Li et al. 2016)	Major depression or other nonbipolar depressive disorder	RCTs of adult cancer patients that compared collaborative care interventions (pharmacological and psychological interventions included) with observation (usual care), placebo or other treatment intervention	*Integrated delivery and follow-up* July 2005–January 2015	25
2	Faller H et al. Germany (Faller et al. 2013)	Emotional distress, anxiety, depression, and quality of life	RCTs of adult cancer patients that compared a psycho-oncologic intervention delivered face-to-face with a control condition	*Post-treatment, ≤ 6 months, and more than 6 months* Electronic searches were performed through May 19, 2010. Search period unclear	198
3	Dieng M et al. Australia (Dieng et al. 2016)	Cost-effectiveness of psychosocial interventions for improving psychological adjustment	All economic evaluation study types that aggregated monetary costs and psychological health outcomes	*Unclear* 1980–May 2015	8
4	Sanjida S et al., Australia (Sanjida et al. 2016)	Antidepressants to improve symptoms of depression	Observational cohort, cross-sectional or case–control studies of adult cancer patients or adult survivors of childhood cancer published in English	*Unclear* 1979–February 2015	38
5	Brebach R et al., Australia (Brebach et al. 2016)	Uptake or adherence to individual psychological supports targeting distress, anxiety, or depression	Research trials offering the chance of psychological interventions targeting distress for cancer patients or survivors	*Unclear* January 1993–May 2014	53
6	Duijts SFA et al., Netherland (Duijts et al. 2011)	Fatigue, depression, anxiety, body-image, stress, and HRQoL	Randomized controlled trials that addressed behavioral techniques or physical exercise for breast cancer patients or survivors	*Unclear* Until March 2009	56

(continued)

Table 1 (continued)

Nr.	Authors	Outcomes	Studies included	Time periods Search period	Number of studies included
7	Fors EA et al., Norway, Sweden (Fors et al. 2011)	Quality of life, fatigue, mood, health behavior, and social function	Randomized controlled trials of female breast cancer patients which aimed to determine effectiveness of psychoeducation, cognitive behavioral therapy, and social support interventions	*During and after primary treatment* Unclear	18
8	Matsuda et al., Japan (Matsuda et al. 2014)	Global health status/QoL scale and subscales of QoL	Randomized controlled trials with early-stage breast cancer patients which compared patients receiving psychosocial support with a control group	*Baseline and 6 months after intervention* September 1988–January 2012	8
9	Simard S et al., Canada, Australia, UK (Simard et al. 2013)	Fear of cancer recurrence	Quantitative studies associated with fear of cancer recurrence in adult cancer survivors; limited data on interventions were available	*Unclear* 1996–2011	130
10	Li Q and AJ Loke, China (Li and Loke 2014)	Explore existing interventions for couples coping with cancer in term of type of intervention, contents, approach, and outcome measurement	Studies related to couple-based interventions	*Unclear* Launch of database (Science Citation Index Expanded (1970 +), PsycInfo (1806 +), Medline (1950 +) via OvidSP, CINAHL database (1982 +))– March 2013	17
11	Nicholls W et al., UK (Nicholls et al. 2014)	Attachment and psychological adjustment to cancer for patients and those close to them	Quantitative studies, which reported attachment and psychological adjustment	*Unclear* Up to June 2013	15

(continued)

Table 1 (continued)

Nr.	Authors	Outcomes	Studies included	Time periods Search period	Number of studies included
12	Parahoo K et al., USA (Parahoo et al. 2015)	Effectiveness of psychosocial interventions in improving quality of life, self-efficacy, and knowledge and in reducing distress, uncertainty, and depression	Comparison of randomized controlled trials about psychosocial interventions that used one or a combination of cognitive behavioral, psychoeducational, supportive and counseling interventions verses. usual care for men with prostate cancer	*Unclear* CENTRAL; The Cochrane Library, 2013, Issue 9), MEDLINE (1946 to October Week 1 2013), EMBASE (1974 to 21 October 2013) and PsycINFO (1806 to October Week 2 2013),	19
13	Sale PMG et al., Brazil Canada, Greeze (Sales et al. 2014)	Potential of psychosocial factors to act as predictors of outcomes, including psychological distress and health-related quality of life	Prospective and intervention studies for patients with colorectal cancer	*Unclear* 1950–September 2013	20
14	Agboola SO et al., USA, Korea (Agboola et al. 2015)	Pain, depression, quality of life	Randomized controlled trials, which evaluate the effect of telehealth for patients with cancer	*Heterogeneous in time and duration* Searched in July 2013, updated in January 2015	20
15	Archer S et al., UK (Archer et al. 2015)	Anxiety and depression, quality of life, coping, stress, anger, and mood	Studies reported effects of creative psychological interventions, including art therapy, music therapy, and dance therapy, for adult cancer patients	*Unclear* Within the last 5 years; search concludes with 31 October 2013	10
16	Brandao T et al., Portugal, USA (Brandão et al. 2016)	Measures used to assess the way to regulate the emotions	Longitudinal studies, randomized controlled trials, quasi-experimental designs, and cross-sectional studies for women with breast cancer	*Unclear* From inception of database to September 2014	59

(continued)

Table 1 (continued)

Nr.	Authors	Outcomes	Studies included	*Time periods* Search period	Number of studies included
17	Bredart a et al., France, Italy, Netherlands (Brédart et al. 2015)	Patient satisfaction instruments developed or used in the cancer outpatient setting	Studies assessing adult cancer patient satisfaction with care received in the outpatient setting or the development and psychometric evaluation of patient satisfaction questionnaire for use in cancer outpatient setting	*Unclear* January 1999–arch 2014	21
18	Kangas M, Australia (Kangas 2015)	Anxiety and/or depression disorders	Randomized controlled trials concerning psychosocial interventions for adult brain tumor patients	*Unclear* From inception of database to December 2014	4
19	Okuyama S et al., USA (Okuyama et al. 2015)	Global assessments of health-related quality of life, including psychosocial functioning as well as content-specific psychosocial assessment	Randomized controlled trials for patients with cancer and survivors related to psychosocial telephone interventions	*Unclear* 1966–March 2013	20
20	Ozga et al., USA (Ozga et al. 2015)	Fear of recurrence	Quantitative studies used cross-sectional design and qualitative studies	*Unclear* 1990–July 2014	15

numerous articles results regarding different psychosocial aspects of cancer are reported. Table 1 gives an overview of several reviews in this field. These reviews go right back to the launch of different databases and examined various outcomes. Some studies analyzed psychological disorders (e.g., No. 1, 2, 6, 13, 15, 18), such as anxiety and depression, symptoms, and various areas regarding health-related quality of life (e.g., No. 7, 8, 12, 13, 19) right through cost-effectiveness of psychosocial interventions (No. 3). The number of studies included range from 4 to 198.

For search strategy, most of them used Preferred Reporting Items for Systematic Reviews (PRISMA) as well as hand search and conducted using important databases such as PubMed, Embase, Web of Science, Scorpus, PsychINFO, Cochrane Library, and CINAHL.

Many psychometric studies did not provide information on item level missing data. However, some reviews failed to show statistically significant effects. Moreover, when beneficial effects were seen, it remained uncertain whether the magnitude of effect was large enough to be considered clinically important. Few authors reflect study limitations like loss to follow-up, study heterogeneity, and small sample size. Most findings of these reviews are encouraging. Additional well-executed and transparently reported research studies are necessary to establish the role of psyche and interventions in patients with cancer. Long-time clinical-controlled studies are to be considered as gold standard. It is very important to implement longitudinal studies. All phases of cancer beginning with diagnosis, treatment from curative to palliative setting, and the corresponding psychological responses should be included.

2.1   Research in Cancer Survivorship

More and more patients live with the disease. In this book, Chapters "Rehabilitation for Cancer Patients" and "Cancer Survivorship in Adults" focus on this issue. To survive the disease also means for many patients a life with manifold limitations. There is a lack of research and effective interventions for the consequences of cancer and its treatment, for example, medical problems (e.g., lymphedema and sexual dysfunction), symptoms (e.g., post-cancer pain syndrome and cancer-related fatigue), psychological distress experienced by cancer survivors and their caregivers (e.g., anxiety, depression, or issues of sexuality, intimacy and fertility), issues of self-management; and quality of life, health behavior and lifestyle, and concerns related to employment, work participation insurance, and disability.

2.2   Intervention Research

Psycho-oncological interventions are effective in reducing anxiety and depression and improving quality of life. For more details, see Chapter "Psychotherapy in the Oncology Setting" in this book. The meta-analyses, however, also show the need for further methodologically high-quality psychotherapies studies in oncology and (early) palliative care. It is noticeable that the majority of the intervention studies were carried out in patients with mixed diagnoses and breast cancer and mainly in early disease phases. In only about 10% of the studies, patients with increased psychological distress were recruited, which assumable reduces the overall effects. Many randomized controlled trials (RCTs) have small case numbers and include comparisons between a single active intervention and an inactive control condition, no treatment or routine care, which is usually undefined. Particularly in the case of individual psychotherapy and relaxation procedures, there appears to be a publication bias (Faller et al. 2013). Future intervention research needs to focus on under-represented patient groups such as patients with head and neck cancer and patients with metastasized cancer receiving palliative care.

In addition to the demand for a better quality of studies, there is an urgent need for research in the development, optimization, and evaluation of manualized psycho-psychological interventions for groups of patients with different problem areas. These include, among others, patients with high psychosocial distress and those who are severely impaired both physically and functionally, such as patients with head and neck cancers, lung cancer, hematologic cancer diseases, or patients in advanced stages of disease. Psychotherapeutic research in physically severely ill patients, however, is associated with a series of difficulties from a methodological as well as from a conceptual perspective. An important question relates, for example, to the expected and realistic outcome of psychotherapeutic interventions in the event of a deteriorating physical condition and correspondingly adequate adaptive coping reactions (including mourning and phases of distress) in the course of the disease. The administrative and organizational efforts of patient recruitment and therapy adherence are not insignificant in the case of a progressive cancer and an uncertain course of disease. Also inactive control group–designs (e.g., waiting group designs) are hardly to realize for ethical reasons.

2.3   Research in Prevention Research

Prevention research in cancer is one of the most neglected areas in psycho-oncology, although it is known that behavioral factors such as health behaviors play an important role in the development of cancer and the recurrence of the disease. Prevention refers not only to the primary prevention, but also to the prevention of recurrent and new or second cancers, and other late effects (secondary and third prevention), cancer surveillance, and the question of how we can use our knowledge of mental and social factors for preventive interventions that help groups that particularly benefit from those programs including socially disadvantaged groups or those with low education and unhealthy lifestyles.

2.4   Healthcare Services Research in Psycho-Oncology

The main topics of healthcare services research in psycho-oncology includes the analysis of structural conditions of psycho-oncological care in the different treatment and rehabilitation settings, epidemiological issues related to the wide range of mental disorders, and subsyndromal distress occurring in cancer patients, as well as in relatives and healthcare professionals, questions of the efficacy and practicability of distress screening among patients and the need for psycho-oncological treatment evaluations under everyday conditions, especially with patient groups that are particularly difficult to approach and include in intervention studies. Healthcare services research in psycho-oncology also include the analysis of barriers and favorable conditions for the implementation of psycho-oncological interventions into the clinical routine, the evaluation of the effectiveness and efficiency of psycho-oncological interventions and programs under routine conditions, and questions about standards for the quality assurance of psycho-oncological services and their implementation (Koch et al. 2016). Many research questions relevant for healthcare services research in oncology require the use of qualitative methods. This approach shows innovative potentials and opportunities.

References

Agboola SO, Ju W, Elfiky A et al (2015) The effect of technology-based interventions on pain, depression, and quality of life in patients with cancer: a systematic review of randomized controlled trials. J Med Int Res 17(3):e65

Archer S, Buxton S, Sheffield D (2015) The effect of creative psychological interventions on psychological outcomes for adult cancer patients: a systematic review of randomised controlled trials. Psycho-Oncol 24(1):1–10

Brandão T, Tavares R, Schulz MS et al (2016) Measuring emotion regulation and emotional expression in breast cancer patients: a systematic review. Clin Psychol Rev 43:114–127

Brebach R, Sharpe L, Costa DSJ et al (2016) Psychological intervention targeting distress for cancer patients: a meta-analytic study investigating uptake and adherence. Psycho-Oncol 25 (8):882–890

Brédart A, Kop JL, Efficace F et al (2015) Quality of care in the oncology outpatient setting from patients' perspective: a systematic review of questionnaires' content and psychometric performance. Psycho-Oncol 24(4):382–394

Dieng M, Cust AE, Kasparian NA et al (2016) Economic evaluations of psychosocial interventions in cancer: a systematic review. Psycho-Oncology:n/a–n/a

Duijts SFA, Faber MM, Oldenburg HSA et al (2011) Effectiveness of behavioral techniques and physical exercise on psychosocial functioning and health-related quality of life in breast cancer patients and survivors-a meta-analysis. Psycho-Oncol 20(2):115–126

Faller H, Schuler M, Richard M et al (2013) Effects of psycho-oncologic interventions on emotional distress and quality of life in adult patients with cancer: systematic review and meta-analysis. J Clin Oncol 31(6):782–793

Fors EA, Bertheussen GF, Thune I et al (2011) Psychosocial interventions as part of breast cancer rehabilitation programs? Results from a systematic review. Psycho-Oncol 20(9):909–918

Holland JC, Weiss TR (2010) History of psycho-oncology. In: Holland JC (ed) Handbook of psycho-oncology. Oxford University Press, Oxford, pp 3–12

Kangas M (2015) Psychotherapy interventions for managing anxiety and depressive symptoms in adult brain tumor patients: a scoping review. Front Oncol 5 (116)

Koch U, Holland JC, Mehnert A (2016) Geschichte und Entwicklung der Psychoonkologie. In: Mehnert A, Koch U (eds) Handbuch Psychoonkologie. Hogrefe Verlag GmbH & Co, KG, pp 13–22

Li M, Kennedy EB, Byrne N et al (2016) Systematic review and meta-analysis of collaborative care interventions for depression in patients with cancer. Psycho-Oncol: n/a–n/a

Li Q, Loke AY (2014) A systematic review of spousal couple-based intervention studies for couples coping with cancer: direction for the development of interventions. Psycho-Oncol 23 (7):731–739

Matsuda A, Yamaoka K, Tango T et al (2014) Effectiveness of psychoeducational support on quality of life in early-stage breast cancer patients: a systematic review and meta-analysis of randomized controlled trials. Qual Life Res 23(1):21–30

Murray CJL, Vos T, Lozano R et al (2012) Disability-adjusted life years (DALYs) for 291 diseases and injuries in 21 regions, 1990–2010: a systematic analysis for the Global Burden of Disease Study 2010. The Lancet 380(9859):2197–2223

Nicholls W, Hulbert-Williams N, Bramwell R (2014) The role of relationship attachment in psychological adjustment to cancer in patients and caregivers: a systematic review of the literature. Psycho-Oncol 23(10):1083–1095

Okuyama S, Jones W, Ricklefs C et al (2015) Psychosocial telephone interventions for patients with cancer and survivors: a systematic review. Psycho-Oncol 24(8):857–870

Ozga M, Aghajanian C, Myers-Virtue S et al (2015) A systematic review of ovarian cancer and fear of recurrence. Palliat Support Care 13(6):1771–1780

Parahoo K, McDonough S, McCaughan E et al (2015) Psychosocial interventions for men with prostate cancer: a Cochrane systematic review. BJU Int 116(2):174–183

Roick J, Danker H, Kersting A et al (2017) Factors associated with non-participation and dropout among cancer patients in a cluster-randomised controlled trial. Eur J Cancer Care:e12645–n/a

Sales PMG, Carvalho AF, McIntyre RS et al (2014) Psychosocial predictors of health outcomes in colorectal cancer: a comprehensive review. Cancer Treat Rev 40(6):800–809

Sanjida S, Janda M, Kissane D et al (2016) A systematic review and meta-analysis of prescribing practices of antidepressants in cancer patients. Psycho-Oncol 25(9):1002–1016

Simard S, Thewes B, Humphris G et al (2013) Fear of cancer recurrence in adult cancer survivors: a systematic review of quantitative studies. J Cancer Surviv 7(3):300–322

Wampold B, Imel Z (2015) What do we know about psychotherapy?—and what is there left to debate? [Web Article]. In: ed

Watson M, Dunn J, Holland JC (2014) Review of the history and development in the field of psychosocial oncology. Int Rev Psychiatry 26(1):128–135

Printed in the United States
By Bookmasters